Clinical Chemistry

DUE DATE	RETURN DATE	DUE DATE	RETURN DATE
MAY 7 1990			
	MAY 7 1990		
MAY 19 1990			
	MAY 17 1990		
JUN 07 1990			
	JUN 20 1990		
JUL 11 1990			
	JUL 15 1990		
APR 18 1994			
	APR 8 1994		

CHEMICAL ANALYSIS

A SERIES OF MONOGRAPHS ON ANALYTICAL CHEMISTRY AND ITS APPLICATIONS

Editor
J. D. WINEFORDNER
Editor Emeritus: **I. M. KOLTHOFF**

Advisory Board

Fred W. Billmeyer, Jr.	Victor G. Mossotti
Eli Grushka	A. Lee Smith
Barry L. Karger	Bernard Tremillon
Viliam Krivan	T. S. West

VOLUME 106

WILEY

A WILEY-INTERSCIENCE PUBLICATION

JOHN WILEY & SONS

New York / Chichester / Brisbane / Toronto / Singapore

R00042 65466

(*continued on back*)

Clinical Chemistry

Edited by

E. HOWARD TAYLOR

Division of Pathology
University of Arkansas for Medical Sciences
Little Rock, Arkansas

WILEY

A WILEY-INTERSCIENCE PUBLICATION

JOHN WILEY & SONS

New York / Chichester / Brisbane / Toronto / Singapore

Copyright © 1989 by John Wiley & Sons, Inc.

All rights reserved. Published simultaneously in Canada.

Reproduction or translation of any part of this work
beyond that permitted by Section 107 or 108 of the
1976 United States Copyright Act without the permission
of the copyright owner is unlawful. Requests for
permission or further information should be addressed to
the Permissions Department, John Wiley & Sons, Inc.

Library of Congress Cataloging in Publication Data:

Clinical chemistry.

(Chemical analysis, ISSN 0069–2883; v. 106)
"A Wiley-Interscience publication."
Bibliography: p.
Includes index.
1. Chemistry, Clinical.   I. Taylor, E. Howard.   II. Title.
III. Series.

RB40.C569   1989   616.07′5   88-33930
ISBN 0–471–85342–9

Printed in the United States of America

10 9 8 7 6 5 4 3 2 1

1178453

CONTRIBUTORS

Bai-Hsiun Chen, University of Arkansas for Medical Sciences, Little Rock, Arkansas

Robert H. Christenson, Durham Veterans Administration Medical Center, Durham, North Carolina

Edward P. Fody, Bethesda Hospital, Cincinnati, Ohio

Dianne Johnson, Baptist Medical Center, Little Rock, Arkansas

Curtis Liu, Memorial Medical Center of Long Beach, Long Beach, California

William H. Porter, University of Kentucky, Lexington, Kentucky

Lawrence M. Silverman, North Carolina Memorial Hospital, Chapel Hill, North Carolina

E. Howard Taylor, University of Arkansas for Medical Sciences, Little Rock, Arkansas

Karen L. Tilley, North Carolina Memorial Hospital, Chapel Hill, North Carolina

Charles P. Turley, University of Arkansas for Medical Sciences, Little Rock, Arkansas

Ronald J. Whitley, University of Kentucky, Lexington, Kentucky

PREFACE

Clinical chemistry is a field which few analytical, organic, or physical chemists are aware even exists. The field has expanded in recent years from traditional teaching areas in schools of medical technology or graduate programs in clinical chemistry to other areas of chemistry. As medically applied chemistry questions begin to enter undergraduate or graduate courses in chemistry or biochemistry, the need exists for a book designed to rapidly familiarize the reader with the essence of clinical chemistry, its potentials, limitations, and medical relevance to diagnosis. Too often the interested reader is overwhelmed with technical theory or an intricate treatise of chemical pathology. This book was written for readers with broad and diverse backgrounds within the field of chemistry who have an interest in rapidly learning more about the field of clinical chemistry. The reader will see an integration of basic analytical concepts in the field of clinical chemistry balanced with the diagnosis of disease.

The practicing clinical chemist must possess not only analytical abilities but also skill in interpreting results and an appropriate balance is maintained in each chapter concerning the areas of electrolytes and acid–base balance, renal function, proteins, enzyme analysis, hormone immunoassays, coagulation, therapeutic drug monitoring, and laboratory evaluation of nutritional status. Important aspects of the field are sample integrity and steps to evaluate quality control and quality assurance, and these areas are covered in the first two chapters.

Although the text is designed for chemists with broad backgrounds, this book was written by practicing clinical chemists and pathologists specializing in the field. Their many years of experience and knowledge are available for reference in areas in which clinical chemists may be less knowledgeable, such as coagulation and nutritional status.

This format is designed for chemists who wish to gain rapid familiarity in the field and the text is dedicated to future clinical chemists who use this as a tool to gain more knowledge into the "practice" of clinical chemistry.

E. Howard Taylor

Little Rock, Arkansas
May 1989

vii

CONTENTS

CHAPTER 1

PREANALYTICAL VARIABLES

EDWARD P. FODY

Bethesda Hospital
Cincinnati, Ohio

INTRODUCTION

All laboratory testing may be divided into three parts: the preanalytical phase, from the time the test is ordered until it is actually performed; the analytic phase, which encompasses the actual determination; and the postanalytical phase, which includes the time from the performance of the test until the result reaches the physician. By far the bulk of a clinical laboratory's time and effort is devoted to the analytical phase. However, errors in the preanalytical phase can render even the most sophisticated analysis worthless.

The preanalytical phase is normally subdivided into patient preparation and specimen handling; the former concerns factors such as fasting, medication, and posture, while the latter deals with the factors affecting the specimen after it leaves the patient. Errors in patient preparation and specimen handling occur frequently and probably represent the most common reason for erroneous laboratory data. Examples include elevated plasma triglycerides collected from an inadequately fasting patient, elevated serum potassium because of hemolysis during blood collection, and decreased serum glucose because of failure to refrigerate a blood collection tube. Only careful attention to these details by both clinician and laboratory will allow the production of valid laboratory data.

ANALYTE STABILITY

Glucose

The same catabolism of glucose which occurs *in vivo* may also take place *in vitro*. In cell-free serum or plasma, glucose is quite stable (*1*). However, when exposed to living cells, such as leukocytes or erythrocytes, glucose may be consumed. It has been stated that glucose levels in whole blood stored at room temperature decrease 7% per hour (*2*). However, the actual rate is quite

1

variable. Erythrocytosis and leukocytosis have been shown to accelerate the catabolism of glucose (3–5).

With the use of serum separator tubes and prompt processing, accuracy of glucose levels can be assured. If this is not feasible, the specimen may be refrigerated. About 20% of available glucose is catabolized at 4°C in 24 hours. Alternatively, an enzymatic inhibitor such as sodium fluoride may be employed. This is usually mixed with oxalate, which serves as an anticoagulant. Blood collection tubes containing these substances have gray stoppers and render glucose stable for 8 hours at 25°C and 3 days at 4°C (6). Most commonly, glucose determinations are performed on separated serum. However, plasma gives equivalent results, provided the anticoagulant does not interfere with the method. Whole blood glucose levels are 10–15% lower than serum or plasma.

Sodium

The sodium level in plasma greatly exceeds that in erythrocytes. For this reason, sodium levels in plasma allowed to remain in contact with cells tend to decrease. Since refrigeration inhibits the action of the erythrocyte membrane pump, which operates to exclude sodium, low temperatures actually accelerate the decrease in plasma (or serum) sodium. Prompt separation of serum or plasma from cells or use of an impermeable gel separator renders sodium quite stable. Pseudohyponatremia may occur in specimens containing large quantities of protein or lipid.

Potassium

Exactly the opposite of sodium, potassium levels in erythrocytes greatly (23 ×) exceed those normally found in serum or plasma. Therefore, even slight amounts of hemolysis occurring during specimen collection or processing may artificially elevate potassium. For example, 1% hemolysis will increase serum potassium almost 25% (8).

In vitro, potassium tends to leak out of erythrocytes, a process which is accelerated by refrigeration. Potassium is also released from cells during the slight erythrocytolysis and thrombocytolysis which occurs during clotting. Leukocytosis may also falsely elevate potassium.

In an unseparated specimen, potassium is most stable at 37°C (9). Lowering the temperature produces an increase in plasma potassium. Elevated potassium levels due to platelet destruction have been documented in specimens with normal (10) and elevated platelet counts (11,12). Hypokalemia, multifactoral in origin, occurs commonly in patients with acute leukemia (13). However, artifactual hypokalemia may be seen in specimens with extreme leukocytosis stored at room temperature (*14*). For these reasons the accurate determination of potassium represents a considerable challenge to both clinician and laboratory. Specimens should be collected into heparin tubes; they should not be refrigerated, but processed and separated as soon as possible. In separated plasma, potassium is stable.

Chloride

The concentration of chloride in erythrocytes is normally about half that found in plasma. Chloride shifts between erythrocytes and plasma tend to occur rapidly to compensate for movement of hydrogen ions and CO_2. Unlike sodium and potassium, the *in vitro* stability of chloride is greater at lower temperatures. Specimens for chloride determination should be kept tightly stoppered to avoid loss of CO_2. Under these conditions, chloride is stable for 2 hours in unseparated or clotted blood (*15*). Serum and plasma levels are equivalent.

Bicarbonate

The term "bicarbonate" is used clinically to represent the total carbon dioxide in the blood. This exists in several different forms: Carbon dioxide (CO_2); bicarbonate ion (HCO_3^-); carbonate ion (CO_3^{-2}); and carbonic acid (H_2CO_3). Their relationship is represented by

$$H_2O + CO_2 \rightleftharpoons H_2CO_3 \rightleftharpoons HCO_3^- + H^+ \rightleftharpoons CO_3^{-2} + H^+$$

Under physiological conditions, all but about 2 mmol/L is present as bicarbonate (*16*).

Since air contains less CO_2 than plasma, rapid diffusion from an open tube will occur. Preservation of anaerobic conditions is obviously important to obtain accurate values. Some loss of CO_2 is inevitable as specimens are transferred to open analyzer cups; however, this loss need not be significant if the analysis is performed quickly. In an open tube or cup, CO_2 losses of up to 6 mmol/L have been reported (*17*). Plasma and serum bicarbonate levels are essentially equivalent. Whole blood and capillary levels are about 3 mmol/L greater than arterial blood.

OVERVIEW: SPECIMEN COLLECTION AND STORAGE FOR ELECTROLYTE DETERMINATIONS

Heparinized plasma is clearly the specimen of choice for electrolyte determinations, due to the artifactual elevation of potassium that occurs with clotting.

For sodium, chloride, and bicarbonate, no difference is seen between serum and plasma. The storage temperature of the specimen must represent a compromise. Sodium–potassium shifts are minimized at 37°C, while chloride is more stable at 4°C. Storage at room temperature (20–25°C) is an acceptable middle ground. Anaerobic conditions should be maintained to minimize loss of CO_2. Plasma should be separated from cells as soon as possible after collection, but, in any event, within 2 hours. Electrolytes in acellular plasma are quite stable if the container is tightly sealed.

Blood Gases

Arterial blood is the specimen most often submitted for blood gas analysis. Occasionally, venous blood is submitted. Blood gas specimens are usually collected in a syringe which has been previously rinsed with heparin, since clotted blood is unacceptable. The needle on the syringe should be capped to prevent gas exchange. Strictly speaking, glass syringes are preferable to plastic ones because gas diffusion can occur through the latter. However, in practice, if the specimen is run promptly, plastic syringes are acceptable. The amount of heparin solution needed is small (0.1–0.2 mL). Care should be taken to expel all air from the syringe before collection. Once drawn, the blood gas specimen must be maintained under anaerobic conditions. Exposure to air will cause a decrease in P_{CO_2} and an increase in P_{O_2} and pH. Often, blood gases are collected under conditions which constitute a clinical emergency, and it is imperative that the laboratory process them immediately. If this is not possible, the stoppered syringe may be maintained on ice for up to one hour, with little change in results (1).

Creatinine and Urea Nitrogen

Both creatinine and urea nitrogen are used to assess renal function. Creatinine is much to be preferred for this purpose, due to the large number of preanalytical factors which alter urea nitrogen.

Creatinine is most frequently determined by the Jaffé reaction, which involves the use of alkaline picrate to form an orange complex. Knowledge of this method is important because of the large number of substances which cause positive interference to varying degrees: cephalothin, cefoxitin, ketone bodies, and others (18). The presence of such substances may cause significant problems in the use of creatinine to measure renal function. This has led to the search for other methods to determine creatinine. One such approach involves the enzymatic hydrolysis of creatinine and the measurement of the ammonium ion formed as a reaction product by colorimetric methods or ion-selective electrode. The reference method is probably high performance liquid chromatography, although this is impractical for everyday use.

Either serum or plasma may be used for the measurement of urea nitrogen and creatinine. If plasma is desired, sodium, potassium, or lithium, heparin, or EDTA is a suitable anticoagulant. Care must be taken not use ammonium-containing anticoagulants. Hemolysis should be avoided, as this will cause the release of Jaffé-reacting chromogens. Removal of the serum from the clot (or plasma from the cells) must be done promptly if a creatinine method that measures ammonium ion is used. Both creatinine and urea nitrogen are stable in separated plasma or serum for one week at 4°C and indefinitely when frozen at −20°C.

Urate

Urate determinations may be performed on serum or heparinized plasma, which give equivalent results. Urate is quite stable (2–3 days at room temperature, 5–7 days at 4–8°C, and up to one year when frozen) (19,20). It presents few preanalytical problems.

Ammonia

Ammonia (or more properly, ammonium ion) is produced by the urea cycle in the liver. The principal causes of true elevators in blood ammonia are urea cycle enzyme deficiencies in children and hepatic cirrhosis in adults. Although ammonia levels are actually of limited use for the diagnosis of hepatic encepalopathy, they are still ordered occasionally for this purpose.

Blood for ammonia is most often collected in heparin anticoagulant (not ammonium heparin, however). EDTA and oxalate are also suitable. Levels are low, and great care is needed to ensure valid results. Closed systems, such as those found on the du Pont aca, are advantageous. Specimens, should be collected with minimum stasis into evacuated blood collection tubes and placed on ice at once. They should then be centrifuged at 4°C and the plasma separated and analyzed immediately. If the specimen is stored at 25°C, plasma ammonia will increase 0.017 μg/mL/min (21).

Bilirubin

Either serum or plasma (any anticoagulant) is suitable for bilirubin determination. The negative interference of hemoglobin with diazo methods has been well described, so hemolysis should be avoided. Since bilirubin is degraded rapidly by light, specimens should be kept in darkness, under which conditions it is stable for 2 days at 25°C, 7 days at 4–8°C, and 3 months at −20°C (7).

Calcium, Magnesium, and Phosphate

Either serum or heparinized plasma may be used for calcium, magnesium, and phosphate determinations. Other anticoagulants are unsuitable. All are stable for several days at room or refrigerator temperatures and for several months if frozen.

It has been well recognized that, especially in patients with acid–base disorders or hypoalbuminemia, total calcium is a poor measurement of the actual calcium status of the blood. New instruments using ion-selective electrodes allow the measurement of the biologically active ionized calcium fraction. The choice of specimen for ionized calcium measurement is controversial. Some authors have favored heparinized plasma, on the grounds that smaller specimens can be used, anaerobic conditions can be maintained more easily, and faster analysis can take place (22). Other authors have favored serum, primarily because of the concern that heparin can bind calcium and thereby distort results. In any event, specimens for ionized calcium need to be collected anaerobically without venous stasis. Specimens should be introduced directly into the instrument with as little delay as possible. However, if immediate analysis is impossible, ionized calcium is stable under anaerobic conditions for 3 days at 4°C or 6 months at −20°C (22).

While anaerobiasis is not needed for determinations of total calcium, phosphate, and magnesium, careful attention to patient preparation is needed. The patient should be supine when these analytes are collected, because an erect posture can elevate them. Tourniquet application time should be minimized (23).

Enzymes

Serum is the specimen of choice for enzyme determinations. If plasma is used, care should be taken that the anticoagulant does not interfere with the assay. The patient should be fasting, and hemolysis must be avoided.

Lactate Dehydrogenase (LDH)

Since erythrocytes are especially rich in lactate dehydrogenase, hemolysis must be avoided. Storage of unseparated specimens at room temperature is preferred to refrigeration, to prevent enzyme leakage from erythrocytes. LDH-5 is the most labile isoenzyme. Although LDH determinations are usually performed on serum, heparinized plasma is also acceptable. LDH is stable in separated serum or plasma for up to 48 hours. However, refrigeration is usually preferred for isoenzyme determinations (24).

Alkaline Phosphatase (AP)

One of the least labile of the commonly measured enzymes, alkaline phosphatase is stable at 4–25°C in separated serum or plasma for up to one week (25).

Amylase

Amylase is the most stable enzyme commonly encountered in the clinical laboratory; it is stable for one week at 25°C and for 3 months at 4°C in either serum or urine (24).

Creatinine Phosphokinase (CPK)

Serum or heparinized plasma may be used. CPK is stable 2–4 hours at 25°C, 12 hours at 4°C, and 3 days at −20°C. Thiol compounds (e.g., Cleland's reagent) were once used to enhance stability, but these are no longer recommended. Many commercial assay systems contain reagents such as EDTA and sulfhydryl compounds, which will reactivate CPK. CPK-1 is the least stable isoenzyme (26).

The Aminotransferases

The aminotransferases aspartate aminotransferase (AST) and alanine aminotransferase (ALT) are usually measured in serum. Hemolysis should be avoided because both enzymes are present in erythrocytes. ALT is more stable than AST, but both may be stored at 4–8°C for several days and at −20°C for several months (26).

Acid Phosphatase (ACP)

Acid phosphatase is most often determined as a tumor marker for prostatic carcinoma. Either immunological or biochemical methods may be employed. Acid phosphatase is extremely unstable at pH values above 6 at room temperature. Stability may be assured by acidification (<pH 6) with acetic acid or disodium citrate. Alternatively, the specimen may be frozen immediately at −20°C. Another acceptable procedure is to collect the specimen directly into an ACD (yellow stopper) vacuum blood collection tube. Under any of these circumstances, ACP is stable for 7 days (27,28).

Lipase

Like amylase, serum lipase is measured to assess pancreatic function. Also like amylase, it is quite stable (1 week at 25°C, 3 weeks at 4–8°C, several months at −20°C) (*26*).

Lipids

While many different lipid assays exist, those most commonly performed in the clinical laboratory include total cholesterol, triglycerides, and high density lipoprotein cholesterol (HDLC). Occasionally other determinations, such as lipoprotein electrophoresis, are requested.

Triglycerides are very sensitive to preanalytical variability. Patients should observe a 12-hour fast, consuming nothing but water; alcohol and all nonessential medications should be withheld. Advancing age, alcohol, pregnancy, and estrogens elevate triglycerides. Analytically, triglycerides undergo slow hydrolysis at 4°C. However, this process will not affect stability for up to 5 days.

Cholesterol values are traditionally said to reflect long-term dietary trends and to be relatively insensitive to recent meals; however, this is untrue for some patients (*29*). Clearly, patients should be fasting for cholesterol measurements. *In vitro*, cholesterol is slowly esterified, but this does not alter total cholesterol measurement. Cholesterol is otherwise stable for several days at room or refrigerator and for months if frozen (*29*).

HDLC stability has recently been studied. This analyte is stable for 1 week at 4°C.

The use of plasma versus for lipid analysis remains controverisal. Both EDTA and oxalate have been shown to lower slightly cholesterol and triglycerides. Heparin has little effect on these values. EDTA stabilizes lipoproteins by binding divalent cations, which catalyzes their chemical transformation. The effects of storage are controversial. Freezing is suitable for cholesterol, triglyceride, and HDLC determination. For lipoproteins patterns, the effects of freezing are variable. Some authors report freezing to be deleterious to lipoprotein patterns (*30*), while others report no change after several months of frozen storage (*31,32*). Repeated freeze–thaw cycles, however, should be avoided.

TOXICOLOGY AND DRUG ANALYSIS

For most drug screening, urine is the specimen of choice. Most drugs are remarkably stable in urine. Flurazepam and secobarbital are stable for 2–3 weeks, and methaqualone is stable for 6 weeks at room temperature, but other drugs are stable for even longer periods. Specimens may be preserved for years by freezing at $-20°C$ or by the addition of fluoride (33). The majority of drugs for which therapeutic monitoring is conducted are quite stable. Cyclosporin is a notable exception, and great care is necessary to ensure that valid specimens are obtained (34). Aminoglycosides are unstable in the presence of β-lactam antibiotics, and prompt analysis or freezing must be carried out to avoid falsely low results.

Tris(butoxyethyl) phosphate, a plasticizer once used in rubber stoppers, displaces highly protein-bound basic drugs (e.g., lidocaine, quinidine, propranolol, tricyclic antidepressants) from serum, causing falsely low values. TBEP now apparently has been eliminated from rubber stoppers by most manufacturers of blood collection tubes.

Except as noted, stability does not appear to be a particular problem with drugs in serum or plasma. Most are stable for several days at 4–25°C and for months at $-20°C$. Quinidine appears to be one of the most labile, however, being stable only 8 hours at 25°C and 24 hours at 4°C (34). Care should be taken to ensure that tubes are kept lightly capped if volatile analytes (ethanol, valproate, ethosuximide) are present.

Metals

While the analytical determination of a large number of metals in blood or urine is technically feasible, only a few are of common clinical interest. These include lead, mercury, arsenic, copper, zinc, and iron. Normal vacuum blood collection tubes, which contain various amounts of trace metals as contaminants, are unsuitable for use for metal determinations (except for iron) because accurate results cannot be assured. Vacuum blood collection tubes (royal blue stoppers) are available for trace metal determinations; however, best results are obtained when specially designed plastic syringes are used. Urine specimens should be collected in glass or plastic bottles cleansed with dilute nitric or hydrochloric acid and rinsed with water of the same quality as is used to perform the analysis (34).

Endocrine Specimens

Since many endocrine studies are related to stimulation, suppression, or diurnal variation, careful attention to patient preparation and timing of specimen collection is crucial in obtaining valid results. Many endocrine analytes, especially peptides, are very unstable. For example, renin and adrenocorticotrophic hormone must be collected in chilled syringes, transported on ice, centrifuged at 4°C and stored at $-70°C$ (35). Other peptide

**Table 1. Recommended Order of Collection for Vacuum Blood
Collection Tubes**

1. Tubes for which sterility is required (blood culture tubes, etc.)
2. Tubes containing no additives
3. Tubes for coagulation studies
4. Other tubes containing additives

hormones, such as insulin and thyrotropin, are stable at 4–8°C for several days. Except for aldosterone, most steroid hormones, including thyroxine and triiodothyroxine, are stable for 2–3 days at 4–8°C and for months at -20°C (*35*). In urine, acidification with boric or hydrochloric acid to $\leq$ pH 2 will ensure stability of analytes such as 17-hydroxysteroids, 17-ketosteroids, and catecholamines (which should be kept in the dark) for several weeks.

Collection Devices

Today the overwhelming majority of blood specimens are obtained using vacuum blood collection tubes, carefully designed to obtain a sample under sterile, anaerobic conditions. These tubes always should be allowed to fill to capacity. Small tubes are available for pediatric use.

Except for blood gas measurements and blood cultures, the use of syringes to collect specimens should be discouraged. They are awkward to manipulate, expensive, and difficult to use for the collection of multiple specimens. If an anticoagulated specimen is required, the blood must be expelled from the syringe into a suitable tube, which allows clotting to take place in the syringe. Vacuum blood collection tubes are much to be preferred over syringes, except in infants and adult patients with extremely poor veins, where it may be necessary to use a butterfly infusion device and syringe for blood collection. However, in such patients, capillary blood collection is often an acceptable alternative, and many suitable tubes, including some with anticoagulant, are available for this purpose. The proper order of collection when multiple tubes are desired from a single venipuncture is shown in Table 1.

Timing of Collection

Whenever possible, specimens should be collected in a fasting state. Ingestion of food causes both physiological and technical interference with many laboratory determinations. Lipemia interferes with the optical measurements

Table 2. Effects of Recent Meals

Analyte	Effect
Sodium	Increase
Phosphate	Increase in men
	Decrease in women
Glucose	Increase
Insulin	Increase
pH	Increase
Bilirubin	Increase
Urate	Increase
Triglycerides	Increase
Lactate	Increase
Cholesterol	Little change
Alkaline phosphatase	Increase

Source: Ref. 34.

in many laboratory instruments. The *in vivo* effects of meals are shown in Table 2.

Timing of specimen collection is especially important for drug levels, especially for drugs with short half-lives, such as the aminoglycoside antibiotics and procainamide. While "trough levels" (those collected immediately before the next dose) are always acceptable, "peak" levels are used as well for certain others, such as antibiotics and antiarrhythmics. If meaningful data are to be obtained, these must be carefully timed in relation to dosing.

Many endocrine analytes (e.g., corticotropin, somatotropin, cortisol) and certain others (e.g., iron) show pronounced diurnal variation. Time of collection must be noted for these specimens. Other endocrine analytes, such as estrogen, progesterone, and the gonadotropins, vary with the stage of the menstrual cycle, and the knowledge of the date of onset of the last menstrual period may be essential for their interpretation. Still other substances, such as testosterone, show wide, unpredictable temporal variations in the same individual, and multiple specimens may be necessary to obtain a true picture of their status.

Posture

A number of changes occur upon standing, including diseases in blood pressure, heart rate, and blood volume. Table 3 lists various analytes that increase upon standing.

Table 3. Analytes That Increase upon Assuming Upright Posture

Protein	Alanine aminotransferase
Albumin	Acid phosphatase
Iron	Sodium
Total lipids	Potassium
Cholesterol	Calcium
Phosphate	Chloride
Urea	Creatinine
Catecholines	Aldosterone
Renin	Vasopressin

Source: Ref. 35.

Table 4. Effects of Vigorous Physical Activity

Analyte	Effect
Creatinine	Increase
Urea	Increase
β-Hydroxybutyrate	Increase
Calcium	Decrease
Magnesium	Decrease
Bicarbonate	Decrease
Lactate	Increase
Potassium	Increase
Urate	Increase
Creatine phosphokinase	Increase
Alkaline phosphatase	Increase
Lactate dehydrogenase	Increase
Aspartate aminotransferase	Increase

Source: Refs. 36–39.

Physical Activity

The effect of physical activity on a number of analytes has been well studied and is shown in Table 4.

Caffeine, Alcohol, and Tobacco

Caffeine, a close chemical relative of theophylline, with which it shares many pharmacological properties, is found in coffee, tea, many cola beverages, and various medications. Table 5 gives the effects of caffeine on laboratory testing.

Table 5. Effects of Caffeine

Analyte	Effect
Triglycerides	Increase
Free fatty acids	Increase
Cortisol	Increase
Cholesterol	Decrease
Catecholamines (urine)	Increase
Glucose	Little change
Insulin	Little change

Source: Refs. 40–42.

Table 6. Effects of Ethanol in Nonalcoholics

Analyte	Effect
Glucose	Increase[a]
Insulin	Decrease
Urate	Increase
Lactate	Increase
Triglycerides	Increase
Free fatty acids	Increase
Calcitonin	Increase
Potassium	Decrease
Phosphate	Decrease
Magnesium	Decrease
Lactate dehydrogenase	Increase
γ-Glutamyl transferase	Increase
Vasopressin	Increase

Source: Ref. 21.

[a] Hypoglycemia may be a late effect.

Patients should avoid alcohol before specimen collection whenever possible. The effects of alcohol ingestion on laboratory results in healthy volunteers are shown in Table 6. About one-third of adult Americans use tobacco, and the effects of this substance are shown in Table 7.

The Specimen Collection Process

In some hospitals, particularly teaching institutions, specimens may be collected by physicians or medical students; most often, hospitalized patients have their blood drawn by employees of the laboratory. In doctors' offices, often a nurse or technician performs this duty. In any event, it is mandatory that the phlebotomist be properly trained. Usually collection of blood specimens is done in response to a written collection slip, which is generated, often by computer, in response to a physician's order. The phlebotomist, whether physician, nurse, medical student, or technician, should have a neat, clean, professional appearance. He or she should introduce himself or herself to the patient and explain the blood collection procedure. The patient should be sitting, or, in the hospital, lying in bed. The phlebotomist should be careful

Table 7. Effects of Tobacco

Analyte	Effect
Nicotine	Increase
Cadmium	Increase
Carbon monoxide	Increase
Cyanide	Increase
P_{O_2}, P_{CO_2}	Little change
Hemoglobin	Increase

Source: Ref. 21.

Table 8. Proper Procedure for Venipuncture Using Vacuum Blood Collection Tubes

Verify that patient identification band matches information on requisition.

Select venipuncture site (generally antecubital fossa). The site should be free of intravenous infusions, skin lesions, etc.

Place patient's arm in downward position. Observe vein.

Select tubes and examine for defects. Additive tubes should be tapped to dislodge clumped powder.

Insert first tube into holder. Push onto needle as far as guide mark.

Cleanse area with gauze soaked in 70% ethanol or isopropanol.

Allow to dry. Do not palpate vein after preparation.

Apply tourniquet, as required.

Perform venipuncture. Push tube to end of holder, puncturing diaphragm.

Remove tourniquet as blood enters tube.

When blood has filled tube, remove and insert next tube (see Table 1 for proper order of tubes).

After blood has been collected, remove needle holder and cover wound with cotton gauze or bandage.

Gently invert additive tubes 10–12 times.

Label tubes with name and identification number of patient, date and time, and phlebotomist's initials.

Source: Ref. 21.

to establish the proper identification, NOT by asking the patient, but by inspecting the armband or, in the case of outpatients, by examining the clinic card. Blood collection tubes should be labeled at the bedside with the patient's name, identification number, time of collection, and phlebotomist's initials.

The use of a tourniquet is controversial. For certain analytes (e.g., ionized calcium, lactate, catecholomines), it is mandatory that a tourniquet not be used. In most other cases, however, use of a tourniquet is acceptable if application time is in the proper sequence of phlebotomy events (Table 8). It cannot be overemphasized that vacuum blood collection tubes are preferable to syringes. The proper order of collection for these tubes was shown in Table 1.

REFERENCES

1. Henry RJ, Cannon DC, Winkelman, J. *Clinical Chemistry: Theory, Analysis, and Correlation*, 2nd ed. New York: Harper & Row, 1974, pp 1265–1326.

2. Weissman M, Klein B. Evaluation of glucose determinations in untreated serum samples. *Clin Chem* 1958;4:420–422.

3. Field JB, Williams HE. Artifactual hypoglycemia associated with leukemia. *N Engl J Med* 1961;79:946–948.

4. Hanrahan JB, Sax SM, Cillo, A. Factitious hypoglycemia associated with leukemia. *Am J Clin Pathol* 1963;40:43–45.

5. Tietz NW. *Clinical Guide to Laboratory Tests*. Philadelphia: Saunders, 1983, p 230.

6. Caraway WT, Watts NB. Carbohydrates, in Tietz NW (ed): *Fundamentals of Clinical Chemistry*. Philadelphia: Saunders, 1986, p 230.

7. Goodman JR, Vincent J, Rosen I. Serum potassium changes in blood clots. *Am J Clin Pathol* 1954;24:111–113.

8. Hultma E, Bergstrom J. Plasma potassium determination. *Scand J Clin Lab Invest* 1962;64: (14 suppl 64) 87–93.

9. Hartman RC, Auditore JV, Jackson DP. Studies on thrombocytosis. I. Hyperkalemia due to release of potassium from platelets during coagulation. *J Clin Invest* 1958;37:699–707.

10. Ingram RH, Seki M. Pseudohyperkalemia with thrombocytosis. *N Engl J Med* 1966;274:369–375.

11. Mir MA, Brabin B, Tang OT, Leyland MJ, Delamore IW. Hypokalemia in acute myeloid leukemia. *Ann Intern Med* 1975;82:54–57.

12. Adams PC, Woodhouse KW, Adela M, Parnham A. Exaggerated hypokalaemia in acute myeloid leukaemia. *Br Med J* 1981;282:1034–1035.

13. Miller WG. Chloride, in Kaplan LA, Pesce AJ (eds): *Clinical Chemistry: Theory, Analysis, and Correlation*. St. Louis: Mosby, 1984, pp 1059–1062.

14. Tietz NW, Pruden EL, Siggaard-Anderson O. Electrolytes, blood gases, and acid–base balance, in Tietz NW (ed): *Textbook of Clinical Chemistry*. Philadelphia: Saunders, 1986, p 1188.

15. Tietz NW. *Fundamentals of Clinical Chemistry*, 2nd ed. Philadelphia: Saunders, 1983, p 880.

16. Rock EC, Walker WG, Jennings CD. Nitrogen metabolites and renal function, in Tietz NW (ed): *Textbook of Clinical Chemistry*. Philadelphia: Saunders, 1986, p 1276.

17. Schultz AL. Nonprotein nitrogenous compounds—Uric acid, in Kaplan LA, Pesce AJ (eds): *Clinical Chemistry: Theory, Analysis, and Correlation*. St. Louis: Mosby, 1984, p 1263.

18. Rock RC, Walker WG, Jennings CD. Nitrogen metabolites and renal function, in Tietz NW (ed): *Textbook of Clinical Chemistry*. Philadelphia: Saunders, 1986, p 1276.

19. Gau N. Nonprotein nitrogenous compounds—Ammonia, in Kaplan LA, Pesce AJ (eds): *Clinical Chemistry: Theory, Analysis, and Correlation*. St. Louis: Mosby, 1984, p 1231.

20. Faser D, Jones G, Kooh SW, et al. Calcium and phosphate metabolism, in Tietz NW (ed): *Textbook of Clinical Chemistry*. Philadelphia: Saunders, 1986, p 1344.

21. Fody EP. General principles of patient preparation and specimen handling, in Howanitz PJ, Howanitz JH (eds): *Laboratory Quality Assurance*. New York: McGraw-Hill, 1986, pp 55–79.

22. Lipoproteins, in Henry RJ, Cannon DC, Winkelman JW (eds): *Clinical Chemistry: Principles and Techniques*, 2nd ed. New York: Harper & Row, 1974, p 1495.

23. Bowers GN, McComb RB. A continuous spectrophotometric method for measuring the activity of serum alkaline phosphatase. *Clin Chem* 1966;12:70–89.

24. Moss DW, Henderson AR, Kachmar JF. Enzymes, in Tietz NW (ed): *Textbook of Clinical Chemistry*. Philadelphia: Saunders, 1986, p 684.

25. Doe RP, Mellinger GT, Seal VA. Stabilization and preservation of serum prostatic acid phosphatase activity. *Clin Chem* 1955;11:943–950.

26. Ellis G, Belfield A, Goldberg DM. Colorimetric determination of serum and phosphatase activity using adenosine 3'-monophosphate as substrate. *J Clin Pathol* 1971;24:493–500.

27. Grafnetter D, Fodor JJ, Teply V, et al. The effect of storage on levels of cholesterol in serum measured by a simple direct method. *Clin Chim Acta* 1967;16:33–37.

28. Fredrickson DS, Levy RI, Lees RS. Fat transport in lipoproteins: An integrated approach to mechanisms and disorders. *N Engl J Med* 1957;276:146–156.

29. Aldersberg D, Bossak ET, Sher IH, et al. Electrophoresis and monomolecular layer studies with serum lipoproteins. *Clin Chem* 1955;1:18–33.

30. Winkelman JW, Wybenga DR, Ibbott FA. Quantitation of lipoprotein components in the phenotyping of hyperlipoproteinemias. *Clin Chem Acta* 1970;27:181–183.

31. Rockerbie RA, Campbell DJ. Effect of specimen storage and preservation on toxicological analyses of urine. *Clin Biochem* 1978;11:77–81.

32. Fody EP, Duby MM, Nadel MS, et al. Fascicle. IV. Therapeutic drug monitoring and toxicology, in College of American Pathologists: *Clinical Laboratory Handbook in Patient Preparation and Specimen Handling.* Skokie, IL: CAP, 1985.

33. Chattoraj SC, Watts NB. Enrocrinology, in *Textbook of Clinical Chemistry* Tietz NW (ed): Philadelphia: Saunders, 1986, pp 997–1171.

34. Young DS. Biological variability, in Brown SS, Mitchell FL, Young DS (eds): *Chemical Diagnosis of Disease,* New York: Elsevier North-Holland, 1979, pp 3–112.

35. Statland BE, Bokeland H. Factors contributing to intraindividual variation of serum constituents. IV. Effects of posture and tourniquet application on variation of serum constituents in healthy subjects. *Clin Chem* 1974;20:1513–1519.

36. Refsum HE, Treit B, Meen HD, et al. Serum electrolyte, fluid and acid–base balance after prolonged heavy exercise and low environmental temperature. *Scand J Clin Lab Invest* 1973;32:111.

37. Refsum HE, Meen HD, Strommee, SB. Whole blood, serum and erythrocyte magnesium concentrations after repeated heavy exercise of long duration. *Scand J Clin Lab Invest* 1973;32:117.

38. Riley WJ, Pyke FS, Roberts AD, et al. The effect of long-distance running on some biochemical variables. *Clin Chim Acta* 1975;65:83.

39. Bunch TW. Blood test abnormalities in runners. *Mayo Clin Proc* 1980;55:113–117.

40. Avogaro P, Capri C, Pais M, et al. Plasma and urine cortisol behavior and fat mobilization in man after coffee ingestion. *Israel J Med Sci* 1973;9:114.

41. Natsmith DJ, Akinyanju PA, Szanto S, et al. The effect in volunteers of coffee and decaffeinated coffee on blood glucose, insulin, plasma lipids and some factors involved in blood clotting. *Nutr Metab* 1970;12:144.

42. Bellet S, Roman L, De Castro O, et al. Effect of coffee ingestion on catecholamine release. *Jpn J Stud Alcohol* 1969;18:288.

CHAPTER 2

QUALITY CONTROL AND QUALITY ASSURANCE

E. HOWARD TAYLOR

University of Arkansas for Medical Sciences
Little Rock, Arkansas

INTRODUCTION

One must define error in terms of the analytical tolerances which are acceptable based on the medical appropriateness of each particular laboratory test. Obviously a 10% error in sodium measurement is *not* at all satisfactory: the reference range is 135–145 meq/L; hence a 10% error would be intolerable. Other tests such as enzyme assays (e.g., creatine phosphokinase (CPK), reference range 50–230 U/L), may better tolerate an error of 10%. In fact, enzyme assays usually do have poorer precision than electrolyte assays, and this is allowable based on the medical interpretation of the test. However, accuracy and precision are most important at medical decision concentrations, that is, at the upper or lower limits of the reference range. Quality control samples which are nearer these decision concentrations are essential to guarantee appropriate results.

Approximately 10–20% of a laboratory's workload is devoted to quality control (QC). This substantial volume influences both the laboratory workload and costs; thus, the selection of a QC program must balance cost effectiveness and statistical accuracy (*1*). To eliminate erroneous results, the criteria for run rejection should have a sound statistical basis.

Not only should a laboratory maintain an internal QC policy, but there *must* exist interlaboratory comparison to further evaluate the accuracy of test results. These proficiency-testing surveys are designed to identify a laboratory's weaknesses and therefore point out any potential problem. This practice is fundamental to all clinical laboratories, which continually undergo peer evaluation to verify the accuracy of test results. The College of American Pathologists (CAP) has developed a very comprehensive system of laboratory standards by documentation of testing methods and laboratory performance on proficiency tests (*2*).

Accuracy is essential in the performance of laboratory analyses that may affect a patient's diagnosis and treatment. How does one guarantee the accuracy of such analytical procedures? A thorough program of quality control (both internal and external) as well as appropriate quality assurance programs are essential. Quality assurance should not be confused with quality control. While quality control tests the laboratory's analytical accuracy, quality assurance tests the medical appropriateness of those results. For example, a patient's result may be erroneous due to a clerical error, although the analytical tolerances for instrumentation and reagents were within defined limits. Results that get to the patient's chart should be monitored as well. This can be accomplished by a computer delta check, which compares the present result to the preceding result and flags results outside a certain range (3). This chapter offers a reasonable approach to internal quality control, external quality control, and quality assurance.

INTERNAL (INTRALABORATORY) QC

Choice of a Control Material

The evaluation of analytical and technical methodology is monitored by analysis of QC material whose concentrations are known. One then assays the QC sample as an unknown and evaluates the result based on the particular laboratory's rules for run acceptance or run rejection. Since the QC sample is analyzed as an unknown and there exists a certain degree of analytical variation, there will be statistical boundaries established to evaluate the accuracy of the run.

Most laboratories purchase commercially available material, which is usually supplied in a lyophilized bottle prepared by addition of a specific diluent or deionized water. Control material is available in both assayed and unassayed form. Assayed material is always more expensive; however, this can be convenient, particularly in evaluation of a new analyzer or method. A list of analytes (as many as 60 may be present) is supplied, and the concentrations (mean and standard deviations) are listed and usually subcategorized by instrument or method. Even when assayed QC material is used, it is advisable to verify these values (mean and standard deviation) in one's own laboratory. Most laboratories purchase unassayed QC material and establish statistical boundaries. These boundaries can be evaluated by examining the precision (reproducibility) of results when the same specimen is analyzed repeatedly to establish a mean and standard deviation. The analytic precision of 31 analytes has been reported (4).

The stability (shelf life) of lyophilized material should be clearly defined by the manufacturer. The stability of commercially available QC material has been summarized (5). Enzymes are usually the least stable; however, variables include control manufacturer, lyophilized versus liquid control, particular enzyme, and analytical method. Analytes with consistent instability include potassium, sodium, chloride, phosphorus, alkaline phosphatase, and creatine phosphokinase (5,6). Lawson et al. (5) have proposed that the definition of instability be 0.5 SD per year. Many manufacturers claim a two-year stability on lyophilized control material; however, one should be aware of decreasing stability, which may appear as increased electrolyte values and decreased enzyme values. This stability is critical because it is necessary to purchase a single lot number that can be assumed to maintain the same value for at least a year. A great deal of time and effort goes into evaluation of a new QC sample to establish the values to be used in the laboratory. The less often a new lot number needs to be evaluated, the more productive the laboratory. The size of vial is also important. Larger sizes (25 or 50 mL) are less expensive per milliliter than smaller sizes (5 or 10 mL), but the unused quantity each day may eliminate the savings.

The matrix should be identical in form to the patient sample (i.e., both should be serum, urine, CSF, etc.). The levels of analyte present should be representative of both the nondiseased state (normal) and the diseased state (abnormal). Many manufacturers have three levels available in which the analyte is present in low, normal, and elevated amounts. The stability over time (day-to-day reproducibility) should be clearly defined for the re-constituted as well as lyophilized material. Some analytes (e.g., enzymes or hormones) may be stable for only a single day while reconstituted, whereas others (e.g., drugs) may be stable for several days. QC material once reconstituted should always be returned to the refrigerator (4°C) throughout the day to maintain stability and to prevent bacterial contamination, which can substantially alter control values (e.g., glucose).

If an in-house frozen pool is used, the expiration date should be determined. If an in-house control is used, under *no circumstances* should the sample be prepared from the standard. Ideally, QC material should be prepared outside the laboratory—for example by a commercial manufacturer. If no outside source is available (e.g., with some unusual therapeutic drugs), a different source of material should be sought. For example, in our laboratory, a standard for pentobarbital is prepared from the powder; however, the QC material is prepared from drug available from the pharmacy in a preparation used for intravenous injection. Although this is an "in-house" control, it is not prepared by someone in our laboratory. Any error in purity or weighing technique that might occur never would be discovered if the QC were simply a "dilution" of the standard. Therefore, quality control material should be prepared from an outside source.

Lyophilized or commercially available QC material is usually stable for at least one year. Lyophilized material offers significant advantages over in-house material, since the former is homogeneous and stable, and has specific levels of analyte at representative concentrations. Ethylene glycol, sometimes used as a preservative in liquid controls, is useful in extending shelf life. Ethylene glycol depresses the freezing point, permitting the material to remain in solution at temperatures above $-20°C$. This allows for increased stability; however, the presence of ethylene glycol can interfere with the determination of electrolytes on some instruments (those which use direct measurement of electrolytes by ion-selective electrode). Once reconstituted, lyophilized material is generally stable for 24 hours, although to prevent unnecessary wastage, one must consider frequency of performing QC analysis and size of QC vial. Thus, stability is an important factor to consider, not only analytically, but also financially.

How Many QC Levels Are Needed?

Commercial manufacturers offer two or three levels of controls, usually physiologically low, normal, and elevated. These values should approximate clinical decision-making levels, although this is not always the case. Different levels can be important to evaluate certain areas of calibration curves. For example, radioimmunoassay (RIA) quantitation is best when percentage bound (B/Bo) is near the center (50% bound), it is particularly difficult when the slope is very steep in a plot of percentage bound versus concentration or when the linearity of the assay is questionable because only a few counts will lead to a large difference in concentration. Similarly, immunoradiometric assays (IRMAs) can vary at the high and low ends of the curve. Multilevel controls would challenge the analytical integrity of calibration curves of these types. In addition, if only one level of control is used, it makes trend analysis very difficult. One may be restricted to a single decision rule (± 2 SD), which may not be sufficiently sensitive to detect errors. Although three levels may not be necessary, two levels are recommended if possible.

Quality Control Rules

One must first establish the statistical boundaries for acceptance of a run. These boundaries can be evaluated by examining the precision (repro-ducibility) of results when the same specimen is analyzed repeatedly to establish a mean (X) and standard deviation (SD). The mean is an evaluation of the accuracy of a method, while standard deviation is a measurement of the precision. The analysis of a QC sample is repeated for at least 30 runs (usually once a day for a month) to evaluate between-run variations. After 30 measurements, an initial estimate of the mean and standard deviation is obtained. This estimate may be reevaluated later if more data points are necessary to give a more representative spread of data.

With any laboratory procedure, it is assumed that there is a randomness associated with the error and therefore the error is Gaussian in distribution. With a Gaussian (normal) distribution, $X \pm 1$ SD accounts for 68% of data, $X \pm 2$ SD, 95%, $X \pm 3$ SD, 99%, etc. Therefore, the error is predictable in terms of how many points should fall above and below and how far they should vary from the mean. The relationship of analytical variation in terms of Gaussian statistics is described extremely well (7). Since the mean and standard deviation are well characterized for each QC sample which is run, it is possible to evaluate graphically the performance of the analysis in terms of run rejection or a warning. These rules for trend evaluation of QC data are described below.

Trend Analysis (Westgard's Multirule Analysis)

There are several strategies for run rejection. The goal is to differentiate a random error from a true analytical problem. This can be best accomplished by following data on quality control charts. The purpose of following data graphically is to observe shifts or trends in data that may uncover a potential problem before it occurs. For example, if all the QC data fall on the same side of the mean, there is no longer randomness, and a bias has been introduced into the system. Even though all these data points may be less than 2 standard deviations away from the mean, clearly something is wrong. Therefore, presentation of data graphically in terms of the deviation from the mean plotted against time clearly has an important value. These QC charts were first described by Levey and Jennings (8).

Many laboratories have set as boundaries on their QC charts 2 standard deviations away from the mean, since 2 SD would encompass 95% of all data, assuming a normal (Gaussian) distribution. However, under this assumption, 5% of QC data should be outside 2 SD or out of control even when no instrument or reagent problem exists. If one uses more than one control, the probability that a false run rejection will occur (based on a single decision rule of ± 2 SD) increases exponentially (Table 1). This idea also applies to performing screening of a disease-free population with a large battery of tests. If one were to run a 10-test profile on disease-free individuals, the chances of all 10 of the patient results falling within the reference range is only 63%. Using 3 SD as a boundary to prevent false rejection due to random error may be too insensitive, since ± 3 SD in a normal distribution would contain 99.7% of QC data. Parameters for a statistical compromise that is neither too insensitive (i.e., likely to overlook an error) nor too sensitive (i.e., likely to

Table 1. Probability of False Rejection Using Only ± 2 SD as Boundary for Run Rejection

No. of Controls	% Within Control[a]	% Out of Control
1	95	5
2	91	9
3	87	13
4	83	17
5	79	21
10	63	37

[a] Based on probability of 0.95^n where n = number of controls.

Table 2. Shewhart Multirule Analysis

QC rule	Description	Action	Example
1_{2s}	One control value exceeds 2 SD	Warning	Figure 1
1_{3s}	One control value exceeds 3 SD	Rejection	Figure 2
2_{2s}	Two consecutive control values exceeds the same 2 SD	Rejection	Figure 3
R_{4s}	Range between two control values exceeds 4 SD	Rejection	Figure 4
4_{1s}	Four consecutive control values exceed the same ± 1 SD	Rejection	Figure 5
10_x	Ten consecutive control values on the same side of mean (x)	Rejection	Figure 6

cause a false run rejection) have been proposed by Westgard et al. (9) and are presented in Table 2.

The multirule Shewhart analysis, a decision tree to decide run rejection, is based on a trend analysis of a Levey–Jennings plot. These rejection rules are illustrated below. Usually two different levels of control material are run with each analysis, and this format is used as an example.

1_{2s} *Rule.* One level of control has exceeded the 2 SD boundary either above or below the mean. This serves strictly as a warning until the other level of control is evaluated (see Figure 1).

1_{3s} *Rule.* One level of control has exceeded the 3 SD boundary either above or below the mean. This constitutes a run rejection no matter what value is obtained for the other control value (see Figure 2).

2_{2s} *Rule.* Both levels of control material exceed either + 2 SD or − 2 SD. The result is rejection (Figure 3).

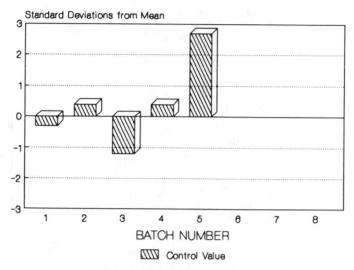

Figure 1. Example of 1_{2s} rule. Batch (run) number 5 exceeds 2 standard deviations.

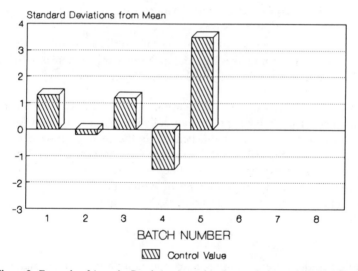

Figure 2. Example of 1_{3s} rule. Batch (run) number 5 exceeds 3 standard deviations.

R_{4s} *Rule.* The range (difference in standard deviations) exceeds 4 SD. This occurs, for example, when level one control exceeds $+2$ SD and the other exceeds -2 SD, indicating that the range between the two is greater than 4 SD (see Figure 4). The result is run rejection.

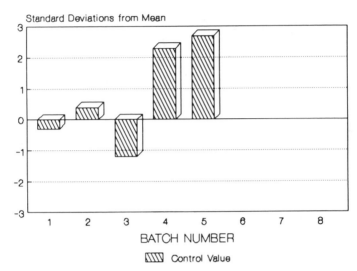

Figure 3. Example of 2_{2s} rule. Batch (run) numbers 4 and 5 exceed 2 standard deviations.

4_{1s} *Rule.* Four consecutive control values exceed the same ± 1 SD (see Figure 5).

10_x *Rule.* Ten consecutive observations fall on the same side of the mean. Clearly the randomness is lost and bias exists somewhere (see Figure 6). The result is run rejection on the tenth observation.

If no run rejection occurs by violation of these rules, then the run is accepted. These rules can be applied manually and scanned visually for trends if QC charts are available at the bench for the technologist to examine. Obviously it does very little good to examine QC charts at a later date after a run has been reported. Ideally, an on-line computer system which compares the recent QC result to an earlier result would be the best form of trend analysis, and run rejection could be made by computer.

Cusum QC Charts

In addition to the Levey–Jennings chart, the cumulative sum (cusum) chart is sometimes used (9,10), although less frequently than the Levey–Jennings chart. With a cusum chart, the sum of the difference between two data points is calculated rather than the individual values. This calculation is done by subtracting the mean value from control value and adding this difference to the cumulative sum. This concept is outlined in the following example. Assume a mean of 110 mg/dL for glucose and an SD of 4.0 mg/dL.

Run Number	Control Value	$X_i - X$	Cusum $X_i - X$
1	113	3	3
2	111	1	4
3	116	6	10
4	114	4	14
5	108	−2	12
6	110	0	12
7	112	2	14
8	104	−6	8

Assuming random error, the control values should fall above and below the mean, resulting in a zero cumulative sum. Should a bias (systematic error) occur, the cusum value will get larger and larger. One can set a boundary to flag a cusum total to indicate that a systematic error has occurred. For example, assume that 2.7 SD is determined to be a satisfactory boundary. In any case, where the cusum exceeds either + or −2.7 SD, the run is rejected. In our example above, $2.7 \times 4.0 = 10.8$, thus run number 4 would be rejected, even though the value 114 is only 1 SD away from the mean. Thus, the cusum chart can also be used to follow trends in control data. Also, cusum charts can be useful to follow patient data to interpret mean values for normal results.

Additional Strategies for Run Rejection

Although the Westgard rules and cusum charts have an excellent statistical basis, these rules are not totally accepted in day-to-day laboratory operation. With increased analytical precision due to automation, the old ±2 SD rule is less frequently used and is being replaced by a combination of some of the Westgard rules and the ±2 SD rule. These modified rules have been described by Haven et al. (11). A run is rejected if

1. patient results appear unlikely regardless of control values,
2. one control value exceeds ±3 SD,
3. one control value exceeds ±2 SD for two successive runs, or
4. both controls exceed ±2 SD.

Evaluating a Run Rejection

When a run is out of control, one asks: Is this a random error? Can a repeat analysis bring the control value within limits? If the answer is no, then a systematic cause for the error should be sought. Systematic errors are often calibration problems, usually in stability (frequency) of calibration, or perhaps

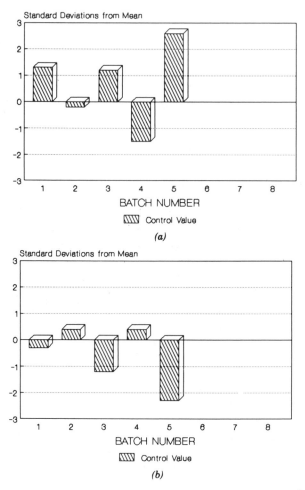

Figure 4. Example of R_{4s} rule. (a) Batch (run) number 5 exceeds $+2$ SD. (b) Batch (run) number 5 exceeds -2 SD from different level of control.

errors in calibrator preparation or value assignment. Also one should check for physical problems associated with an instrument (e.g., clogged tubing or short sample due to sampler probe misalignment). If the problem is not easily identified as instrument related or calibration related, a method evaluation may be necessary. Perhaps it is the control material, an interference, recovery, or linearity problem. If a method comparison is performed, the slope and intercept may allow one to quantify the proportional or constant error, respectively.

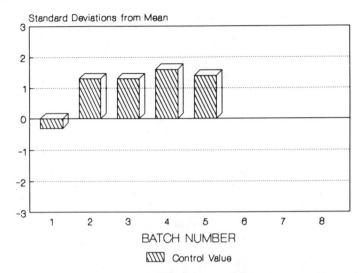

Figure 5. Example of 4_{1s} rule. Batch (run) numbers 2 through 5 all fall greater than $+1$ SD but less than 2 SD.

To identify a random error, precision may be a problem. Within-run and between-run means and standard deviations may be necessary to compare to earlier runs. Whatever is done, there should exist a written procedure to clearly define run rejection and to further document what was done to correct any problem that results in run rejection. Documentation is essential to verify for inspectors (e.g., CAP checklist) that corrective action was taken.

INTERLABORATORY (EXTERNAL) QUALITY CONTROL

The discussion of Levey–Jennings charts, Westgard's multirules, cusum charts, and other QC rules has been directed at evaluation of a QC material in one's own laboratory. How does one compare results relative to other laboratories that analyze the same QC material? This external comparison is interlaboratory quality control in which the same samples (proficiency tests) are analyzed nationwide. Both intra- and interlaboratory QC programs are essential to maintain effective QC. Intralaboratory QC evaluates the daily accuracy and precision of the method, and interlaboratory QC is necessary to maintain the accuracy of the particular analytical method by means of peer evaluation.

The comparison of quality from one lab to another is extremely important in maintaining the overall proficiency of the laboratory. Interlaboratory

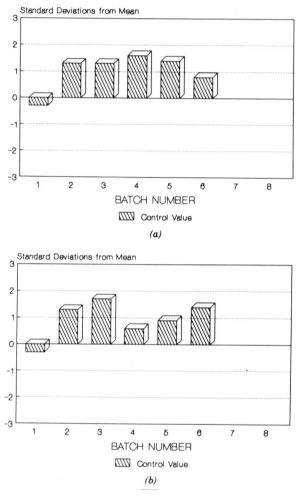

Figure 6. Example of 10_x rule. (*a*) Batch (run) numbers 2 through 6 all fall on same side of the mean. (*b*) Batch (run) numbers 2 through 6 all on the same side of the mean for a different level of control.

proficiency testing (surveys) involves the evaluation of unknown samples sent to many laboratories; these surveys are a means of comparing one's lab to those of peers who have evaluated the same material. The College of American Pathologists (2) has done an outstanding job in providing material and also establishing a standardized, easy-to-read computer format for evaluation of results. Sample computer printout of CAP proficiency test results is shown in Figure 7. The result of each test is compared with a mean and standard deviation for the particular method as well as all other methods for that particular test. The number of labs performing each method and also the standard deviation index (SDI) are also shown. The format for evaluating SDI is a very convenient method of evaluating results, since it determines the number of standard deviations that the results vary from the mean. Usually, plus or minus 2 standard deviations (± 2 SDI) is acceptable, since this would compare with 95% of laboratories. Therefore, a quick scan of the SDI looking for values outside 2 standard deviations can be used to rapidly evaluate the results. The cumulative SDI shows a Levey–Jennings plot of data accumulated for the entire year, and one can apply the multirule trend analysis methods as discussed previously for intralaboratory QC. As shown in Figure 7, with albumin, there exists a problem since all four survey sets fell below the mean. In the cases of bilirubin, calcium, chloride, cortisol, and creatinine there is a randomness above and below the mean, and all values fall between $+2$ SD and -2 SD.

Proficiency tests exist for nearly all tests done in a clinical laboratory. The specimens that are used are prepared in excess; after the survey is completed, the excess is made available to laboratories. This material, which is survey-validated reference material, is available to help laboratories troubleshoot particular analytical methods.

In addition to programs such as CAP, which are used for are used for accreditation, there are interlaboratory quality control programs sponsored by commercial manufacturers of QC material. Bio-Rad laboratories (12) sponsors such a program in which many laboratories use the same lot number of QC material in the internal QC program and submit their analytical results to a central facility. Later, a computer summary shows a statistical summary comparison of all labs which use the same QC material. These commercially available interlaboratory comparisons serve the same purpose: a check of accuracy and precision when compared with one's peers.

Without interlaboratory comparison, one might never detect a systematic error which occurred consistently on the days the QC samples were run and evaluated. Thus, systematic errors are detected only when operating parameters were different from the "original" parameters when the QC was evaluated. It is the purpose of interlaboratory proficiency tests to evaluate data and to assure that systematic errors are not present before the internal QC mean and standard deviation are assigned. Also, before placing a new instrument or method in service, one would perform a method comparison to identify any systematic errors that might occur (13). The interlaboratory surveys provide an ongoing method comparison with one's peers and are essential to assure that systematic errors do not creep into a laboratory or perhaps go undetected by internal QC methods.

EVALUATION STATISTICS / **CUMULATIVE S.D.I.**

CONSTITUENT / UNIT OF MEASURE / YOUR LABORATORY'S METHOD/SYSTEM / COMPARATIVE METHOD	SPECIMEN NUMBER	CODE	YOUR RESULT	MEAN	S.D.	NO OF LABS	YOUR SDI	87 C C-11	87 C C-12	87 B C-6	87 B C-7	87 A C-1	87 A C-2	86 D C-16	86 D C-17
ALBUMIN GM/DL — DYE BINDING-BCG / OLYMPUS DEMAND	C-11	13	3.7	3.99	.14	160	-2.1								
	C-12	13	2.9	3.08	.11	158	-1.6								
DYE BINDING-BCG W/RA — ALL INSTRUMENTS	C-11			3.99	.23	743	-1.3			.3		.8		1.3	
	C-12			3.04	.18	739	-.8		1.6		.2		1.6		3.7
BILIRUBIN, TOTAL MG/DL — DIAZO J-G W/O BLANK / DUPONT ACA	C-11	12	4.8	4.61	.16	373	+1.2								
	C-12	12	1.1	1.04	.12	375	+.5								
ALL METHOD PRINCIPLES — ALL INSTRUMENTS	C-11			4.73	.36	5715	+.2	1.2		.8		.6		.3	
	C-12			.96	.15	5715	+.9		.5				.5		.2
CALCIUM-SERUM MG/DL — CRESOLPHTHALEIN COMPL / BECKMAN ASTRA 4 & 6	C-11	14	12.1	12.11	.29	333	-.0								
	C-12	14	9.3	9.76	.25	342	-1.8								
ATOMIC ABSORPTION — ALL ATOMIC ABSORP SPEC	C-11			12.40	.33	28	-.9	.0		.2		.8		.6	
	C-12			10.08	.30	27	-2.6		1.8		.1		.4		.7
CHLORIDE MMOL/L — COULOMETRIC-AMPEROMETR / BECKMAN ASTRA 4 & 8	C-11	14	110	111.3	1.7	1285	-.8								
	C-12	14	98	98.6	1.5	1285	-.4								
ALL CHLORIDE COMMON GP — ALL AUTO CHEM INSTR	C-11			110.5	2.8	3461	-.2	.8		1.2		.5		.0	
	C-12			98.4	2.4	3459	-.2		.4		1.1		.1		.5
CORTISOL - SERUM MCG/DL — ABBOTT TDx	C-11	12	14.2	12.63	1.20	633	+1.3	1.3		.7		.0			
	C-12	12	10.7	9.36	.88	633	+1.5		1.5		.5		.4		
NO COMPARATIVE METHOD														MTH/SYS CHG	
	C-11													.0	
	C-12														.0
CREATININE-SERUM MG/DL — KINETIC ALK. PICRATE / BECKMAN ASTRA 4 & 8	C-11	14	4.9	4.80	.10	1031	+1.0								
	C-12	14	1.1	1.04	.06	1043	+1.0								
ALL METHOD PRINCIPLES — ALL INSTRUMENTS	C-11			4.92	.31	6497	-.1	1.0		1.8		1.6		1.0	
	C-12			1.09	.13	6529	+.2		1.0		.7		2.1		.7

Figure 7. Example of interlaboratory proficiency test survey results provided by the College of American Pathologists (CAP).

QUALITY ASSURANCE

Internal quality control that has been done properly and interlaboratory comparison proficiency tests still do not guarantee that the correct answer will appear on the patient's chart. The biggest fear in any laboratory is a clerical error or transcription error, either in demographic data or in the actual laboratory result. There must be some means of verifying a result before it goes to the chart. Obviously, one cannot double-check every result by calling the physician to see whether all values are medically appropriate.

The most common clerical errors are transpositions of digits and decimal errors. A method of checking for absurd values and also comparing the results to previous results can go far in preventing, but not necessarily eliminating, clerical errors. Absurd values can be checked by computer when defining limits of possible values. If a result entered into the computer does not seem possible, the computer should challenge that result. For example, sodium of 195 meq/L is probably not realistic; if it were supposed to be 159, a transposition of digits has occurred. If the true value is 195, however, a double-check on the computer screen is certainly appropriate. Each laboratory should define "absurd values" for most tests to check for clerical errors.

Another check for clerical errors is the delta check, which subtracts the present value from the most recent previous value to determine the delta or difference. Table 3 lists the values used for delta checks for the most common analytes. Some authors (14) suggest a percentage difference instead of absolute value in evaluation of the "delta." Percentage difference may work well for an analyte such as sodium (reference range 135–145 meq/L) but poorly for bilirubin (reference range 0–1.0 mg/dL). A change of bilirubin from 0.1 to 0.2 mg/dL represents a 100% increase in the difference of the values, but it is not clinically or analytically significant. When given a choice of a value or percentage difference in the computer format for delta checks, it is better to

Table 3. Delta Check Values in Use at the University of Arkansas for Medical Sciences

	Value		Value
Sodium	20 meq/L	Calcium	3.0 mg/dL
Potassium	2.0 meq/L	Phosphorus	2.5 mg/dL
Chloride	20 meq/L	Osmolality	20 mosm
CO_2	20 meq/L	Ammonia	30 μg/dL
BUN	50 mg/dL	Protein	3.0 g/dL
Creatinine	10 mg/dL	Albumin	3.0 g/dL

Table 4. Panic (Critical) Values in Use at the University of Arkansas for Medical Sciences

	Less than	Greater than
Sodium	120 meq/L	160 meq/L
Potassium (adult)	3.0 meq/L	6.5 meq/L
Potassium (newborn)	3.0 meq/L	8.0 meq/L
Glucose (adult)	50 mg/dL	500 mg/dL
Glucose (newborn)	30 mg/dL	500 mg/dL
Ionized calcium	3.0 mg/dL	6.5 mg/dL
CO_2	10 meq/L	40 meq/L
Chloride	80 meq/L	120 meq/L

choose the absolute value, since it is more versatile, as shown in the example of sodium and bilirubin above.

If the delta exceeds a certain value, the most recent value is flagged to the attention of the technologist for evaluation. It is possible that there exists a physiological explanation (e.g., patient receiving IV potassium); however, it is worth the few moments to investigate a potential problem. Usually the delta is sufficiently large to catch transcription errors, not analytical errors. To the delta check values used in our laboratory (Table 3) could be added other tests. However, large physiological fluctuations can occur with some tests (e.g., enzymes), and may not lend themselves to an appropriate delta check.

Also as part of our quality assurance program, we monitor some variables which originate on the nursing station. Examples of these variables are number of mislabeled samples from each nursing station, error in proper tube for collection, and hemolyzed samples. Although seemingly trivial, these variables can affect the final result, and controlling for them is just as important as doing internal and external QC. Also in our laboratory we have developed critical values called panic values: results that are either life threatening or extremely toxic to the patient, requiring that the physician be notified immediately. Table 4 lists some analytes and their panic values.

CONCLUSIONS

The combination of quality control and quality assurance is essential for quality laboratory work. Accuracy depends on quality in preanalytical, analytical, and reporting aspects of test procedures. Thus, quality control and quality assurance constitute a management tool to verify the validity of results. Laboratories accredited by the CAP meet very strict guidelines to satisfy requirements in quality control. Many states also maintain licensure requirements which necessitate strict adherence to quality control practices. Laboratory practices should be rigorous to ensure that the most reliable, cost-effective result is produced to provide maximum benefit to the physician and the patient.

REFERENCES

1. Howanitz PJ. Old vs. new quality control rules: Which rules are more cost effective? *Pathologist* Feburary 1985, pp 8–10.

2. College of American Pathologists. *Clinical Laboratory Handbook in Patient Preparation and Specimen Handling.* Skokie, IL: CAP, 1985.

3. Wheeler LA, Sheiner LB. A Clinical evaluation of various delta check methods *Clin Chem* 1981;27:5–9.

4. Ross JW, Fraser MD, Moore TD. Analytic clinical laboratory precision—State of the art for thirty-one analytes. *Am J Clin Pathol* 1980;74:521–530.

5. Lawson NS, Haven GT, Williams GW. Analyte stability in clinical chemistry quality control materials. *CRC Crit Rev Clin Lab Sci* 1982;17:1–50.

6. Lawson NS, Haven GT, Moore TD. Long-term stability of enzymes, total protein, and inorganic analytes in lyophilized quality control serum. *Am J Clin Pathol* 1977;68:117–129.

7. Westgard JO, Klee GG. Quality assurance in Tietz NW (ed): *Textbook of Clinical Chemistry*, Philadelphia: Saunders, 1986, pp 424–458.

8. Levey S, Jennings MJ. The use of quality control charts in the clinical laboratory. *Am J Clin Pathol* 1950;20:1059–1066.

9. Westgard JO, Barry PC, Hunt MR, et al. A multi-rule Shewhart chart for quality control in clinical chemistry. *Clin Chem* 1981;27:493–501.

10. Westgard JO, Groth T, Aronsson T. deVerdier CH. Combined Shewhart–cusum control chart for improved quality control in clinical chemistry. *Clin Chem* 1977;23:1881–1887.

11. Haven GT, Lawson NS, Ross JW. Quality control outline. *Pathologist* 1980;34:619–621.

12. Bio-Rad Laboratories, Anaheim, CA.

13. Westgard JO, Hunt MR. Use and interpretation of common statistical tests in method comparison studies. *Clin Chem* 1973;19:49–57.

14. Ladenson JH. Patients as their own controls: Use of the computer to identify laboratory error. *Clin Chem* 1975;21:1648–1653.

CHAPTER 3

ELECTROLYTES AND ACID–BASE DISORDERS

BAI-HSIUN CHEN and E. HOWARD TAYLOR

University of Arkansas for Medical Sciences
Little Rock, Arkansas

ELECTROLYTES

Electrolytes are ions that exist in body fluids. They can affect metabolic events such as osmolality, state of dehydration, and pH of both intracellular and extracellular fluid (ICF and ECF). They are also important for regulation of membrane potential and normal functioning of nervous tissue and muscle. This section examines the major electrolytes: sodium, potassium, and chloride.

Sodium

Sodium (Na^+) is the major cation in ECF, while chloride (Cl^-) and bicarbonate (HCO_3^-) are the major anions. Sodium plays a central role in maintaining the normal distribution of water and the osmotic pressure in the extracellular fluid compartment. The normal range of serum sodium concentrations in healthy subjects is 135–145 mmol/L. Although sodium can be excreted via the gastrointestinal tract and through the skin, the kidney is still the major regulator for sodium excretion. When the intake of sodium is increased, with the transient expansion of the plasma volume and interstitial fluid volume, there is inhibition of renin release, followed by inhibition of aldosterone; thus there is decrease of sodium reabsorption in the distal convoluted tubule and cortical collecting duct. All these factors increase the excretion of sodium and return the extracellular volume to normal.

Hyponatremia

Low serum sodium (hyponatremia) occurs when there is a greater excess of extracellular water than of sodium or a greater deficit of sodium than of water. Generally, changes in total body sodium are not necessarily associated with similar changes in serum sodium concentration. The sodium concentration reflects the relative balance of extracellular sodium and water. That is why, actually, hyponatremia is found in sodium-retentive states, such as congestive heart failure, liver cirrhosis, or nephrotic syndrome, while water excess is greater than sodium excess (dilutional hyponatremia). The symptoms of hyponatremia depend on the cause, magnitude, and rate of fall in serum sodium. At 115 mmol/L or lower, the patient may have mental confusion, fatigue, headache, nausea, or vomiting. Below 110 mmol/L, the patient may have convulsions, semicoma, or coma.

The syndrome of inappropriate antidiuretic hormone (SIADH) is another condition of dilutional hyponatremia. The main diagnostic criteria include hyponatremia, hypoosmolar plasma (<275 mosm/kg), urine osmolality that slightly exceeds plasma (300–400 mosm/kg), and a urine sodium concentration that is neither high nor low (often 40–80 mmol/kg) (1,2). The SIADH can be seen in (1) ectopic, autonomous secretion of ADH, such as bronchogenic carcinoma or adenocarcinoma of the pancreas, (2) increased secretion of ADH by the hypothalamus in the absence of appropriate osmolar or volume stimuli, such as central nervous system disorders (intracranial hemorrhage, hydrocephalus), hypothyroidism, or drugs (morphine, barbiturates, cyclophosphamide, carbamazepine), or (3) increased secretion of ADH by the hypothalamus secondary to "regional hypovolemia" such as asthma, pneumothorax, or chronic obstructive pulmonary disease (3). The condition of sodium deficit greater than water deficit (depletional hyponatremia) can be seen in prolonged vomiting, chronic diarrhea, salt-losing enteropathies or excessive renal loss due to diuretics, adrenal insufficiency, hypoaldosteronism, and chronic renal disease, especially tubulointerstitial disease.

There is also another condition of dilutional hyponatremia, due to analytical artifacts of flame photometry or diluting ion-selective electrode (ISE) techniques, in which plasma water is replaced by lipids, protein, or glucose. This condition, called pseudohyponatremia, occurs in hyperlipidemia; the value for serum sodium is falsely lowered because less water volume is available for sodium to dissolve. This topic is discussed under "Analytical Methods for the Determination of Sodium and Potassium."

Hypernatremia

Increased serum sodium concentration occurs when there is a greater deficit of extracellular water than of sodium or a greater excess of sodium than of water. A water deficiency greater than sodium deficiency can be seen in excessive sweating (due to exercise, fever, hot environment), burns, hyperventilation, and diabetes insipidus (either nephrogenic or due to ADH deficiency). In nephrogenic diabetes insipidus, the amount of ADH is adequate or elevated, but the renal receptor is absent or ineffective.

Sodium excess greater than water excess is an unusual phenomenon and occurs occasionally in ingestion of large amounts of sodium or administration of hypertonic NaCl or $NaHCO_3$. The clinical cause of hypernatremia is primary hyperaldosteronism in which increased concentrations of aldosterone result in a decreased plasma renin activity. The main diagnostic points for primary hyperaldosteronism are hypernatremia, hypokalemia, decreased serum chloride, and increased CO_2 content.

Potassium

Potassium is the major intracellular cation. About 98% of the total body potassium is found in the intracellular water space, reaching a concentration there of about 150–160 meq/L. In the extracellular water space, the concentration of potassium is only 3.5–5 meq/L. On the average, we can consume about 100 mmol of potassium daily. Potassium is present in most foods, with higher concentrations in bananas and oranges. The major means of potassium excretion is through the kidney. The kidney is capable of regulating the excretion of potassium to maintain body potassium homeostasis. Potassium is freely filtered by the glomerulus. Almost all the filtered potassium is reabsorbed in the proximal tubules and ascending limb of Henle's loop; thus only about 10% of the filtered potassium reaches the distal convoluted tubule.

Hypokalemia

Decreased serum potassium concentration can be due to decreased intake, redistribution of extracellular K^+ into intracellular fluid, and increased loss of potassium-rich body fluids. Situations of decreased intake include low potassium diet, alcoholism, and anorexia nervosa. Redistribution can be seen in insulin therapy of diabetic hyperglycemia, while cell uptake of glucose is accompanied by uptake of potassium. Increased gastrointestinal losses can be seen in vomiting, diarrhea, fistula, and malabsorption. Increased urinary loss can be seen in (1) increased aldosterone conditions such as primary hyperaldosteronism or adrenal hyperplasia, (2) adrenogenital syndrome, (3) renal disease, such as renal tubular acidosis or Fanconi's syndrome, (4) overusage of diuretics, and (5) alkalosis. Clinically, hypokalemia is characterized by muscle weakness, irritability and paralysis, fast heart rate and specific conduction effects in electrocardiogram (U wave), and eventual cardiac arrest. Serum potassium below 3.0 mmol/L is associated with marked neuromuscular symptoms and is evidence of a critical degree of intracellular depletion.

Hyperkalemia

Hyperkalemia can be grouped into conditions resulting from increased potassium intake, shift from intracellular fluid to extracellular fluid, and decreased potassium loss. Increased potassium intake is usually seen iatrogenically (i.e., patients receiving too much potassium intravenously). It is also due to high potassium diet, high dose potassium penicillin, or transfusion of aged blood. The shift of potassium from the ICF to the ECF can be seen in acidosis, crush injury, tissue hypoxia, insulin deficiency, and digitalis overdose. Conditions of decreased urinary loss include renal failure, hypoaldosteronism, diuretics such as spironolactone and triamterene, that block distal tubular potassium secretion, and primary defects in renal tubular potassium secretion. The clinical signs and symptoms of hyperkalemia include changes in the electrocardiogram, cardiac arrhythmias, muscle weakness, and paresthesias. A serum potassium level higher than 7.5 mmol/L may be associated with cardiac arrhythmias.

The reference range for serum potassium of adults is 3.5–5.0 mmol/L; Serum values for newborns are higher than for adults: 3.7–5.9 mmol/L. The specimens for serum or plasma potassium must be collected to minimize hemolysis, because release of potassium as few as 0.5% of the erythrocytes can increase the serum level by 0.5 mmol/L. Thrombocytosis (*4*) and leukocytosis (*5*) also can affect measured potassium levels.

ANALYTICAL METHODS FOR THE DETERMINATION OF SODIUM AND POTASSIUM

Flame Photometry

As metal atoms of Na and K are heated in a flame, they will become excited and reemit this energy at a wavelength characteristic for the element. Alkali metals are easy to excite in a flame. Sodium produces a yellow emission, while potassium produces a red-violet color. Light emitted from the thermally excited ions is directed through separate interference filters to corresponding photodetectors. The lithium or cesium emission signal is taken as a reference (internal standardization) against which sodium and potassium signals are individually composed.

The dilution of sample is usually fixed at 100- or 200-fold by a manual dilution procedure, by a diluting accessory on the instrument or, as in continuous-flow analysis, by dialysis of prediluted sample into a recipient stream. The dilution ratio is chosen to optimize linearity of detector response and to bring the signal within the range of sensitivity of the detector. The

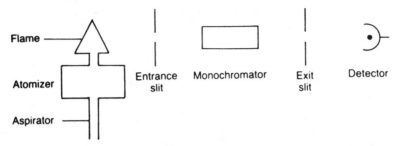

Figure 1. Diagram of components of a flame photometer. [From Burtis CA, in Tietz NW (ed): *Textbook of Clinical Chemistry.* Philadelphia: Saunders, 1986, p 74.]

choice of flame depends largely on the temperature desired; for sodium and potassium determinations, a propane compressed air flame is required. Figure 1 shows a schematic of the basic parts of a flame photometer.

Ion-Selective Electrode (ISE)

In principle, flame photometry measures the substance concentration, sodium or potassium, and the ISE measures ion activity (6–10). The activity is more important from a biochemical or physiological point of view than the substance concentration because tissue cells "see" the activity, not the protein-bound, complex-bound, or electrostatically "bound" ions (6). The principle of potentiometry is the determination of changes in electromotive force (*E*, potential) in the potential measuring circuit between a measurement electrode (the ISE) and a reference electrode, as the selected ion interacts with the membrane of the ISE (Figure 2). The measuring system is calibrated with solutions containing Na^+ and K^+, and the unknown concentration is interpolated from their measured potentials.

There are two kinds of ISE method: direct and indirect. The former is exemplified by measurements made on undiluted blood samples, such as the Nova system (Nova Biomedical, Newton, MA 02164). Measurement with ion-selective electrode cell assemblies that have been calibrated with activity standards offers the unique possibility of assaying the physiologically most relevant fraction of an ion in blood (ion activity) (*11*). For the indirect methods, sample is introduced into the measurement chamber and mixed with a rather large volume of diluent of high ion strength, as in the Astra systems (Beckman Instruments, Brea, CA 92621). In recent years, single-use, thin-film ion-selective electrodes for Na^+, K^+, and CO_2 determinations are unique applications of a direct method (Ektachem, Eastman Kodak Company, Rochester, NY 14650).

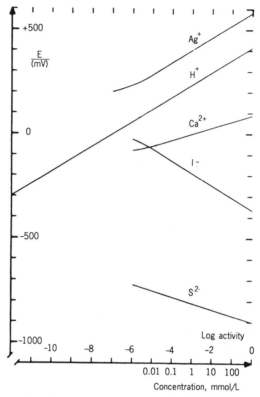

Figure 2. Illustration of the Nernst equation: the relationship between electromotive force of an ion-selective electrode (E), and the logarithm (base 10) of the activity of the ion ($\log a$)

$$E = E' + \frac{2.3RT}{zF} \cdot \log a$$

where E' is constant at constant temperature and z is the charge for the ion, R is the gas constant (8.3143 J/K mol), T is the absolute temperature (298 K), F is the Faraday constant (96,487 C/mol). The slope is ± 59.16 mV for monovalent ions and ± 29.58 mV for divalent ions. [From Siggaard-Anderson O, in Tietz NW (ed): *Textbook of Clinical Chemistry*. Philadelphia: Saunders, 1986, p 118.]

The ion-selective membrane electrodes can be classified as glass, solid-state, and liquid ion-exchange electrodes. Glass electrodes are made from specially formulated glass consisting of a melt of SiO_2 with added oxides of various metals. Na^+ glass membranes have found a widespread application and are routinely used in clinical analyzers. For the past 20 years, all the K^+-selective membrane electrodes in clinical analyzers have relied on valinomycin, a neutral carrier that binds K^+ in the center of a ring of oxygen atoms. The membrane is highly selective for potassium. The only drawback has been observed during measurement of undiluted urine, where PVC membranes suffer from some anion interferences (*12*). The problem was eliminated by the incorporation of valinomycin into the silicone rubber membrane.

Generally for normal serum, the ISE result for sodium is almost the same as the results obtained by the flame photometry. But large differences arise when the water concentration of the serum changes—for example, because of severe hyper- or hypoproteinemia or severe hyperlipemia (*13*). For example, if the mass concentration of water has decreased by 15% to 0.80 kg/L, the ISE result may be 140 mmol/L, whereas flame photometry gives only 120 mmol/L (*6*). Thus the results obtained with severely hyperlipemic sera need to be accompanied by an explanatory remark to the effect that the flame photometry result is spuriously lower than an ISE result (although both flame photometer and ISE produce pseudohyponatremia, as discussed above).

CHLORIDE

Chloride is the major anion in the extracellular water space. Sodium and chloride together represent most of the osmotically active constituents of plasma. Chloride plays an important role in maintenance of water distribution, osmotic pressure, and anion–cation balance in the extracellular fluid component. Chloride is excreted mainly through the kidney, and then other small amounts of chloride are excreted through the gastrointestinal tract and the skin.

Hypochloremia is observed in salt-losing nephritis, prolonged vomiting, burns, over-hydration, and thiazide therapy; usually the conditions are the same as with sodium depletion except for the presence of metabolic alkalosis, in which with the bicarbonate excess requires the loss of chloride to maintain electrical neutrality. Hyperchloremia occurs when chloride accumulates in the body because intake exceeds output. The conditions of chloride retention are the same as those of sodium retention except for the presence of metabolic acidosis, in which extracellular bicarbonate is depleted; thus extracellular chloride increases for the maintenance of electrical neutrality. The reference range for serum chloride is 99–108 mmol/L. Symptoms are not directly attributable to hypochloremia or hyperchloremia. Rather, symptoms that occur in patients with an abnormal serum chloride concentration are caused by the associated abnormality in serum sodium or pH. Determination of chloride concentration in sweat is useful in diagnosing the exocrine glandular disorder cystic fibrosis. Infants affected usually have concentration greater than 60 mmol/L. The patient is induced to sweat by iontophoresis or by the introduction of pilocarpine into the skin (*14*).

Analytical Methods for the Determination of Chloride

Measurement of chloride concentration can be done by mercurimetric titration, by coulometric titration, by colorimetry using $Hg(SCN)_2$, and by the use of ion-specific electrodes (*15*). In the mercurimetric method, the soluble complex $HgCl_2$ forms after the Cl^- combines with Hg^{2+}. Excess Hg^{2+} combines with indicator diphenylcarbazone to form a blue color. In coulometric–amperometric determination of chloride, Ag^{2+} generated from a silver electrode at a constant rate reacts with chloride ion in the sample to form insoluble AgCl. As soon as the stoichiometric point is reached, continued generation of Ag^+ triggers shutdown of the system. A timing device records the elapsed time between start and stop of silver ion generation. The technique is very suitable for pediatric use because small volumes are required. For the thiocyanate method, $Hg(SCN)_2$ is added to the sample and dissociates owing to the complexing of Hg^{2+} with Cl^-. The free thiocyanate ion (SCN^-) reacts with added Fe^{3+} to form the colored complex $Fe(SCN)_3$, which is measured photometrically. Cl^- electrodes are solid-state electrodes using membrane composed of AgCl. The Orion AgCl membrane electrode is used for measurement of the activity of chloride in sweat by direct measurement on the skin surface (Orion Company, Boston). The ion-specific electrodes offer the most precise method, although all the other methods provide comparable clinical data from surveys (*16*).

BLOOD GASES AND ACID-BASE DISORDERS

The maintenance of a relatively constant internal environment is one of the major physiological functions of the organ systems of the body. The average person in Western society consumes an acid diet and has a daily acid load of approximately 0.8 meq per kilogram of body weight per day (*17*). The major sources of acid in the diet are sulfur-containing amino acids and organic phosphoric acids.

The body buffer can be divided into three major components: bicarbonate, protein, and phosphates. The predominant feature of the bicarbonate, carbonic, and carbon dioxide buffer system is the property of volatility (*18*). The buffer of significance is between bicarbonate and carbonic acid, the level of carbonic acid is a function of the partial pressure of carbon dioxide (P_{CO_2}). The reaction $CO_2 + H_2O \rightarrow H_2CO_3$ is catalyzed by carbonic anhydrase and is one of the fastest reactions in metabolism (*19*). The relation between P_{CO_2} and H_2CO_3 in body fluids is such that $H_2CO_3 = 0.03 \times P_{CO_2}$ (mmHg). It is important for the equilibrium between carbon dioxide and H_2CO_3 because carbon dioxide is highly permeable throughout the body and no significant cellular barriers to carbon dioxide are known to exist. A second important aspect of the bicarbonate–carbonic acid buffer is that bicarbonate may be generated by the kidney, as well as being reabsorbed (20).

The imidazole groups in the histidine residues of the peptide chains have pK values in the pH range encountered in the blood. The protein present in the greatest quantity in the blood is hemoglobin. Of the 540 amino acid residues in hemoglobin, 36 are histidine, with pK values ranging from 7 to 8. Thus, as oxygen leaves hemoglobin in the tissue capillaries, the imidazole group removes hydrogen ions from the erythrocyte interior, allowing more carbon dioxide to be transported as bicarbonate. The process is reversed in the lungs.

The phosphate pool is comprised of intracellular and extracellular phosphate and is regulated by vitamin D and parathyroid hormones acting on bone, kidney, and gut. The phosphate pool includes serum in organic phosphate (3.5–5.0 mg/dL), intracellular phosphate, and calcuim phosphate in bone. The phosphate buffer system mainly consists of the buffer pair of the dihydrogen phosphate ($H_2PO_4^-$) and the monohydrogen phosphate (HPO_4^{2-}).

$$H_2PO_4^- \rightleftharpoons H^+ + HPO_4^{2-}$$

Since the pK_a of the acid form is 6.8, when the pH ranges near 7.0, the acid form can readily donate a proton and the base form can accept a proton. Many organic phosphates found in the body also have pK_a's within ± 0.5 pH unit of 7.0, and these compounds also can function as buffers under physiological conditions. A buffer commonly consists of a weak acid (HA) and its conjugate base (A$^-$). The equilibrium reaction of a hypothetical buffer solution would be

$$HA \rightleftharpoons H^+ + A^-$$

with the following equilibrium equation

$$K_a = \frac{[H^+][A^-]}{[HA]}$$

where K_a is the dissociation constant for the weak acid of the buffer solution. One can rearrange the equation as

$$[H^+] = \frac{K_a[HA]}{[A^-]}$$

take the negative logarithm of both sides

$$-\log[H^+] = -\log K_a - \log \frac{[HA]}{[A^-]}$$

and rearrange it to the Henderson–Hasselbach equation of

$$pH = pK_a + \log \frac{[A^-]}{[HA]}$$

The reactive equation for the bicarbonate–carbonic acid buffer system is

$$pH = pK_a + \log \frac{[HCO_3^-]}{[H_2CO_3]}$$

In the normal condition, the pK_a is 6.11 at 37°C, and the ratio of HCO_3 to H_2CO_3 is 20:1. Thus

$$pH = 6.11 + \log 20 = 7.4$$

Acid–Base Disorders

Acid–base disorders resulting in a blood pH of less than 7.4 are termed acidosis, and those resulting in a blood pH greater than 7.4 are termed alkalosis. The range of arterial pH compatible with life is from 6.80 to 7.80 ± 0.1 unit (21). In normal individuals, arterial pH is maintained between 7.35 and 7.45. Acid–base disorders are most readily classified in terms of their immediate cause with respiratory or metabolic oxygen. The acid–base disorders were based on the modified Henderson–Hasselbach equation.

$$pH = pK_a + \log \frac{[HCO_3^-]}{[P_{CO_2}]}$$

The term P_{CO_2} is called the respiratory component, and the bicarbonate concentration of serum is called the metabolic component of acid–base status. The pH of serum depends on the ratio of the concentration of bicarbonate to P_{CO_2} rather than the absolute concentration of these components.

Metabolic Acidosis

Metabolic acidosis occurs as a result of a marked increase in endogenous acid production (such as lactate and ketoacids), loss of bicarbonate stores (diarrhea), or progressive accumulation of endogenous acids. There exist two types of clinical metabolic acidosis: elevated anion gap acidosis and normal anion gap or hyperchloremic acidosis (23–25). The anion gap (AG) is defined as follows:

$$AG = Na^+ - (Cl^- + HCO_3^-)$$

The anion gap represents those unmeasured anions normally present in serum and is equal to 10–12 meq/L. For most of the clinical disorders, an increase of the anion gap can be seen with an accumulation of acid in extracellular fluid. When there is invasion of strong acid in extracellular component, it is buffered by HCO_3^-. Then in a pure simple anion gap acidosis, the increase in the anion gap above the normal value should be approximately equal to the decrease in HCO_3^- below the normal value; but in patients with acid–base disorder due to diabetic ketoacidosis with protracted vomiting, we may see an elevated anion gap that exceeds the bicarbonate deficit. Increased anion gap metabolic acidosis can be seen in ketoacidosis (induced by diabetes mellitus, starvation, or alcohol), lactic acidosis, chronic renal failure, methyl alcohol, and salicylate overdose. Lactic acidosis is a common cause of metabolic acidosis. It can occur in a variety of clinical conditions (25), such as shock, systemic disorders, drugs, and inborn errors of metabolism. It is necessary to know that it is not the lactic anion itself which is responsible for the acidosis, but the hydrogen ion produced by the sequence of reactions leading to lactate accumulation (26). The normal anion gap (hyperchloremic) metabolic acidosis can be seen in gastrointestinal disorders, diarrhea, fistula, ileostomy, ingestion of acid, or renal tubular acidosis. Gastrointestinal bicarbonate loss due to diarrhea is a common cause of hyperchloremic acidosis. Liver disease that impairs the formation of urea and ammonia will also result in a metabolic acidosis because of retention of H^+. The laboratory finding in metabolic acidosis (Table 1) includes a decrease in both pH and HCO_3^-. Initially the P_{CO_2} may be

Table 1. Summary of Various Laboratory Tests in Acid–Base Disorders

Disorder	Test[a]			
	pH	P_{CO_2}	HCO_3^-	Base Excess
Metabolic acidosis	↓	N	↓	↓
Respiratory acidosis	↓	↓	N	N
Metabolic alkalosis	↑	N	↓	↑
Respiratory alkalosis	↑	↓	N	N

Source: Reproduced by permission from Sherwin JE, Bruegger, in Kaplan LA, Pesce AJ (eds): Clinical Chemistry. St. Louis: Wosby, 1984, p. 400.

[a] N = initially normal.

normal, but it will decrease as a result of the respiratory response for maintenance of the ratio of HCO_3^- to H_2CO_3. A base deficit (negative base excess) will also be present. The medical treatment is to correct the cause of the acidemia (e.g., by the insulin treatment of diabetes).

Metabolic Alkalosis

Metabolic alkalosis is characterized by a primary elevation of serum bicarbonate concentration and a reciprocally reduced serum chloride concentration and elevated arterial pH (27). The arterial P_{CO_2} (P_{aCO_2}) is usually elevated as well, by about 0.7 mmHg for each milliequivalent-per-liter increment in the bicarbonate concentration (17). Metabolic alkalosis may be seen in excessive, chronic ingestion of bicarbonate of soda, or ingestion of large quantities of alkali antacids for treatment of peptic ulcer, or vomiting. Nasogastric aspiration is frequently a cause of metabolic alkalosis because of loss of gastric hydrochloric acid.

Renal loss of hydrogen ions is attributable to factors that augment distal hydrogen ion secretion, notably increased mineralocorticoid activity such as primary hyperaldosteronism, or Cushing's syndrome. Other factors that can contribute to accelerated distal acidification include increased tubular flow and sodium delivery by diuretics, delivery of nonabsorbable anions that accentuate the lumen-negative potential difference, hypercapnia, and possibly hypoparathyroidism and hypercalcemia. The use of loop or thiazide diuretics is probably the most common cause of metabolic alkalosis (27).

To compensate the increase of the HCO_3^-/H_2CO_3 ratio, the respiratory system slows in order to raise the P_{CO_2} and the carbonic acid concentration in the blood. The P_{CO_2} rises more rapidly than the HCO_3^-, thereby decreasing the pH. The treatment of metabolic alkalosis involves administration of NaCl or KCl, depending on the degree of hypokalemia, and perhaps also administration of NH_4Cl if the alkalosis is severe and persistent.

Respiratory Acidosis

Respiratory acidosis is a systemic acid–base disorder in which there is a rise in P_{CO_2} which lowers pH and a secondary increase in serum concentration of HCO_3^-. Any disorders that interfere with the normal ability of the lungs to expel CO_2 can cause respiratory acidosis. These disorders include pulmonary edema, bronchoconstriction, pneumonia, emphysema, apnea, and bradycardia. Morphine ingestion and barbiturate poisoning can cause an immediate respiratory depression resulting in respiratory acidosis (27).

Diseases that produce hypercapnia with hypoxemia to a level compatible with prolonged existence with or without oxygen therapy produce chronic respiratory acidosis. Chronic obstructive pulmonary disease (COPD) is the most common cause of chronic respiratory acidosis (28). The mechanisms for failure to maintain normal excretion of carbon dioxide may include an alteration in the respiratory excretory component and an alteration in the respiratory control system (decreased sensitivity of the chemoreceptors to carbon dioxide) (29). Many premature infants, who lack the surfactant to allow the alveoli to exchange gases smoothly, have respiratory acidosis.

The treatment of respiratory acidosis is not like metabolic acidosis, which is usually given with sodium bicarbonate for deficit in bicarbonate. Adequate oxygenation is the first priority and includes establishing a patent airway using artificial ventilation and administering oxygen. After the restoration of oxygenation, treatment is directed to correcting the underlying cause of the respiratory failure. This is usually possible for causes of acute respiratory acidosis but impossible for causes of chronic respiratory acidosis.

Respiratory Alkalosis

Respiratory alkalosis is a systemic acid–base disorder generated by a fall in arterial P_{CO_2} which raises pH and produces secondary reductions in serum concentrations of HCO_3^-. Usually hyperventilation is the main cause of respiratory alkalosis, and the hyperventilation conditions include hysteria, excessive crying, pregnancy, salicylate intoxication, impairment of the central nervous system's control of the respiratory system, asthma, fever, pulmonary embolism, and excessive use of a mechanical respirator. Respiratory alkalosis is a common finding in hospitalized patients who undergo arterial blood gas sampling. Mazzara et al. (30) demonstrated 46% respiratory alkalosis in 8289 sets of arterial blood gas studies from patients in intensive care units.

The kidneys respond to the alkalosis by excreting increased amounts of bicarbonate under the conditions of lower P_{CO_2} that occur during respiratory alkalosis. In response to the alkalosis, the proximal tubules of the kidney decrease the reabsorption of bicarbonate. This renal response to respiratory alkalosis is termed compensatory metabolic acidosis.

Salicylates stimulate the medullary respiratory centers to increase the rate and depth of ventilation. In Gabow's study of 67 adult patients with salicylate intoxication (31), 22% had simple respiratory alkalosis and another 56% had a mixed respiratory alkalosis and metabolic acidosis; about 46% had a P_{CO_2} level of 20 mmHg or less. The preferred treatment for acid–base disorders is to treat the underlying cause. Usually the degree of alkalemia produced by the respiratory alkalosis is not dangerous and need only be noted. Sometimes it is corrected by lowering the respiration rate with drugs, such as sedatives, or by having the patient breath air with a higher CO_2 content.

Table 2. Prediction of Compensatory Responses in Simple Acid–Base Disturbances

Disorder	Prediction of Compensation
Metabolic acidosis	$P_{aCO_2} = (1.5 \times HCO_3^-) + 8 \pm 2$
Metabolic alkalosis	$P_{aCO_2} = (0.9 \times HCO_3^-) + 9 \pm 2$
Respiratory alkalosis	$\Delta HCO_3^- = \dfrac{\Delta P_{aCO_2}}{10} \times 4$
Respiratory acidosis	$\Delta HCO_3^- = \dfrac{\Delta P_{aCO_2}}{10} \times 2.5$

Source: Ref. 21, p. 802.

Clinical Approach to Patients with Acid–Base Disorders

The most commonly encountered clinical acid–base disturbances are simple acid–base disorders. More complicated clinical situations, especially in severely ill patients, may give rise to mixed (*32,33*) conditions. To appreciate and recognize a mixed acid–base disturbance, it is important to understand the physiological compensatory responses that occur in simple acid–base disorders.

The limit of the compensatory response to simple acid–base disorders are outlined in Table 2. To illustrate, a patient with metabolic acidosis due to ketoacidosis and having a serum bicarbonate concentration of 12 mg/L would be expected to have an arterial P_{CO_2} between 24 and 28 mmHg. Values for arterial P_{CO_2} below 24 or greater than 28 mmHg define a mixed disturbance (metabolic acidosis and respiratory alkalosis, or metabolic acidosis and respiratory acidosis, respectively). Compensation is a predictable physiological consequence of the primary disturbance and does not represent a "secondary" acidosis or alkalosis. A patient with primary metabolic acidosis should have a low arterial P_{CO_2}. The demonstration of an arterial P_{CO_2} in the usual normal range indicates a failure of the compensatory response and defines the presence of a superimposed respiratory acidosis.

Collection, Processing, and Measurement of Blood Gas

Generally the brachial and radial arteries are the preferred vessels for arterial puncture. The artery to be punctured is identified by its pulsations, and the skin site is cleaned, whereupon an unanesthetized arterial puncture provides an accurate measurement of resting pH and P_{CO_2}. If it is impractical or impossible to get arterial blood for analysis, the venous blood can be used, but the venous blood yields incorrect values for arterial oxygen saturation and alveolar P_{CO_2}. A blood specimen for blood gas analysis should be placed in ice water immediately after it has been obtained from the patient. The P_{O_2} will decay 2.7 mmHg/min at 37°C when the P_{O_2} of the original blood is above 150 mmHg (*34*).

The modern blood gas instrument usually contains pH, P_{CO_2}, and P_{O_2} electrodes. The pH reference electrode is a calomel or silver–silver chloride electrode filled with saturated KCl, which contacts the sample through a port, thus forming a salt bridge. The Severinghaus electrode is used commonly for P_{CO_2}. This is a pH electrode surrounded by an electrolyte solution separated from the blood by a membrane permeable to carbon dioxide; the membrane can be of silicone rubber or Teflon. For O_2 determination, the polarographic Clark oxygen electrode is used. The blood is separated by an oxygen-permeable membrane of polypropylene or polyethylene (Figure 3). Oxygen is reduced at the electrode, and the potential change is proportional to the rate

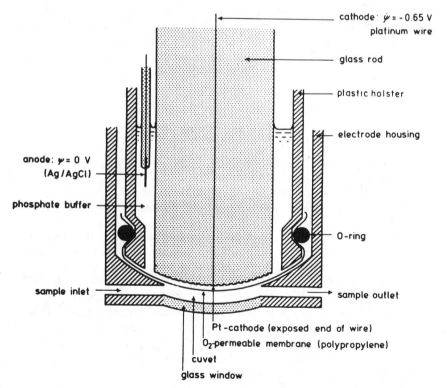

Figure 3. Schematic of a P_{CO_2} electrode. [From Siggard–Anderson O, in Tietz NW (ed): *Textbook of Clinical Chemistry*. Philadelphia: Saunders, 1986, p 122.]

of oxygen reduction. This rate varies directly with the oxygen tension of the blood.

To calibrate P_{O_2} and P_{CO_2} electrodes, either a gas or a liquid of known oxygen partial pressure must be used. The commercially available "low gas" mixture for calibration usually has a fractional composition of 5% CO_2, 0% O_2, and 95% N_2; the "high gas" mixture has fractional composition of 10% CO_2, 20% O_2, and 70% N_2. These compositions correspond roughly to a calibration range of 38–76 mmHg for P_{CO_2} and 0–152 mmHg for P_{O_2}.

Although temperature correction of pH and P_{CO_2} measured at 37°C is still the subject of considerable clinical controversy (*35*), most blood gas instruments, by keyboard entry of the patient's real body temperature, can calculate temperature-corrected pH and P_{CO_2}, as well as primary data. The algorithms of blood gas for temperature correction usually are rather complicated.

Ashwood's studies (*36*) reveal that $\Delta pH/\Delta T = 0.0147 \times °C^{-1}$ and $\Delta \log P_{CO_2}/\Delta T = 0.021 \times °C^{-1}$ appear to be reasonable estimates over the range of 25–42°C. Thus the magnitude of correction to 40°C for pH would be +0.045 and for P_{CO_2} would be +13%. Prudent policy for the laboratory might be to generate and report temperature-corrected results for pH and P_{CO_2} only upon specific request of the physician. However, reports of temperature-corrected always should be accompanied by the original result measured at 37°C.

REFERENCES

1. Chattoraj SC, Watts NB. Endocrinology, in Tietz NW (ed): *Textbook of Clinical Chemistry*. Philadelphia: Saunders, 1986.

2. Streeten DHP, Moses AM, Miller M. Disorders of the neurohypophysis, in Braunwald (ed): *Harrison's Principles of Internal Medicine*. New York: McGraw-Hill, 1987.

3. Kleiman LI, Lorenz JM. Physiology and pathophysiology of body water and electrolytes, in Kaplan LA, Pesce AJ (eds): *Clinical Chemistry*. St. Louis: Mosby, 1984.

4. Ingram RH, Seki M. Pseudohyperkalemia with thrombocytosis. *N Engl J Med* 1962;267:895–900.

5. Adams PC, Woodhause KW, Adela M, et al. Exaggerated hypokalemia in acute myeloid leukemia. *Br Med J* 1962;282:1034–1035.

6. Maas AH, Siggaard-Anderson D, Weisberg HF, et al. Ion-selective electrodes for sodium and potassium: A new problem of what is measured and what should be reported. *Clin Chem* 1985;31:482–485.

7. Ladenson JH. Direct potentiometric analysis of sodium and potassium in human

plasma: Evidence for electrolytic interaction with a non-protein, protein-associated substances. *J Lab Clin Med* 1977;90:654–655.

8. Ladenson JH. Evaluation of an instrument (NOVA-1) for direct potentiometric analysis of sodium and potassium in blood and their direct potentiometric determination in urine. *Clin Chem* 1979;25:757–763.

9. Levy GB. Determination of sodium with ion-selective electrodes. *Clin Chem* 1981;27:1435–1438.

10. Langhoff E, Steiness I. Potentiometric analysis for sodium and potassium in biological fluids. *Clin Chem* 1982;28:170–172.

11. Desch U, Ammann D, Simon W. Ion-selective membrane electrodes for clinical use. *Clin Chem* 1986;32:1448–1459.

12. Anker P, Jenny HB, Wathier U, et al. Determination of K^+ in blood serum with a valinomycin-based silicone rubber membrane of universal applicability to body fluids. *Clin Chem* 1983;29:1447–1448.

13. Creer MH, Laderson J. Analytic errors due to lipemia. *Lab Med* 1983;14:351–355.

14. Littlewood JM. The diagnosis of cystic fibrosis. *Practitioner* 1980;224:305.

15. Tietz NW, Pruden EL, Siggaard-Anderson O. Electrolytes, blood gases, and acid–base balance, in Tietz NW (ed): *Fundamentals of Clinical Chemistry*. Philadelphia: Saunders, 1987.

16. Geisinger KR. Serum chloride: A CAP survey. *Am J Clin Pathol* 1980;74 (suppl):546.

17. Cozan MG, Rector FC, Seldin DW. Acid–base disorders, in Brenner BM, Rector FC (eds): *The Kidney*. Philadelphia: Saunders, 1981.

18. Laski ME. Normal regulation of acid–base balance. *Med Clin North Am* 1983;67:771–780.

19. Maren TH. Carbonic anhydrase: Chemistry, physiology and inhibition. *Physiol Rev* 1987;47:595–725.

20. Pitts RF. Renal regulation of acid–base balance, in *Physiology of Kidney and Body Fluids*. Chicago, Year Book Medical Publishers, 1968, pp 179–212.

21. Dubose TD, Jr. Clinical approach to patients with acid–base disorders. *Med Clin North Am* 1983;67:799–813.

22. Oh MS, Carroll HJ. The anion gap. *N Engl J Med* 1977;297:814.

23. Walmsley RN, White GH. "Normal" anion gap: (hyperchloremic) acidosis. *Clin Chem* 1985;31:309–313.

24. Walmsley RN, White GH. Mixed acid–base disorders. *Clin Chem* 1985;31:321–325.

25. Cohen RD, Woods HF. *Clinical and Biochemical Aspects of Lactic Acidosis*. London: Blackwell, 1976.

26. Frommer JP. Lactic acidosis. *Med Clin North Am* 1983;67:815–829.

27. Cogan MG, Liu FY, Berger BE, et al. Metabolic alkalosis. *Med Clin North Am* 1983;67:903–914.

28. Kaehney WD. Respiratory acid–base disorders. *Med Clin North Am* 1983;67:915–928.

29. Murray JF. Respiratory structure and function, in Wyngaarden JB, Smith LH, Jr. (eds): *Cecil Textbook of Medicine*, 16th ed. Philadelphia: Saunders, 1982, pp 339–349.

30. Mazzara JT, Ayres SM, Grace WJ. Extreme hypocapnia in the critically ill patient. *Am J Med* 1974;56:450–456.

31. Gabow PA, Anderson RJ, Pottz DE, et al. Acid–base disturbances in the salicylate-intoxicated adult. *Arch Intern Med* 1978;138:1481–1484.

32. Narins RG, Emmett M. Simple and mixed acid–base disorders: A practical approach. *Medicine* 1980;59:161–187.

33. Narins RG, Gardner LB. Simple acid–base disturbances. *Med Clin North Am* 1981;65:321–346.

34. Newball H. Arterial blood samples should be stored in ice for gas analysis. *JAMA* 1973;223:696–697.

35. Hansen JE, Sue DY. Should blood gas measurement be corrected for patient's temperature? *N Engl J Med* 1980;303:341.

36. Ashwood ER, Kost G, Kenny M. Temperature correction of blood gas and pH measurement. *Clin Chem* 1983;29:1877–1885.

CHAPTER 4

EVALUATION OF RENAL FUNCTION

DIANNE JOHNSON

Baptist Medical Center
Little Rock, Arkansas

INTRODUCTION

The kidneys are two bean-shaped organs located under the lowermost ribs in the retroperitoneal space. Combined, they weigh approximately 300 grams, and they consist of three main functional components: the vascular supply beginning with the renal arteries, renal parenchyma, and the collecting system. Each renal artery divides into posterior and anterior portions with subsequent divisions into interlobar, arcuate, and finally interlobular arteries, which ultimately terminate in the afferent arterioles, each supplying a single glomerulus. The renal arteries deliver about 1200 mL of blood per minute to the parenchyma, which is composed of about 2 million nephrons, the true functional units of the kidney. Each nephron consists structurally of the glomerulus, a spherical epithelial space invaginated by a capillary tuft that connects the afferent and efferent arterioles, and a tubule of epithelial cells which is continuous with the glomerular epithelial space and ultimately leads to collecting ducts that empty into the major collecting system composed of the renal pelvis, ureters, and finally the urinary bladder (*1*).

The kidneys convert more than 1700 liters of blood per day into about 1 liter of urine, which is then excreted through the collecting system. In so doing, the kidney performs some of the most critical functions necessary for survival. These functions may be characterized as excretory, regulatory, and endocrine. The excretory function is responsible for the elimination of waste products of metabolism as well as any excess inorganic substances ingested in the diet. Waste products include the nonprotein nitrogenous compounds urea, creatinine, and uric acid. The regulatory function of the kidney plays a major role in ion and water homeostasis. The mechanisms of differential reabsorption and secretion of various ions located in the tubule of the nephron regulate the body's concentration of water and salt and maintain the appropriate acid–base balance of the plasma. The endocrine functions of the kidney may be regarded either as primary (because the kidney is an endocrine

55

Table 1. Renal Function Laboratory Tests

Function	Laboratory Test
Excretory	Serum and urine creatinine
	Creatinine clearance
	Serum urea nitrogen
Regulatory	
Ion homeostasis	Serum and urine electrolytes
	Blood pH
	Serum calcium
	Serum phosphorus
	Serum magnesium
Water balance	Urine specific gravity
	Serum and urine osmolality
Endocrine	Serum erythropoietin
	Serum renin
	1,25-dihydroxycholecalciferol

organ producing hormones) or as secondary (because the kidney is a site at which hormones produced elsewhere are activated). In its primary endocrine function the kidney produces renin, prostaglandins, and erythropoietin. In its secondary endocrine function, the kidney is a site of degradation of insulin, glucagon, and aldosterone. In addition, the kidney is the location of the hydroxylation of 25(OH)-D3 to produce $1,25(OH)_2$–D3, the most active form of vitamin D.

Table 1 summarizes the various functions of the kidney and the corresponding laboratory tests for their evaluation.

TESTS OF RENAL EXCRETORY FUNCTION

Excretion of Nonprotein Nitrogenous Compounds: Renal Clearance Studies

The majority of clinical laboratory tests used to assess kidney function are related to the measurement of the kidney's ability to clear waste products, usually nitrogenous compounds, from the body. When the kidney fails to function normally, the waste products accumulate in the blood in increasing concentrations. The two most commonly measured compounds are serum urea and serum creatinine. However, it is well known that there must be advanced renal failure before a significant increase in concentration of either of these substances occurs in the blood. To detect earlier stages of kidney disease, the clearance of certain substances by the kidney must be evaluated.

Clearance is defined as the quantity of blood or plasma completely cleared of a substance per unit of time and is expressed mathmatically as (2)

$$C_s = \frac{U_s \times V}{P_s}$$

where U_s is urinary concentration of the substance S, P_s is its plasma concentration, V is urine flow rate (mL/min), and C_s the clearance in units of milliliters of plasma cleared of the substance per minute. Different chemical substances have different clearances.

The clearance of paraamino hippurate (PAH), an exogenous substance almost completely cleared from the blood by the tubules, is a measure of tubular excretory function. The small amount that is not removed is in the blood, perfusing nonfunctional regions of the organ such as the pelvis and peripelvic fat. Most substances are not as efficiently cleared as PAH. The clearance of substances that are filtered exclusively or predominantly by the glomerulus but neither reabsorbed nor secreted by other regions of the nephron can be used to measure the glomerular filtration rate (GFR) (3). Inulin, a plant polysaccharide, is such an exogenous substance, and thus the GFR may be determined by inulin clearance.

$$GFR = \frac{U_{inulin} \times V}{P_{inulin}}$$

Creatinine, a useful endogenous metabolic substance that is released into body fluids in such a way that plasma levels remain constant over a 24-hour period, may also be measured as an indicator of GFR. However, a small quantity of creatinine is reabsorbed by the tubules, and a small quantity of creatinine appearing in the urine (7–10%) is due to tubular secretion. As a result, creatinine clearance is approximately 7% greater than inulin clearance (4) when creatinine is measured with a method of high specificity. However, most methods for measuring creatinine used in the clinical laboratory are nonspecific, and this difference is often smaller. Creatinine clearance is approximately equal to a normal GFR of 125 mL/min.

Plasma and urine assays for inulin and PAH are too difficult and too time-consuming to be practical in routine clinical laboratories. In addition, measuring clearance of PAH and inulin would involve the expense and discomfort of infusing them intravenously over a long enough time to maintain a stable blood concentration. Therefore, creatinine clearance is almost universally used for the clinical assessment of GFR. Plasma and urine creatinine are easily and conveniently measured by either manual or automated methods.

Urea is another major endogenous product of human metabolism that is easily and inexpensively measured by laboratory methods. Because urea is partially reabsorbed, it is not as rapidly cleared from the blood as creatinine. Approximately 50% of the urea filtered by the glomerulus is returned via the tubules to the blood. Thus, the clearance of urea would be expected to be about half that of creatinine, or 70 mL/min. However, the production of urea in the body is not constant over time and is too dependent on several nonrenal variables such as diet and hepatic synthesis to make it useful as a measure of GFR.

Creatinine

Biochemistry and Physiology

Creatinine is predominantly synthesized in the liver from arginine, glycine, and methionine (5). It is then transported in blood to other organs such as muscle and brain, where it is phosphorylated to phosphocreatine, a high energy compound. Approximately 1–2% of muscle creatine is converted to creatinine daily. This production varies with age and sex because the amount of endogenous creatinine is proportional to muscle mass. Daily excretion of creatinine may be increased as a result of dietary intake of creatine and creatinine in meats. However, these dietary fluctuations of creatinine intake cause only minor variation in daily creatinine excretion by the same individual. In the absence of kidney disease, the excretion rate in any one individual is constant and parallels endogenous production. Intraindividual variation tends to be less than 15% from day to day. Most of the variations in creatinine excretion among healthy individuals are attributed to differences in age, sex, and lean body mass.

Measurement of Creatinine

The methods for measuring creatinine most widely used today are based on the Jaffé reaction, which has the distinction of being the oldest clinical chemistry method still in common use (6). The assay is based on the reaction of creatinine with an alkaline solution of sodium picrate to form a red-orange complex of uncertain structure called the Janovsky complex (5,7). The absorbance of this compound is measured between 510 and 520 nm, although its maximum absorbance is reported to be 485 nm (5). This is because sodium picrate, one of the reagents of the reaction that is present in excess, absorbs significantly at wavelengths below 500 nm.

It is well known that the original Jaffé reaction is nonspecific for measurement of creatinine in plasma. The noncreatinine Jaffé-reacting chromogens include protein, glucose, ascorbic acid, guanidine, acetone, cephalosporins, and α-ketoacids such as acetoacetate and pyruvate (8,9). Numerous modifications of the Jaffé method have therefore been created to improve the specificity for creatinine in plasma. Because urine contains an insignificant amount of these interfering substances, the nonspecificity of the reaction is not a problem for measurement of urine creatinine.

Manual methods based on the Jaffé reaction have traditionally been endpoint methods with 10–15 minutes allowed for color development. When serum or plasma is to be analyzed in an endpoint reaction, a protein-free filtrate is used, since the α-ketomethyl or α-ketomethylene groups found in protein react with alkaline picrate, and the resulting complexes are highly colored. The reaction is performed at a constant temperature of less than 30 °C; at higher temperatures, glucose, uric acid, and ascorbic acid can have an unacceptably high reductive reactivity for picrate, resulting in formation of picramate, which has a maximum absorbance at 482 nm and causes an overestimation of creatinine (10). Maintenance of a constant temperature is also important because both the absorbance of the picrate ion and the creatinine picrate reaction product increase with increasing temperature.

Floridin (fuller's earth) has been used to increase the specificity of the Jaffé reaction by adsorbing the creatinine present in the protein-free filtrate, thus isolating it from potential interferents. Other materials with comparable properties are Lloyd's reagent and bentonite (11,12). These materials are porous aluminum silicate clays that form colloidal suspensions with natural adsorptive power. A small amount of the adsorbent is added to a protein-free filtrate at room temperature; adsorption is essentially complete after 1 minute. Creatinine is adsorbed with approximately 92% efficiency and, after centrifugation and decanting of the interferent-containing supernatant, one can add the alkaline picrate directly to the creatinine-adsorbent pellet. Most potential interfering substances are not adsorbed. Only pyruvate in excess of 0.9 mmol/L and 2-oxoglutarate in excess of 0.5 mmol/L are adsorbed and can thus cause interference (11). A similar purification has been described using an ion-exchange resin that adsorbs creatinine from an acid solution to the sodium form of the resin. Results from the cation-exchange resin are reported to compare well with those obtained using fuller's earth (13). Treating a protein-free filtrate with these various adsorption techniques may improve specificity somewhat but is generally considered to be an excessively time-consuming procedure and tends to increase method imprecision (5).

Kinetic assays, which measure the rate of the pseudo-first-order reaction that forms the red-orange Janovsky complex, were developed as a means to improve specificity and to automate the procedure. The kinetic method gained popularity with the availability of instruments capable of making accurate absorbance readings at precise, reproducible intervals (*14–16*). In addition, to centrifugal analyzers, the du Pont aca and the Beckman creatinine analyzer use this technique. In the kinetic modification, formation of the picrate–creatinine complex is monitored after a 10–60 second delay after mixing of the reactants. This allows the fast-acting interfering substances to be eliminated before the initial absorbance reading is made. Before the creatinine reaction has gone to completion and before the more slowly reacting interfering substances have reacted significantly, additional measurements are made. Deproteinization need not be done, since the reaction between the protein and alkaline picrate is slow and thus does not occur during the usual kinetic reaction interval. However, a critical evaluation of kinetic methods in 1980 pointed out that many of the kinetic methods are still subject to positive interference by α-keto compounds and to negative interference by bilirubin and its metabolites (*16*, see also Ref. 9). Many drugs have also been shown to increase the results (*17*). The most common of these are methyl dopa and cefoxitin (*18*).

Enzymatic assays for creatinine were first attempted in 1937 (*18*). Enzymatic methodology has only recently become commercially feasible for routine clinical use. The major obstacle has been the availability of pure enzymes. Creatinine amidohydrolase (EC 3.5.3.10), also called creatinase or creatine hydrolase, has been used to convert creatinine to creatine, coupled to an indicator reaction as follows.

$$\text{creatinine} + H_2O \xrightarrow[\text{amidohydrolase}]{\text{creatinine}} \text{creatine}$$

$$\text{creatine} + ATP \xrightarrow[\text{kinase}]{\text{creatine}} \text{creatine phosphate} + ADP$$

$$ADP + PEP \xrightarrow[\text{kinase}]{\text{pyruvate}} ATP + \text{pyruvate}$$

$$\text{pyruvate} + NADH + H^+ \xrightarrow{\text{lactate}} \text{lactate} + NAD^+$$

The disappearance of NADH is continuously monitored. The second enzyme system used for creatinine quantitation is creatinine diminase (EC 3.5.4.21), also known as "creatinine imminohydrolase." This enzyme converts creatinine to *N*-methyl-hydantoin and ammonia. The ammonia is quantitated colorimetrically after its reaction with α-ketoglutarate and the monitoring of NADPH disappearance (*19*), or by use of an ammonia electrode (*20*).

Methods using this enzyme system are subject to interference with high levels of endogenous ammonia. Therefore, a correction for endogenous ammonia must be made, and the reaction mixture must be free of ammonia-producing and ammonia-consuming materials. Substantial amounts of ammonia can appear by protein deamination if blood is left at room temperature. Enzymatic methods have been adapted for both manual and automated use (21).

Separation and quantitation of creatinine has been accomplished with high performance liquid chromatography (HPLC), by use of cation-exchange stationary phase with citrate buffer mobile phase, or with a reversed-phase (22) column and phosphate–sodium lauryl sulfate–methanol mobile phase (23). Although the HPLC assay is impractical for routine analysis of creatinine, its specificity qualifies it as a reference method and for validating other methods.

Other methods of creatinine analysis involve reaction of creatinine with 3,5-dinitrobenzoic acid or its derivatives (24), with 1-4 naphthoquinone-2-sulfonate (25), and with o-nitrobenzaldehyde (26). In addition, mass fragmentography has been proposed as a reference method (27).

Choice of Methods

Several factors must be considered in the choice of methodology for analysis of creatinine in the clinical laboratory. These include, of course, specificity, which I have discussed in some detail, as well as availability and sample size. Of prime importance is specificity, particularly when analyzing specimens from patients with kidney dysfunction, in which numerous interfering substances are likely to be present. The analysis of creatinine must be available in a timely fashion 24 hours a day, since it is the most commonly ordered laboratory indicator of renal function. Sample size must be kept to an absolute minimum, especially when ordered on pediatric and/or dialysis patients.

The Jaffé reaction with pretreatment using fuller's earth seems to meet the foregoing requirements more successfully than other methods. This particular method, which has a high level of specificity and is readily adaptable to standard instrumentation, can be available with minimal delay. Only pyruvate and oxoglutarate, when present at high enough concentrations, remain potential sources of interference (11). However, pretreatment of the specimen with fuller's earth involves a manual procedure, and therefore the sample requirement is larger than for other automated methodologies. The Jaffé reaction with fuller's earth is considered to be a reference method for the reasons listed above and is not used in routine automated analysis.

The unmodified, original Jaffé reaction has major disadvantages related to its lack of specificity. Substances reported to give a falsely increased value include ascorbic acid, pyruvate, acetone, acetoacetic acid, levulose, glucose, aminohippurate, uric acid, protein, and cephalosporin antibiotics (*17*). Conversely, bilirubin or other hemoglobin degradation products cause a falsely decreased value (*8*). Without modifications, approximately 20% of the "creatinine" in serum or plasma and 5% of the "creatinine" in urine is caused by noncreatinine materials when the original Jaffé reaction is used. Despite these drawbacks, this methodology has been widely used for a long time because of its low cost and adaptability to automation.

A second modification of the Jaffé reaction that is also highly adaptable to automation is the kinetic method. But even though this methodology reduces error caused by both fast- and slow-reacting materials, no correction is made for noncreatinine reactants that have reaction rates comparable to that of creatinine. Pyruvate, α-ketoglutarate, and oxaloacetate have reaction rates that fall into this range. However, this method offers the advantages of speed, easy adaptation to automation, and small sample size.

Enzymatic methods recently have been adapted for automation with the availability of a pure enzyme reagent (*19*). These procedures have the potential to replace the chemical creatinine assays now in common use once the specificity of such procedures has been thoroughly evaluated under varying circumstances.

Specimen Requirements for Creatinine Determination

Serum, plasma, or urine specimens may be used. Creatinine in serum or plasma is stable for at least 7 days at 4°C and indefinitely when frozen. Creatinine is stable in urine for 2–3 days at room temperature and at least 5 days if refrigerated.

Common anticoagulants do not generally cause interference in most modifications of the Jaffé reaction, although heparin, which can be formulated as the ammonium salt, must be avoided in enzymatic methods that measure ammonia production. Significant hemolysis should be avoided because red cells contain nonspecific chromagens, which may cause spuriously elevated values. Lipemic and icteric samples may give falsely decreased results.

Reference Range for Serum or Plasma Creatinine

Reference ranges for serum or plasma creatinine as determined by specific reference methods are given in Table 2. Values in the elderly individual increase only slightly, since the decreased excretion of creatinine is partially compensated for by the decreased production of creatinine as a result of decreased muscle mass.

Table 2. Reference Ranges for "True" Creatinine

| | | True Plasma Creatinine | | | |
| | | mg/dL | | μmol/L | |
Age	Height (cm)	Mean	Range[a]	Mean	Range[a]
Cord blood		0.75	0.51–0.99	66.3	45.1–87.5
0–2 weeks	50	0.50	0.34–0.66	44.2	30.0–58.3
2–26 weeks	60	0.39	0.23–0.55	34.5	20.3–48.6
26–52 weeks	70	0.32	0.18–0.46	28.3	15.9–40.7
2 years	87	0.32	0.20–0.44	28.3	17.7–38.9
4 years	101	0.37	0.25–0.49	32.7	22.1–43.3
6 years	114	0.43	0.27–0.59	38.0	23.9–52.2
8 years	126	0.48	0.31–0.65	42.4	27.4–57.4
10 years	137	0.52	0.34–0.70	46.0	30.1–61.9
12 years	147	0.59	0.41–0.78	52.2	36.2–69.0
Adult, male	174	0.97	0.72–1.22	85.7	63.6–108
Adult, female	163	0.77	0.53–1.01	68.1	46.8–89.3

Source: Ref. 2, p.1279.

[a] ± 2 SD.

Creatinine Clearance

The creatinine clearance is determined by mathmatically relating the concentration of serum creatinine to the total quantity excreted in the urine over a period of time. To perform a creatinine clearance, both a timed urine specimen (usually 24 hours) and a sample of serum collected during this time period are required. The patient must maintain adequate fluid intake during the collection period to maintain a urine flow of 2 mL/min and also must avoid heavy exercise, coffee, tea, and drugs, which may spuriously affect results (*28*).

The concentration of creatinine is measured in both serum and urine by any one of the methods discussed above. Creatinine clearance is calculated as follows:

$$C_{cr} \text{ (mL/min)} = \frac{U_{cr} \text{ (mg/dL)} \times V_{urine} \text{ (mL/24 hours)}}{P_{cr} \text{ (mg/dL)} \times 1440 \text{ min/24 hours}}$$

where C_{cr} = creatinine clearance
V_{urine} = volume of urine excreted in 24 hours
U_{cr} = concentration of creatinine in urine
P_{cr} = concentration of creatinine in serum
Creatinine clearance rates for various age groups are shown in Table 3 (*29*).

Table 3. Creatinine Clearance (mL/min 1.73 m^2)^a

Age (years)	Males	$\bar{x}$	Females	$\bar{x}$
20–30	88–146	117	81–134	107
30–40	82–140	110	75–128	102
40–50	75–133	104	69–122	96
50–60	68–126	97	64–116	90
60–70	61–120	90	58–110	84
70–80	55–113	84	52–105	78

Source: Ref. 2, p. 1281.

^{a} Calculated from a nomogram for ascertaining age-adjusted percentile rank in creatinine clearance.

Clinicopathological Correlations of Creatinine and Creatinine Clearance

The constancy of creatinine formation and excretion makes creatinine a useful index of renal function, primarily of glomerular filtration. Because it is not significantly influenced by such variables as diet, degree of hydration, and protein metabolism, the plasma creatinine is a significantly more reliable screening test or index of renal function than is the blood urea nitrogen (BUN). The plasma creatinine tends to increase somewhat more slowly with hemodialysis. The serum creatinine level has been used in combination with the BUN to differentiate between prerenal and renal causes of azotemia (30). The normal ratio of BUN to creatinine is 10:1. Values higher than this suggest that the cause of an elevated BUN is prerenal rather than renal or postrenal. For a more in-depth discussion of BUN/Cr, see "Urea Nitrogen," below.

The clearance of creatinine is an even more sensitive method of estimating GFR. The linear decrease of creatinine clearance over time, as renal function decreases, has been thoroughly documented for several forms of chronic glomerulonephritis (including chronic membranous glomerulonephritis), diabetic nephropathy, chronic interstitial nephritis, and at least some cases of chronic pyelonephritis. Graphic representation (Figure 1) of creatinine clearance as a function of time has prognostic value as it allows the physician to estimate when the severity of renal failure makes dialysis necessary.

Serum Urea Nitrogen

Biochemistry and Physiology

Urea constitutes the major excretory product of protein metabolism and is thus the predominant nonprotein nitrogenous substance in the blood,

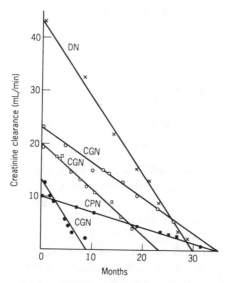

Figure 1. Changes in creatinine clearance with time for some diffuse renal diseases. CGN: chronic glomerulonephritis; DN: diabetic nephropathy; CPN: chronic pyelonephritis. Sequential determinations of creatinine clearance over periods ranging from 10 to 30 months illustrate clearly the linear decrease in renal function in progressive renal disease. (From Ref. 2, p. 1273.)

comprising more than 75% of the nonprotein nitrogen eventually excreted. Urea is synthesized in the liver from carbon dioxide and ammonia by hepatic enzymes of the urea cycle. After synthesis in the liver, urea is transported to the kidney, where it is filtered by the glomerulus. Much of the urea in the glomerular filtrate is excreted in the urine. However, in the normal kidney, 40–70% of the highly diffusable urea moves passively out of the renal tubule and into the interstitium, ultimately to reenter plasma. Consequently, urea clearance underestimates GFR. Additionally, the level of urea in the plasma is too dependent on such nonrenal variables as the protein content of the diet, hepatic synthesis, and the level of protein catabolism to make it a useful marker of GFR. However, the measurement of plasma or serum urea may provide useful clinical metabolic information in certain circumstances. See "Clinicopathological Correlations. . . ," on page 68.

Determination of Urea Nitrogen

Two analytical approaches have traditionally been used to determine the concentration of urea: either a direct chemical analysis or an indirect analysis, whereby urea is hydrolyzed to ammonia, which is subsequently quantitated. The oldest methods involve the indirect measurement of ammonia nitrogen after treatment of specimens with elevated temperatures (125°C) or the enzyme urease.

$$2H_2O + O=C\begin{smallmatrix}NH_2\\NH_2\end{smallmatrix} \xrightarrow[\text{urease}]{125°C} (NH_4)_2CO_3$$

In these older methods, the ammonia released from urea was quantitated either by acid titration or colorimetrically, using the Nesslerization or Berthelot reactions (31,32). These procedures could be performed directly on serum, blood, or urine samples. Although these methods are adequate and inexpensive, they are too sensitive to ammonia contamination, and endogenous NH_3 must be removed from urine samples before assaying.

The most common method for measuring NH_4 produced after treatment of the sample with urease uses a coupled-enzyme system with an NAD/NADH indicator reaction. These reactions, which are very useful as measures of urine urea at normal levels of endogenous ammonia, are monitored kinetically at 350 nm, and the rate of decrease in absorbance is proportional to concentration of urea. The endogenous urine ammonia is rapidly consumed in the initial seconds of the reaction, and the subsequent changes in absorbance at 340 nm are due primarily to ammonia generated by the urease reaction with urea. This method demonstrates good specificity and sensitivity when done as a kinetic assay and is currently the most popular on automated systems such as the du Pont aca and the Hitachi 705 by BMC.

The direct chemical analysis of urea involves condensation with diacetyl monoxime in the presence of strong acid and an oxidizing agent to form a yellow diazine derivative (31–33). Chemicals that have been used to enhance and stabilize the color produced in this reaction include thiosemicarbazide, ferric ions and potassium persulfate. Many other compounds containing urea residues (e.g., citrulline, alloxan, and allantoin) will also produce a colored product. However, these compounds rarely cause a significant problem with interference because they normally are in such low concentrations in serum. The major advantage of this method is that it measures urea directly and ammonia does not interfere. Direct chemical analysis has been successfully automated on the Technicon SMA (34) and some other discrete analyzers but has two disadvantages: it uses dangerous and noxious reagents, and it has limited linearity.

Two decades ago, a method was reported for quantitating urea by using an electrode to measure the rate of increase in conductivity of a sample after hydrolysis by urease to the ionic species NH_4 and HCO_3. Because the rate of change in conductivity is measured, contamination with endogenous NH_3 is not a problem with this method. Therefore one can analyze both serum and urine specimens for urea concentration. This technique has been adapted for automated analysis by Beckman on their BUN and Astra analyzers (35).

The most widely used method for the analysis of serum urea is the coupled enzymatic assay. Quality assurance surveys by the College of American Pathologists (CAP) indicate that approximately 50% of clinical laboratories use this method. Approximately 21% use the direct diacetyl monoxime procedure, and 16% use the conductivity technique. The majority of these procedures are automated, whereas only a few laboratories use the Nesslerization and Berthelot reactions manually.

Choice of Method

Along with nonspecificity, the inability to automate the quantitation of urea by the Nesslerization and Berthelot reactions discourages the use of these methods in the modern clinical laboratory. Both are end-point reactions subject to incomplete conversion of urea to ammonia, and both require relatively long incubation times. Also, clinical laboratories using the Berthelot and Nesslerization reactions report higher coefficients of variation than do laboratories using other methods.

Conversely, users of the direct diacetyl monoxime reaction report relatively low coefficients of variation, and the reaction is readily adaptable to automated analysis. The major disadvantages to this method include instability of the colored product, limited linearity, and the use of hazardous reagents.

Methods with the highest degree of specificity are the coupled-enzyme procedures and the conductivity method. These methods also are easily and quickly performed and provide excellent precision. It is not surprising then that these are the most commonly used on automated instruments.

Specimen Requirements for Urea Nitrogen Determination

Either serum, heparinized plasma, or urine specimens are suitable for the diacetyl monoxime, coupled-enzyme, and conductivity methods. Anticoagulants containing either ammonium or fluoride salts cannot be used in specimens analyzed by the urease methods.

Urea is stable in urine at pH < 5.0 for several days at 4–6°C. However, contamination of urine with bacteria that hydrolyze urea will result in a loss of urea and formation of ammonia (36).

Reference Range for Blood Urea Nitrogen

The references range for BUN in an adult is 6–21 mg/dL.

Note. BUN (blood urea nitrogen) continues to be the terminology for the plasma or serum urea nitrogen, even though the analysis of blood for urea is no longer performed. However, reporting and expressing results of a urea assay in units of urea nitrogen is too entrenched in this country to be discontinued. But urea nitrogen concentration can be converted to urea concentration as follows:

$$\frac{\text{mol wt of urea}}{\text{at. wt of N} \times 2} = \frac{60}{40} = 2.14$$

$$(\text{urea N, mg/dL}) (2.14) = \text{urea mg/dL}$$

Clinicopathological Correlations of Urea Nitrogen and Urea Nitrogen Clearance

Numerous renal and nonrenal disorders may result in an increased blood urea nitrogen (plasma urea concentration). An elevated level of urea in the blood is called azotemia. The conditions causing azotemia are traditionally divided into three main categories: prerenal, renal, and postrenal.

The major causes of prerenal azotemia are related to decreased perfusion of the kidneys that prevents filtration of urea from the blood. Disorders that result in decreased blood flow to the kidneys included congestive heart failure (CHF), shock, hemorrhage, and dehydration. In fact, in most hospital populations, CHF is overwhelmingly the most common cause of an elevated urea (37). Increased protein metabolism will also cause prerenal azotemia. Thus a high protein diet, fever, major illness, and stress may result in increased urea levels because of increased breakdown of protein.

Renal causes of azotemia include acute and chronic renal failure of various etiologies, glomerular nephritis, and tubular necrosis. An extreme level of plasma urea caused by renal failure and accompanied by clinical symptoms is referred to as uremia. This condition is eventually fatal if not treated by dialysis.

Postrenal azotemia is caused by conditions that obstruct urine outflow through the ureters, bladder, or urethra. These include nephrolithiasis, prostatism, and tumors of the genitourinary tract.

The principal clinical use of the determination of plasma urea is in combination with the plasma creatinine as a urea nitrogen-to-creatine ratio used to discriminate between prerenal and postrenal azotemia. A normal individual on a normal diet will have a ratio ranging between 8 and 21. Significantly lower ratings occur in cases of low protein intake, starvation, and severe liver disease. High ratios with normal creatinine levels may be seen with catabolic states of tissue breakdown, high protein intake, and gastrointestinal hemorrhage. High ratios associated with elevated creatinine values indicate either postrenal obstruction or prerenal azotemia superimposed on renal disease. Since, however, this ratio may be affected by the methodology used to determine urea and creatinine and can show significant variability, it should be used as a rough indicator of disease states, not as a precise quantity.

Uric Acid

Biochemistry and Physiology

Uric acid is the major product of the catabolism of purine nucleosides in higher animals such as humans and apes. Conversion of both dietary and endogenous nucleic acids takes place primarily in the liver. Uric acid is then transported via the plasma to the kidney, where it is filtered by the glomerulus. Approximately 98–100% of the filtered uric acid is reabsorbed in the proximal convoluted tubules, secreted into the lumen of the distal part of the proximal tubule, and further reabsorbed in the distal tubule. Following this complex process, the net urinary excretion of uric acid is only 6–12% of the amount filtered. Renal handling of uric acid accounts for the majority of the daily uric acid excretion. The balance is excreted into the gastrointestinal tract and degraded by bacterial enzymes.

The first pK_a of uric acid is 5.75. Above this pH (as occurs in plasma), uric acid exists primarily as urate ion, which is more soluble than uric acid (*38*). However, at a pH below 5.75 (as may occur in the urine), uric acid is the predominant form.

Measurement of Uric Acid

Methodology in current use for the determination of uric acid encompasses two categories: spectrophotometric assays using phosphotungstic acid and enzymatic assays using uricase.

Reacting an alkaline solution of uric acid with phosphotungstic acid to get a blue color (tungsten blue) was first used in 1912. The basis of this test is the oxidation of uric acid (*39*) to allantoin and carbon dioxide. Allantoin then reduces the phosphotungstic acid to tungsten blue, which has a maximal absorption at 700 nm. The presence of protein causes both turbidity and an unpredictable quenching of the absorbance, necessitating removal of the protein before color development. The most popular method of this type, the "Caraway" method, uses a protein-free filtrate as well as sodium carbonate to provide the alkaline pH necessary for optimal color development (*40*). The blue color can be stabilized by the addition of cyanide to the reaction mixture. However, proper adjustment of the pH will provide adequate color. Although this method is widely used, it is nonspecific. Phosphotungstic acid assays are subject to many interferences, including endogenous compounds such as glucose and ascorbic acid in plasma or urine, and glutathione, ergothionine, and cysteine from hemolyzed erythrocytes, and exogenous compounds such as acetaminophen, acetylsalicylic acid, caffeine, theobromine, and theophylline. All these compounds reduce phosphotungstic acid and therefore cause falsely elevated values. Numerous modifications of the phosphotungstic acid assay have not improved their specificity.

To increase the specificity of the laboratory determination of uric acid, the enzyme uricase was employed. Uricase methods are based on the specificity of the uricase-catalyzed oxidation of uric acid to allantoin with subsequent production of hydrogen peroxide. The simplest of these methods is based on the differential absorption of uric acid versus allantoin. Uric acid has a significant UV absorbance band at 290–293 nm, whereas allantoin does not. The difference in absorbance before and after incubation with uricase will be proportional to the uric acid concentration (41,42). This method is currently used on several automated instruments to include GEMSAEC (ENI) and the du Pont aca. Another approach to the enzymatic measurement of uric acid is the quantitation of the hydrogen peroxide produced when uric acid is oxidized in the uricase-catalyzed reaction (43,44).

In these methods either peroxidase, a phenol derivative, and 4-aminoantipyrine are used and the absorbance is measured at 500 nm, or catalase, NADH, and ADH are added and the reaction is monitored at 340 nm. These methods are readily adaptable to automation. In fact, Technicon uses a peroxidase-coupled method on the SMA II.

Yet another enzymatic approach uses a polarographic oxygen sensor to detect the rate of oxygen consumption, which is a measure of the rate of the uricase-catalyzed oxidation of uric acid and is proportional to the uric acid concentration (45). In addition, a colorimetric method has been used with the uricase technique (46). This method measures the total reducing substance produced by the colorimetric titration with iodine before and after reaction with uricase.

A high performance liquid chromatographic procedure for the measurement of uric acid have also been used. The HPLC methods use either an ion-exchange separation followed by amperometric detection in a thin-layer, flow-through electrochemical cell (47) or reversed-phase chromatography with spectrophotometric detection (48).

Choice of Methods

The preferred method for measurement of uric acid in a routine clinical laboratory is an automated coupled enzymatic procedure, available commercially from various sources. This method is easily adapted to a variety of discrete automated analyzers. It is both more sensitive and precise, as well as easier to perform, than is the differential absorption enzymatic assay, which has the major disadvantages of requiring an ultraviolet spectrophotometer and the problem of high background absorbance with the presence of proteins in the serum.

Polography is not widely used even though it is reported to have good precision. Unfortunately it is subject to interference by allopurinol, xanthine, and hypoxanthine (45). The colorimetric assay is also rarely used because the instrumentation required for such an assay is not readily available. High performance liquid chromatography is proposed by some to be the best suited for a reference method in that it is more sensitive and specific than the other methods (47–49). However HPLC is much too cumbersome a procedure for routine use.

In a recent comprehensive chemistry survey in which the College of American Pathologists polled approximately 6000 laboratories, 62% of the participants reported use of uricase methods, 34% used phosphotungstic acid methodology, less than 1% used polography, and 3% used other assays (50).

Specimen Requirements for Uric Acid Determination and Reference Range

Suitable specimens for determination of uric acid can be obtained from serum, urine, or heparinized plasma. EDTA and sodium fluoride should be avoided as anticoagulants/preservatives, since they will falsely elevate values when the uricase coupled-enzyme methodology is used. Uric acid is stable in serum for 48–72 hours at room temperature, for 3–7 days at 4–6°C, and for at least 6 months when frozen ($-20°C$). Uric acid is stable in urine for several days at room temperature. However, specimens should always be stored at 4–6°C to avoid bacterial growth and the effect of microbial uricase. To prevent urate precipitation in urine, sodium hydroxide is added to the collection bottle before collection of the specimen. The reference range for uric acid is shown in Table 4.

Table 4. Reference Range for Uric Acid

Subjects	Range (mg/dL)
Adult females	2.5–6.2
Adult males	3.5–8.0
Children (1 month–12 years)	2.0–7.0

Source: Ref. 30, p. 427.

Clinicopathological Correlations of Uric Acid and Uric Acid Clearance

The elevation of serum or plasma uric acid is referred to as hyperuricemia. Table 5 lists the major causes of hyperuricemia. Because uric acid is filtered by the glomerulus and secreted by the tubules, renal disease interfering with these functions will cause elevated levels of uric acid. Renal retention of uric acid may occur in acute or chronic renal failure or as a consequence of drug therapy. Diuretics in particular will cause hyperuricemia. Organic acidemia due to increased acetoacetic acid in diabetic ketoacidosis or to lactic acidosis may interfere with tubular secretion of urate. The measurement of uric acid in the evaluation of kidney function is not very useful, however, since so many other factors affect its plasma level.

Table 5. Major Causes of Hyperuricemia

Gout
Hematological conditions
    Leukemia
    Lymphoma
    Hemolytic anemia
    Megaloblastic anemia
    Infectious mononucleosis
    Polycythemia vera
Chronic renal disease (renal failure)
Drug-induced
    Thiazides
    Salicylates
    Pyrazinamide (PZA)
    Cytotoxics
Tissue necrosis
Malnutrition of all types
Therapeutic radiation
Alcohol
Lead poisoning
Glycogen storage, type I
Lactic acidosis
Toxemia of pregnancy
Psoriasis (active)
Lesch–Nyhan syndrome

Source: Ref. 30, p. 427.

TESTS OF RENAL REGULATORY FUNCTION

The kidneys are primarily responsible for maintenance of fluid and electrolyte composition of the body. Since changes that occur in the electrolyte composition are discussed elsewhere in this book, we confine our discussion to the role of the kidney in maintaining water homeostasis.

Water is the most abundant component of the human body, constituting approximately 60% of body weight. Body water, and therefore body weight, remains fairly constant from day to day in normal persons despite wide fluctuations in fluid intake. The concentrating and diluting mechanisms of the kidney contribute largely to the homeostasis of total body water, and the rate (51) of urine flow normally can be varied within a very wide range. The kidney has the ability to elaborate urine that is either more concentrated or more dilute than the plasma from which it is derived. It is this capacity of the kidney to form urine of greatly varying osmolality that enables the kidney to regulate within narrow physiological limits the solute concentration and therefore, the osmolality of body fluids, despite wide fluctuations of intake of salt and water (52). Water balance is controlled primarily through voluntary intake, which is regulated through the thirst center in the hypothalamus, and urinary loss. The control of urinary water loss by the concentrating and diluting ability of the kidney is the most important automatic mechanism by which body water is regulated. Factors affecting the urinary water loss include ADH, aldosterone, arterial pressure receptors, and nervous reflexes.

The determination of reduction in concentrating and diluting ability of the kidney can provide a very sensitive means of detecting early impairment in renal function. Urinary specific gravity and osmolality, two common laboratory parameters used as a measurement of this function, are both conveniently and economically quantitated.

Measurement of Urine Specific Gravity

Biochemistry and Physiology

Specific gravity is the ratio of the mass of a solution to the mass of an equal volume of water (53). Since this is a comparison of weights, it is not an exact measurement of the number of solute particles. However, there is good correlation between specific gravity and osmolality as long as the urine does not contain appreciable amounts of protein, sugar, or exogenous material such as contrast dye (54). In the healthy individual, urea, sodium chloride, and phosphate contribute most to the specific gravity.

Several methods are available for measuring specific gravity in the routine clinical laboratory. These include the refractometer, hydrometer (urinometer), and reagent strip methodologies.

Refractometer Method

The refractive index and the specific gravity of a urine specimen are related to the content of dissolved solids present. Each substance contributes differently to the refractive index and also to the specific gravity. Because various urine specimens are likely to contain dissolved substances of similar types and proportions, the refractive index (RI) and the specific gravity may be correlated. However, increased amounts of abnormal substances such as glucose and protein may partially invalidate this correlation. The RI is the ratio of the velocity of light in air to the velocity of light in a solution. This ratio varies directly with the number of dissolved particles in solution. Measurement of the RI of urine became feasible and convenient with the development of a clinical refractometer. The device requires only a few drops of urine, and scale readings of the instrument have been calibrated in terms of specific gravity. The specific gravity reading on the refractometer is slightly larger than a urinometer reading by about 0.002 (55).

Urinometer (Hydrometer) Method

The urinometer is a hydrometer designed for the measurement of urinary specific gravity at room temperature. When the hydrometer is placed in the urine specimen, which is contained in a cylinder, it sinks to the level characteristic of the specific gravity of the specimen. The value may then be read directly from the calibrations on the stem. These readings may be in error if the urinometer is not allowed to float freely. It must not adhere to the sides of the tubes, and no bubbles should cling to the stem. Erroneous readings may also occur if compensation is not made for temperature, gross proteinuria, or glycosuria. Because temperature influences the specific gravity, urine should be allowed to come to room temperature before a reading is made, or a correction of 0.001 should be made for each 3°C above or below the calibration temperature indicated on the urinometer. Similarly, 0.003 should be subtracted for every gram per 100 mL of either glucose or protein.

Reagent Strip Methodology

With increasing electrolyte concentration in the urine, reagents in the strip release hydrogen ions, causing a lowering of the pH of the reagent strip and a subsequent color reaction proportional to the ionic strength. The solute urea, which occurs in large amounts in urine, does not contribute to the reagent strip result as it does for the urinometer and refractometer.

Alkaline urines neutralize the released acid, causing a lower specific gravity reading. Thus, for a urine pH of 6.5 or more, 0.005 should be added to the reading. High levels of protein, contributing to the anions in the urine, may cause an elevation of up to one color block on the strip. Glucose and radiographic media do not cause an alteration in the specific gravity recorded on the reagent strip as they do with the urinometer and the refractometer.

Specimen Required

Specific gravity is most often determined as a part of a routine urinalysis on a random urine specimen. Less frequently, however, specific gravity is measured on timed specimens after water restrictions, in which case more exact information is derived. (See "Clinicopathological Correlation," below.)

Reference Range

Normal values for a 24-hour urine specimen are 1.015–1.025. Values after fluid restriction should exceed 1.025. If a random urine specimen has a specific gravity of 1.023 or more, concentrating ability can be considered to be normal.

Measurement of Urine and Serum Osmolality

Biochemistry and Physiology

The term "osmolality" describes the physical property of a solution based on the concentration of solute (expressed as millimoles) per kilogram of solvent. Increased serum osmolality is usually due to a change in the sodium concentration, because sodium and its associated actions account for 90% of the osmotic activity in plasma. The sensation of thirst, which is stimulated by the hypothalamic thirst center, is generated in response to increased osmolality of the blood. The natural response to the thirst sensation is to consume more fluids, therefore increasing the water content of the extracellular fluid, diluting out the elevated sodium levels and decreasing the osmolality of the plasma (56). Another method of maintaining normal osmolality is to control the excretion of water via the kidneys or the loss of water from the body via the lungs, sweat, and feces. The hypothalamus controls the loss of water through the kidneys in response to changes in the osmotic pressure of plasma. For example, increased plasma osmolality, occurring when the water concentration is decreased relative to the concentration of sodium and other electrolytes, causes the stimulation of antidiuretic hormone (ADH) secretion from the posterior pituitary. ADH acts on the cells of the collecting ducts in the kidneys to increase water reabsorption. Water is subsequently conserved, the plasma osmolality decreases, and secretion of ADH stops (57). Aldosterone has an opposite effect. Low serum osmolality results in a high water content presented to the kidneys and therefore, an increased renal blood flow. This causes activation of the renin–angiotensin system, leading to aldosterone secretion. Aldosterone blocks water reabsorption thus increasing plasma osmolality.

The measurement of urine osmolality is used to demonstrate the kidneys' ability to concentrate urine. In the glomerulus, an ultrafiltrate is extracted from the bloodstream and passed to renal tubules. The osmolality of the ultrafiltrate is nearly equal to that of the plasma. As it completes its passage through the nephron, most of the ultrafiltrate, including water, is reabsorbed into the bloodstream. Urine that is delivered to the bladder is approximately 3–4 times more concentrated than the plasma.

Methods of Measuring Serum and Urine Osmolality

Methods for determining osmolality are based on the colligative properties of a solution, that is, those properties that depend on the number of molecules of solute per kilogram of solvent rather than on their size or molecular weight. Such properties include freezing point, boiling point, vapor pressure, and osmotic pressure. As an osmotically active substance is added to water, the osmolality of the water increases. The increase in osmolality causes a decrease in the freezing point temperature and the vapor pressure and an increase in the boiling point temperature. The two most commonly used methods of analysis of osmolality are the freezing point depression and vapor pressure (58). Osmometers are used in the clinical laboratory to measure these properties.

Freezing Point Depression

The use of salt to melt ice and snow is an example of freezing point depression. The salt increases the osmolality, thereby lowering the freezing point of the solution compound to that of the pure solvent (ice or snow). Temperature at equilibrium is a function of the number of particles in solution. The temperature is depressed 1.86°C for each mole of particles dissolved per kilogram of water. The normal osmolality of blood is about 0.3 osm/kg (300 mosm/kg), and the freezing point is $-0.62°C$. Changes in the osmolality can be estimated by measuring the freezing point depression using an osmometer. Serum, plasma, or urine may be used. The specimen is supercooled (i.e., cooled below its freezing point) in an insulated freezing bath and then crystallized, using a vibrator which agitates the solution. As crystalliniz-ation occurs, heat of fusion is produced and the temperature of the solution increases, reaching a plateau which is slightly below the freezing point. This temperature is compared with plateau temperatures obtained with known standards; therefore, no correction factor is necessary. The temperature changes are measured by a thermistor and converted to milliosmoles per kilogram of water.

To achieve adequate precision in freezing point depression osmometry, a number of factors, which include bath temperature, fluid composition, and fluid volume, must be considered. Both fluid composition and volume change as moisture condenses from the room air. Thickness of the container and the amount of sample must be standardized. Osmolality values obtained by the freezing point depression methodologies will be invalid when other osmot-ically active substances, such as lipids, alcohol, or mannitol, are present in the sample.

Vapor Pressure

An alternative method for measuring osmolality is to use a vapor pressure (or dew point) osmometer. The sample to be tested is absorbed into a small disc of filter paper, which is inserted into a sample holder and sealed in an enclosed chamber. A temperature-sensitive thermocouple is incorporated into the chamber. The vapor pressure of the sample is directly proportional to the thermocouple voltage and is calibrated in (again in mosm/kg H_2O) by use of known standards.

Vapor pressure osmometers are simpler in design than freezing point depression osmometers and use smaller volumes of sample. If specimens do not contain any particulate matter, freezing point depression and vapor pressure osmometers will give identical results. However, there is a positive bias with vapor pressure instruments if the serum is lipemic (59). Studies have also indicated that vapor pressure instruments are less precise than freezing point osmometers. More important, vapor pressure osmometers cannot detect the pressure of volatiles (alcohols), whereas freezing point instruments can (47,60). This difference is due to the ability of a volatile solute to increase the total vapor pressure of solutions, eliminating the direct solute depression of vapor pressure (62).

Specimen Required

Osmolality may be measured in serum, urine, or plasma. The use of plasma is not recommended, however, because of the possibility of introducing osmoti-cally active substances to the specimen from the anticoagulant. Blood should be collected by venipuncture with a minimum of stasis, and the serum should be separated by centrifugation soon after collection. If serum is not to be analyzed soon after centrifuging, it should be refrigerated or frozen.

A random urine specimen is sufficient to screen the kidney's ability to concentrate urine. Urine should be collected in a clean, dry container without preservatives and centrifuged at high enough speed to remove all particulate material. The specimen should be refrigerated if the analysis cannot be carried out soon after collection.

Reference Range

Serum	275–295 mosm/kg
Urine (24-hour specimen)	300–900 mosm/24 hours
Urine/serum ratio	1.0–3.0

Clinicopathological Correlation of Specific Gravity and Osmolality

The measurement of urine specific gravity may be a useful screening test for renal concentrating ability as long as the limitations of the procedure are recognized. However, measurements of osmolality are considered to be more valid. Studies have compared the values for specific gravity (63) and osmolality in normal individuals and in unselected patients with renal disease. In healthy individuals, these values were shown to have a good correlation. However, the correlation was much less pronounced in patients with renal disease, presumably because the presence of heavy molecules, such as protein, glucose, or iodine-containing compounds, affects specific gravity significantly more than osmolality.

Osmolality of a healthy individual may vary widely according to the state of hydration. Individuals on an average fluid intake, will maintain a urine osmolality of 300–900 mosm/kg. However, after excessive fluid intake, the osmotic concentration may fall as low as 1 mosm/kg, while individuals with severely restricted fluid intake may have a urine osmolaltiy of up to 1200 mosm/kg.

If a random urine specimen has a specific gravity of 1.023 or more and/or a urine osmolality of 600 mosm/kg or more, renal concentrating ability is considered to be normal. However, if the random urine specimen is dilute, no conclusion about concentrating ability can be made. A definitive follow-up test requires overnight water restriction. A specific gravity of 1.025, or more or an osmolality of 850 mosm/kg or above, is evidence of normal concentrating ability. In chronic progressive renal failure, the concentrating ability of the tubules is decreased until the specific gravity and the osmolality of the urine approach those of the plasma ultrafiltrate. Clinically, this fixation in specific gravity and osmolality is manifested by nocturia and polyuria.

In diabetes insipidus, which might arise from inadequate ADH production or from insensitivity of the renal tubules to ADH, the urine specific gravity and osmolality are extremely low. In this disease, the baseline urine might have a specific gravity of less than 1.005 and an osmolality of 50 mosm/kg. A clinically more useful set of data can be obtained by relating urine and serum osmolality values as a ratio. After fluid restriction, the ratio is 3.0 or above. In patients with renal tubular disease, the ratio will be less than that observed in normal individuals. In polyuria from diabetes insipidus, the ratio will be between 0.2 and 0.7 even after fluid restriction. This will differentiate this type of polyuria from that seen in other conditions such as diabetes mellitus. In polyuria of neurogenic origin, the ratio may be normal without fluid restriction, increasing after fluid restriction (*64*).

REFERENCES

1. Robbins SC, Cotran RS, Kumar V. *Pathologic Basis of Disease*, 3rd ed. Philadelphia: Saunders, 1984.

2. Tietz NW (ed.) *Textbook of Clinical Chemistry*. Philadelphia: Saunders, 1986.

3. Blau EB, Haas JE. Glomerular sialic acid and proteinuria in human renal disease. *Lab Invest* 1973;28:477–481.

4. Miller BT, Winkler AW. The renal excretion of endogenous creatinine in man. Comparison with exogenous creatine and insulin. *J Clin Invest* 1938;17:31–40.

5. Narayanau S, Appleton HD. Creatinine: A review. *Clin Chem* 1980;26:1119–1126.

6. Jaffé M. Über den Nierderschalg welchen Pikrensäre in normalem Harn erzeugt an über eine neue reaktion des Kreatinins. *Z Physiol Chem* 1886;10:391.

7. Butler AR. The Jaffé reaction. Identification of the coloured species. *Clin Chim Acta* 1976;59:277–232.

8. Smith CH, Landt M, Steelman M. The Kodak Ektachem 400 Analyzer evaluated for automated enzymatic determination of plasma creatinine. *Clin Chem* 1983;29:1422–1425.

9. Solden SJ, Hill JG. The effect of bilirubin and ketones on reaction rate methods for the measurement of creatinine. *Clin Biochem* 1978;11:82–86.

10. Heinegard D, Tederstrom G. Determination of serum creatinine by direct colorimetric method. *Clin Chim Acta* 1973;43:305–310.

11. Haeckel R. Assay of creatinine in serum with the use of fuller's earth to remove interferents. *Clin Chem* 1981;27:179–183.

12. Owen JA, Igyo B, Schandutt. The determination of creatinine in plasma or serum, and urine; a critical examination. *Biochem J* 1954;58:426.

13. Polar E, Metcoff J. "True" creatinine chromogen determination in serum and urine by semiautomated analysis. *Clin Chem* 1965;11:763–770.

14. Spencer K, Price CP. A review of non-enzyme-mediated reactions and their

application to centrifugal analyzers, in Price CP, Spencer K, (eds): *Centrifugal Analyzers in Clinical Chemistry*, New York: Praeger, 1980, pp 213–253.

15. Bowers CD. Kinetic serum creatinine assays. I. The role of various factors in determining specificity. *Clin Chem* 1980;26:551–554.

16. Bowers CD, Wong ET. Kinetic serum creatinine assays. II. A critical evaluation and review. *Clin Chem* 1980;26:555–561.

17. Young DS, Pestaner LC, Gibberman V. Effects of drugs on clinical laboratory tests. *Clin Chem* 1975;21:5.

18. Miller BF, Dubos R. Determination by a specific enzymatic method of the creatinine content of blood and urine from normal and nephritic individuals. *J Biol Chem* 1937;121:457–467.

19. Tangelli E, Principe L, Bassi D. Enzymatic assay of creatinine in serum and urine with creatinine iminohydrolase and glutamate dehydrogenase. *Clin Chem* 1982;28:1461–1462.

20. Thompson H, Redenitz GA. Ion electrode based enzymatic analysis of creatinine. *Anal Chem* 1974;46:246–249.

21. Fernandey P, Cox M. Banc' concepts of renal physiology, in *The Kidney vs. Anesthesia*, vol. 22. Boston: Little, Brown, 1984.

22. Brown ND, Sing HC, Neeley WE, et al. Determination of "true" serum creatinine by high performance liquid chromatography combined with a continuous-flow microanalyzer. *Clin Chem* 1972;23:1281–1283.

23. Solden SJ, Hill GJ. Micromethod for determination of creatinine in biological fluids by high performance liquid chromatography. *Clin Chem* 1978;24:747–750.

24. Langley WD, Evans M. The determination of creatinine with sodium 3,5-dinitrobenzoate. *J Biol Chem* 1936;115:333–341.

25. Sullivan MS, Irrevere F. A highly specific test for creatinine. *J Biol Chem* 1958;223:530–538.

26. Van Pilsum JF, Martin RP, Kito E, et al. Determination of creatinine, creatine, arginine, guanidineacetic acid, guanidine, and methylguanidine in biological fluids. *J Biol Chem* 1956;222:225–236.

27. Bjorkhem, Blomstrand IR, Ohman G. Mass fragmentography of creatinine proposed as a reference method. *Clin Chem* 1977;23:2144–2151.

28. Tietz NW (ed). *Clinical Guide to Laboratory Tests*. Philadelphia: Saunders, 1983, pp 154–155.

29. Serisbock-Nielson K, Molholm-Hansen J, Kampmann J. Rapid evaluation of creatinine clearance. *Lancet* 1971;1(part 2):1133–1134.

30. Bakerman S. *ABC's of Interpretive Laboratory Data*. Greenville, NC: Interpretive Laboratory Data, Inc, 1983.

31. Natelson S. *Techniques of Clinical Chemistry*, 3rd ed. Springfield, IL: Thomas, 1971, pp 728–745.

32. Henry RJ, Cannon DC, Winkelman J. *Clinical Chemistry: Principles and Techniques*, 2nd ed. New York: Harper & Row, 1974, pp 504–506.

33. Faulkner WR, Mertis S. *Selected Methods of Clinical Chemistry*, vol 9. Washington DC: American Association of Clinical Chemistry, 1982, pp 365–373.

34. Hallett CJ, Cook KGH. Reduced nicotinamide adenine denucleotide–coupled reaction for emergency blood urea estimation. *Clin Chim Acta* 1971;35:33–37.

35. Paulson G, Ray R, Sternberg J. A rate sensing approach to urea measurement. *Clin Chem* 1971;17:644.

36. Patton CJ, Crouch SR. Spectrophotometric and kinetics investigation of the Berthelot reaction for determination of ammonia. *Clin Chem* 1977;49:464–469.

37. Morgan DB, Carver ME, Payne RB. Plasma creatinine and urea: Creatinine ratio in patients with raised plasma urea. *Br J Med* 1977;2:929–932.

38. Watts RWE. Purines and nucleotides, in Brown SS, Mitchell FL (eds): *Chemical Diagnosis of Disease*. Amsterdam: Elsevier/North Holland, 1979.

39. Felix O, Denis W. A new method for the determination of uric acid in blood. *J Biol Chem* 1912;13:469–475.

40. Caraway WT. *Standard Methods of Clinical Chemistry*, vol 4. New York: Academic Press, 1963, pp 239–247.

41. Humienny SJ. Personal communication, 1983.

42. Ishihard A, Kurakasi K, Nehard H. Enzymatic determination of ammonia in blood and plasma. *Clin Chim Acta* 1972;41:255.

43. Kabasakalian P, Kalliney S, Wescott A. Determination of uric acid in serum with the use of uricase and a tribromophenol–aminoantipyrine chromogen. *Clin Chem* 1973;19:522.

44. Kingsley GR, Tager HS. Ion exchange method for the determination of plasma ammonia nitrogen with the Berthelot reaction, in MacDonald RP (ed): *Standard Methods of Clinical Chemistry*, vol 6. New York: Academic Press, 1970; p 115.

45. Bell R, Ray RA. A rate-sensing approach to the measurement of uric acid in serum and urine. *Clin Chem* 1971;17:644.

46. Troy RJ, Purdy WC. The colorimetric determination of uric acid in serum and urine. *Clin Chim Acta* 1970;27:401–408.

47. Pachla LA, Kissinger PT. Measurement of serum uric acid by liquid chromatography. *Clin Chem* 1979;25:1847–1852.

48. Kiser EJ, Johnson GF, Witte DL. Serum uric acid determined by reversed-phase liquid chromatography with spectrophotometric determination. *Clin Chem* 1978;24:536–540.

49. Hansen A, Fuchs D, Konig K, et al. Quantitation of urinary uric acid by reversed-phase liquid chromatography. *Clin Chem* 1981;27:1445–1456.

50. Comprehensive Chemistry Survey, Set C-A. College of American Pathologists, Skokie, IL, 1982.

51. Kokko JP. Renal concentrating and diluting mechanism. *Hosp Practice* 1979;14:110–116.

52. Rose BD. *Clinical Physiology of Acid–Base and Electrolyte Disorders*. New York: McGraw-Hill, 1977, pp 336–340.

53. Henry JB. *Clinical Diagnosis and Management by Laboratory Methods*, 17th ed. 1984, p 121.

54. Wau F. Renal function tests, a guide to interpretation. *Hosp Med* 1981;9:77–92.

55. Wolfe AV. Urinary concentrative powers. *Am J Med* 1962;32:329.

56. Zilva JF, Pannall PR. *Clinical Chemistry in Diagnosis and Treatment* 3rd ed. Chicago: Year Book Medical Publishers, 1979.

57. Natelson S, Natelson E. *Principles of Applied Clinical Chemistry*, vol 1. New York: Plenum, 1975.

58. Lee LW, *Elementary Principles of Laboratory Instruments*, 4th ed. St. Louis: Mosby, 1978.

59. Mercui DC. Comparison of dewpoint and freezing point osmometry. *Am J Med Technol* 1978;44:1066.

60. Weisburg HF. Osmolality-calculated delta and more formulas. *Clin Chem* 1975;21:1182.

61. Rocco WV. Volatiles and osmometry. *Clin Chem* 1976;22:399.

62. Barlowe LK. Volatiles and osmometry (continued). *Clin Chem* 1976;22:1230.

63. Holmes JH. Measurement of osmolality in serum, urine and other biological fluids by the freezing point determination, in Workshop on Urinalysis and Renal Function Studies, Commission on Continuing Education, American Society of Clinical Pathologists, 1962.

64. Davidson I, Henry JB. *Clinical Diagnosis and Management by Laboratory Methods*, 16th ed, vol 1. Philadelphia: Saunders, 1979.

CHAPTER 5

PROTEINS

KAREN L. TILLEY and LAWRENCE M. SILVERMAN

North Carolina Memorial Hospital
Chapel Hill, North Carolina

ROBERT H. CHRISTENSON

Durham Veterans Administration Medical Center
Durham, North Carolina

INTRODUCTION

Current laboratory evaluation of the countless number of proteins in the human body is generally limited to those found in blood, cerebrospinal fluid (CSF), urine, and other major body fluids. In most cases, the proteins in these materials were originally derived from blood plasma. This discussion is limited to the current clinical methods used in evaluating these proteins and their clinical significance. Since disease alters the proportion and concentration of plasma proteins in characteristic ways, protein electrophoresis often is used as a screening procedure to detect abnormalities in serum, urine, and CSF. Follow-up procedures often include quantitation of specific proteins and typing of immunoglobulin disorders by immunoelectrophoresis and/or immunofixation.

PROTEIN ELECTROPHORESIS

Principle

In 1937, Tiselius (*1*) first demonstrated the migration of charged particles in a liquid medium under the influence of an electric field, a process known as moving-boundary electrophoresis. *Zone electrophoresis*, the technique used in modern protein separation methods, uses a porous, stabilized support medium for the separation of proteins into zones based on their electrical charges. The support media most often used today are forms of cellulose acetate, agarose, and polyacrylamide gels.

Proteins, which are composed of amino acids, are called *ampholytes* because they exhibit both positive and negative charges. They also have an *isoelectric point* (pI), which is the pH value at which the sum of all the positive and negative charges of a molecule is zero. The relationship of the pH of the solution to the pI of the molecule determines the direction in which the protein molecule migrates. The rate of migration depends on the net electric charge of the molecule, the size and shape of the molecule, the strength of the electric field, the type of support medium used, and the temperature at which the reaction takes place.

The liquid medium, the buffer, carries the electric current and establishes the pH at which the reaction takes place. Because the buffer ions cluster around the charged molecule, the ionic strength of the buffer affects the mobility of the protein. The higher the concentration of ions (*ionic strength*), the slower the movement of the protein. Although high ionic strength buffers yield sharper bands, they also generate more heat, which can damage heat-labile proteins. Barbital buffers with a pH of 8–9 and ionic strength of 0.025–0.075 are used today for most electrophoretic methods.

The appropriate supporting medium is determined by several factors including pore size, degree of *electroòsmosis*, and application needs. Pores should be large enough to allow the protein molecules to move through the medium but sufficiently restricted in size to cut off bulk flow of the buffer. *Electroosmosis* is the movement of the buffer in the opposite direction under the influence of an electric field. Supporting media such as agarose have counterions, which allow for the net flow of buffer in only one direction.

Most electrophoretic methods use a chamber containing two buffer-filled troughs. A wire running the entire length of the chamber attaches to posts at the ends of each trough. These wires connect to an external power supply and function as anode and cathode. Between the two troughs lies the supporting medium. In some procedures that use higher voltages, the medium may rest on a coolant-filled plate to decrease the temperature in the chamber. If the sides of the medium itself do not extend into the buffer, paper wicks are used to complete the circuit.

When the supporting medium is under an electric current, heat is generated because of its resistance to the current, and evaporation occurs. To counteract this evaporation, buffer flows from either trough toward the center of the medium. The rate of flow is constant and greater at the sides of the medium than at the center. This *wick flow* influences the rate of protein migration, since some proteins near the anode will be moving against the flow of buffer and others near the cathode will be moving with it. Because of this factor, samples are generally applied cathodic of the center of the support.

Because the concentration of immunoglobulin G in CSF is normally in the range of 0.8–4.2 mg/dL, specimen preconcentration is necessary prior to electrophoresis and treatment using most conventional stains. Fortyfold preconcentration is sufficient to allow visualization of oligoclonal bands and is easily done with commercially available devices based on centrifugal ultrafiltration (Amicon Corporation, Danvers, MA). For urine samples, a 50-fold concentration using a 15,000-MW cutoff filter is suggested for most conventional electrophoresis procedures.

After electrophoresis, proteins are visualized by staining with a dye chosen according to the sensitivity needed and the electrophoretic medium used. Amido Black and Bromphenol Blue are popular choices for agarose gel electrophoresis. Ponceau S, a less sensitive but more specific red protein dye, is often used with cellulose acetate methods. Coomassie Brilliant Blue R-250 is frequently used in polyacrylamide gel–isoelectric focusing (PAGE-IEF) procedures and can detect less than 0.2 μg of protein. More recently, convenient methods using silver nitrate have been developed for the detection of oligoclonal banding in CSF. Since these silver stains are 10–50 times more sensitive than other stains, CSF preconcentration before electrophoresis is not necessary (2). On the other hand, these stains are technically more difficult to perform and their use can result in artifactual banding, which may complicate interpretation.

For most electrophoretic procedures, a pooled normal human serum can be used as a control. Commercial control material is available but expensive. For the detection of oligoclonal bands in CSF, a pooled control of sera with monoclonal proteins of varying mobilities can be diluted to the desired concentration. Both the serum and CSF controls can be aliquoted and frozen at $-20°C$ for long-term storage.

Methods and Media

Cellulose Acetate

Although cellulose acetate has long been a popular choice for electrophoresis in clinical laboratories, it is now being replaced by commercial agarose gel methods. Cellulose acetate comes packaged as a thin, dry, opaque film. When the dry film has been soaked in buffer, the air spaces within the interlocking cellulose fibers fill with buffer and the membrane becomes pliable. Samples are applied with a wire microapplicator. After electrophoresis and staining with Ponceau S, the membranes are cleared for densitometry and storage by treating with a methanol–glacial acetic acid mixture and heating until they become clear (like cellophane). The cleared membrane can now be put in a clear plastic protective envelope for scanning and long-term storage.

Cellulose acetate is easy to use and relatively inexpensive, and once cleared, the final product may be stored indefinitely. It has a fast speed of separation,

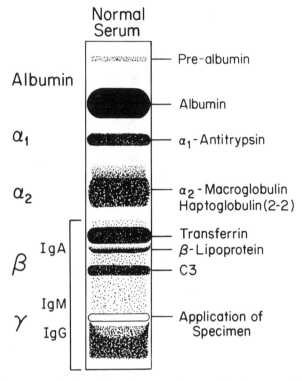

Figure 1. Serum protein electrophoresis pattern demonstrating five zones of separation.

usually 20–60 minutes. The proteins separate into five general zones: albumin, and the α_1, α_2, β, and γ globulins. On CSF samples, prealbumin is frequently observed. The patterns may be scanned on a densitometer and the percentages for the five zones reported. Since only five regions of proteins are seen by this method giving poor sensitivity, some minimonoclonal and oligoclonal bands may be missed. Figure 1 shows the five zones of separation of a protein electrophoresis pattern.

Agarose Gel

Agarose gel has been rapidly replacing cellulose acetate as the medium of choice for protein electrophoresis. Two types of agarose gel method are available commercially. The first separates proteins into five zones, and the pattern is comparable to that of cellulose acetate. A modified version, high resolution agarose, may show 10 or more fractions. Agarose has low

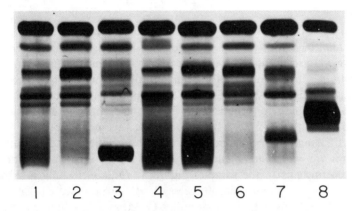

Figure 2. Protein patterns obtained by high resolution agarose gel electrophoresis: 1, normal; 2, acute inflammatory; 3, IgG monoclonal; 4, polyclonal increase in immunoglobulins; 5, acute and chronic inflammatory; 6, acute inflammatory with decreased immunoglobulins; 7, IgG monoclonal; 8, IgA monoclonal with decreased IgG and IgM.

electroosmosis, and its large pore size makes it suitable for many immunoelectrophoretic techniques. Because agarose can be poured after reheating to about 50°C, antiserum can be added to make immunodiffusion plates. Figure 2 shows various protein patterns obtained by agarose gel electrophoresis.

Polyacrylamide Gels and Isoelectric Focusing

Polyacrylamide gel electrophoresis (PAGE) is not routinely used in clinical situations for serum protein electrophoresis, since it may yield up to 20 or more fractions. On the other hand, PAGE is useful for the study of individual proteins in serum and other fluids and for the detection of genetic variants such as α_1-antitrypsin and alkaline phosphatase isoenzymes. These gels are composed of three gel layers that vary in composition and pore size. They are clear, easy to prepare, and have low electroosmosis.

Isoelectric focusing (IEF) is the separation of proteins based on their pI by movement through a medium that has a stable pH gradient, with the pH changing in the direction of migration. The protein molecules will move to the zone in which the pH equals the pI. This procedure uses a very high voltage because of the high concentration of carrier ampholytes (small synthetic peptides which establish the pH gradient). The major advantage to this procedure is the high resolving power, which separates proteins into very sharp zones.

PROTEIN IDENTIFICATION

When a band is seen in the γ region of the serum protein pattern, it may be further identified and typed by either of two methods: *immunoelectrophoresis* or *immunofixation*. Both approaches use the basic principle of electrophoresis. In immunoelectrophoresis (IEP), serum is applied to a plastic-backed agarose gel and electrophoresed. After the electrophoresis is completed, specific antisera are applied to troughs that parallel the electrophoretic patterns and allowed to incubate for 18–24 hours. During this incubation time, simultaneous diffusion of the serum proteins and specific antisera results in a precipitin arc whose shape and position are characteristic of the individual separated proteins in the sample (Figure 3). Often screening is done with polyvalent antisera and then, if necessary, it can be repeated using monovalent antisera for the immunoglobulins G, M, and A, κ light chains, and λ light chains. The gel can then be photographed or stained and dried for a permanent record.

A newer technique that has been gaining wide acceptance is immunofixation (IFE). This method, which combines electrophoresis and immunoprecipitation, was first described in a practical form by Alper and Johnson in 1969 (*3*) and has been used for the study of immunoglobulins since 1976 (*4*). An aliquot of a serum or concentrated urine sample is first electrophoresed on an agarose gel. After electrophoresis, specific monovalent antisera are applied to each protein pattern. This was originally done by dipping cellulose acetate strips in the antisera and then overlaying the agarose gel. Commercial kits now have precut antisera templates that allow for direct application of the antisera to the gel surface without contamination of the other patterns. This direct application allows for a more rapid and even distribution of the antisera

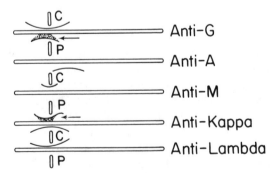

Figure 3. Diagram of an immunoelectrophoresis pattern for IgG$_\kappa$: C = normal control and P = patient sera.

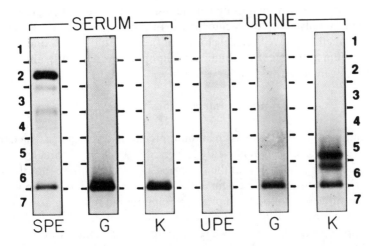

Figure 4. Immunofixation protein electrophoresis of serum and urine: serum (SPE), IgG$_\kappa$; urine (UPE), one IgG$_\kappa$ band with two free κ.

and also decreases the amount needed. After the excess antisera has been washed off the gel, the gel may be stained and the patterns compared visually (Figure 4). Only the protein that has complexed with the antisera will precipitate into the gel surface; the rest will wash off.

Immunofixation has become popular because it can be performed in a much shorter time ($1\frac{1}{2}$ hours) than is possible with IEP (18 hours). This method offers good sensitivity and resolution, even at low concentrations, and requires no special equipment other than what is needed to perform protein electrophoresis. Its patterns are analogous to the protein electrophoresis patterns and are therefore easier to interpret. Another advantage of IFE over IEP is that IFE is better for detecting monoclonal bands in the presence of polyclonal immunoglobulins. One disadvantage of immunofixation is that it is more prone to antigen excess than IEP. If the protein concentration is too great for the antisera titer used, the stained pattern will show prozoning, a condition in which staining occurs at the margins but there is little stain in the central area. IEP also requires less hands-on technical time and expertise than IFE.

PROTEIN QUANTITATION

Besides typing the monoclonal proteins observed on the protein electro-phoresis, it is often desirable to quantitate the amount of protein present. The proteins most frequently quantitated in the clinical lab are IgG, IgM, IgA, and the proteins involved in the acute phase response (see below). Recently commercial methods have been developed for the quantitation of κ and λ light chains in serum and urine, prealbumin, apolipoproteins AI and B, and other which are not included in this discussion.

Radial Immunodiffusion

Radial immunodiffusion (RID) is an immunoprecipitin technique in which the antibody to a specific protein is evenly dispersed in a gel. Small circular holes are punched out in the agar and the sample is allowed to diffuse into the gel over a period of time. As the protein in the serum reacts with the antibody in the gel, the antigen–antibody complexes precipitate out in a ring around the sample application. In 1965, Mancini (5) demonstrated that there is a linear relationship between the area of the precipitate and the concentration of the antigen at equilibrium. In the same year, Fahey (6) demonstrated that the plates could be read at 24 hours and the ring diameters of the standards could be plotted against their concentration to measure the concentration of unknowns.

In current practice, the square of the diameter of the standard is plotted on a linear graph against the concentration of the standard, and the squared diameter of the unknown is interpolated from the linear graph. This procedure requires excellent technical skill for achieving reproducible results. Adding sample to the wells without nicking the agar is critical to avoid getting elliptical rings. Accurate measurements are essential, since the rings must be read to the 0.1 mL scale. This procedure is still used as the reference method for most quantitative protein procedures. Although difficult to perform well, it does have the advantage of not requiring any expensive or complicated equipment.

Nephelometry and Turbidimetry Principles

In an attempt to automate and shorten the reaction time for measuring proteins, two major new methods evolved. Most of the protein procedures used in the clinical laboratory today are a modification of either nephelometry or turbidimetry. Both methods measure light scatter: nephelometry is the measurement of light scattered by particles in solution, and turbidimetry is the measurement of the decrease in light transmitted through a particulate solution. Turbidimetry is readily adaptable to many of the modern chemistry analyzers available today. The use of microprocessors on these instruments has greatly improved our ability to measure turbidity with high accuracy and precision.

There are two general classes of nephelometers: end-point and kinetic (also known as rate). The end-point nephelometers measure the sum total of light scattered by the formation of antigen–antibody complexes over a set time period, usually 30–60 minutes. This measurement requires a blank to be read with every sample. Rate nephelometers, on the other hand, measure the rate at which light scatter is progressing in a solution (does not require a blank). The rate of formation of light-scattering complexes increases until the antigen concentration reaches a certain maximum known as the *equivalence point.* Once the solution has reached a condition of *antigen excess,* the rate decreases. Figure 5 plots the immunoprecipitin curve. Instruments such as the Beckman ICS and Array (Beckman Instruments, Inc., Brea, CA 92621) can measure this rate of light scatter and, using a microprocessor, convert to concentration by comparison against a previously programmed standard curve. Rate nephelometers have some advantages over end-point nephelometers: the blank measurement has been eliminated, they offer rapid analysis (<60 seconds), and since they are more sensitive to change, they can detect and quantitate immunocomplexes that cannot be detected by end-point instruments. Nephelometry is usually more sensitive at low concentrations than turbidimetry because of the low signal-to-noise ratio. However, modern turbidimeters have excellent discrimination and can quantify small changes in signal.

Most nephelometers use either a laser or a tungsten–halogen light source. The laser provides a stable, highly collimated, and intense band of light. The Beckman ICS uses a tungsten light source with a broadband filter for wavelength selection. This broad range gives good performance, with the

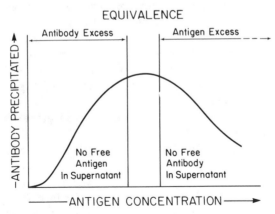

Figure 5. The immunoprecipitin curve. (Adapted from Beckman Instruments, Inc., ICS-8 monograph.)

particle sizes being measured in most situations. Polymers that are added to the reaction buffer used in these instruments (polyethylene glycol 8000 in a 3–5% concentration is a popular choice) increase the solubility of the protein by reducing a significant amount of water in the solution. This additive increases the linearity of the reaction.

CLINICAL SIGNIFICANCE OF THE SERUM PROTEINS

The material on acute phase reactants that follows is taken from the *Journal of Medical Technology* as part of a special issue on inflammation (7).

Acute Phase Reactants

The acute phase response (APR) involves the host's adaptation to tissue injury (*8–11*). APR proteins are synthesized by the liver and function, in various ways, to protect the host against further damage and to prevent the loss of constituents such as hemoglobin. In the hours and days that follow the initial injury, most of these proteins' levels are increased in the serum or plasma. However, a few proteins are actually found to be decreased. These proteins are referred to as *negative* acute phase proteins. In this group are albumin, transferrin, and prealbumin. Explanations for this decrease include (1) compensatory shunting of amino acids into the synthesis of positive acute phase proteins and (2) a relative hemodilution secondary to APR. Even though the exact cause for negative APR proteins is unclear, combining positive and negative APR proteins provides the most useful clinical data.

APR proteins rise or fall in the period immediately following an acute insult. However, some APR proteins are found to be increased in serum within hours while others are increased days afterward. In combination with this differential time of release, each protein has a characteristic half-life ($t_{1/2}$) which reflects the time at which the protein is cleared from the circulation. Together, the release and clearance patterns result in a clinically useful *time window*, or period of time during which certain APR proteins provide maximal clinical information.

Generally, APR proteins can be grouped into early (6–24 hours), mid (2–3 days), and late (3–7 days) stages following an insult.

Table 1 summarizes the most widely accepted data concerning half-lives and groupings of the APR proteins. In addition, Figure 6 graphically represents the same data in a different format. Representative proteins from each stage can be further grouped into panels, which can then provide information concerning the status of a specific patient with respect to the time of the acute event.

Table 1. Changes in Acute Phase Protein Levels after Injury

Acute Phase Protein[a]	$t_{1/2}$	Early	Mid	Late
1. C-Reactive protein	24 hours	+ + + +	+	−
2. Amyloid A protein	??	+ + +	+	−
3. α_1-antitrypsin	4 days	+ + +	+ +	+
4. α_1-acid glycoprotein	5 days	+ + +	+ +	+
5. Haptoglobin	2 days	+ +	+ +	−
6. Fibrinogen	2 days	+	+ +	+
7. Ceruloplasmin	4 days	−	+ +	+ +
8. Complement component 3	??	−	+ +	+ + +
9. Complement component 4	??	−	+ +	+ + +
10. Albumin (neg)	17 days	−	−	−
11. Transferrin (neg)	7 days	−	−	−
12. Prealbumin (neg)	12 hours	−	−	−

[a] Negative acute phase reactants (albumin, transferrin, and prealbumin) decrease, rather than increase, following injury.

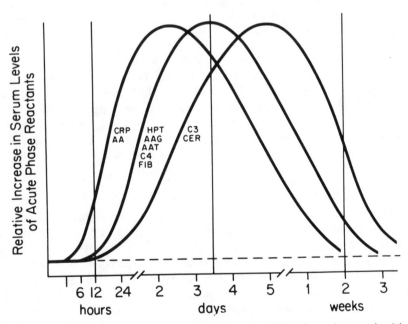

Figure 6. Changes in serum levels of acute phase proteins: CRP = C-reactive protein, AA = Amyloid A Protein, HPT = haptoglobin, AAG = α_1-acid glycoprotein, AAT = α_1-antitrypsin, C3 and C4 = complements 3 and 4, FIB = fibrinogen, and CER = ceruloplasmin.

Clinical Utility of APR Proteins

While APR proteins can be used as early indicators of inflammation, their clinical utility is limited because of nonspecificity with respect to the *cause* or source of the acute event. Nonetheless, APR proteins are frequently used to *confirm* inflammation, even if the cause is not known; moreover, APR proteins are also used to monitor the course and/or treatment of the underlying cause or symptoms. Several of the APR proteins are measured indirectly; for example, an estimate of fibrinogen can be made from the erythrocyte sedimentation rate. However, with the availability of highly specific antisera, immunoassays are currently available which are accurate, rapid, and relatively inexpensive.

Specific APR Proteins and Panels

C-Reactive Protein (CRP). CRP was the first APR protein to be discovered (1930) and is recognized as the most sensitive, and perhaps least specific APR. CRP can rise up to 1000-fold in the first 24 hours after insult and remains elevated for 2 to 3 days. CRP activates the classic complement pathway and initiates opsonization, phagocytosis, and lysis of invading cells. Because of its extreme nonspecificity, CRP levels should be interpreted only with a complete clinical history and, whenever possible, by comparison with previous values.

α_1-Antitrypsin (AAT). AAT is a protease inhibitor whose deficiency is associated with both liver and lung disease. While AAT's name implies antitrypsin activity, actually AAT is not particularly effective against trypsin because of the low pH of intestinal secretions in which trypsin is active. AAT is most effective at a neutral pH and has its most clinically significant inhibition against neutrophil elastase and collagenase. While CRP is increased earlier and rises more significantly, AAT is often used either in combination with or as a substitute for CRP because of better specificity.

Haptoglobin (HAP). HAP binds free hemoglobin in serum, thus serving both a conservation and a protective role. The heme moiety is preserved, and the deleterious effects of massive hemolysis on the kidney tubule are prevented. The HAP–hemoglobin complex is rapidly removed by the reticuloendothelial system, resulting in a decreased level of circulating HAP. Thus, a decreased HAP level is an excellent indicator of recent intravascular hemolysis. This effect must be considered when interpreting HAP levels, since APR changes can be masked in individuals with concomitant intravascular hemolysis.

Ceruloplasmin (CER). CER is a mid-to-late APR protein which binds copper and also functions as an antioxidant. CER measurements are most useful in diagnosing and/or confirming Wilson's disease, which is associated with a deficiency of CER. However, as with HAP, the presence of the APR in an individual at risk for Wilson's disease can complicate interpretation.

Complement Components C_3 and C_4. C_3 and C_4 may actually share a common evolutionary origin because of their similarity in structure and function. Both C_3 and C_4 are late APR proteins, sometimes called the "subacute phase reactants." Both C_3 and C_4 participate in the classic complement pathway; however, only C_3 takes part in the alternative pathway. As with HAP and CER, interpretation of C_3 and C_4 can be complicated in individuals in whom both the APR and complement consumption occur.

Negative APR Proteins

Transferrin (TRF). TRF is the major iron-transporting protein in serum but also possesses antioxidant activity, in many ways similar to CER. TRF levels decrease following APR; however, TRF levels are also decreased as the result of malnutrition and/or decreased hepatic synthesis secondary to liver disease. TRF levels are associated with the host's susceptibility to certain bacteria, which need iron as a growth factor. High circulating transferrin levels bind more of the available iron, leaving less for the bacteria. Conversely, low TRF levels bind less iron, resulting in more available iron. Individuals with TRF deficiency or decreased TRF levels secondary to malnutrition and/or liver disease are more susceptible to bacterial infections. As with other APR proteins (CER, HAP, C_3, and C_4), interpretation of TRF levels may be complicated by concomitant conditions, which can either increase or decrease serum TRF.

Albumin (ALB) and Prealbumin (PRE). ALB and PRE are multifunctional proteins which primarily serve as carriers for hormones, drugs, anions, cations, and so on. Both are synthesized in the liver and are decreased following malnutrition and/or liver disease. PRE has been used as a particularly sensitive indicator of nutritional status because of its very short half-life (< 12 hours). As with TRF, these negative APR proteins are decreased following an acute event, although the exact reason for the decrease is unknown.

APR Panels

Effective APR panels generally include representative proteins which are markers for the early, mid, and late stages. For example, one might group CRP, HAP, C_3, and C_4 together as an APR panel. If one also includes the immunoglobulins, the panel covers both acute and chronic inflammation. Since albumin is frequently ordered, one has a negative APR protein for confirmation. As mentioned above, AAT is commonly used in combination with, or substituted for, CRP. Often serum protein electrophoresis, which usually includes chemical determinations of total protein and albumin, serves as an effective screen for APR. Patterns consistent with APR can be visualized by electrophoresis; specific APR proteins can then be ordered, if necessary, as a means of assessing the patient's status or for monitoring therapy. Also, electrophoresis can save money, since for many electrophoretic patterns, no additional tests will be required.

IMMUNOGLOBULINS

Together with the APR proteins, immunoglobulins are the most commonly ordered proteins to be measured by either electrophoresis or light-scattering techniques. While the recognized classes of immunoglobulins include IgG, IgA, IgM, IgD, and IgE, only IgG, IgA, and IgM are discussed in this section.

IgG

IgG is the major immunoglobulin (molecular weight 160,000) produced by the plasma cells, comprising approximately 70% of the total circulating immuno-globulin pool. IgG participates in the chronic inflammtory response to most invading bacteria and viruses. It appears to cause aggregation of small antigens and to activate complement-mediated events.

IgM

IgM accounts for approximately 5–10% of the total circulating immuno-globulins. It is the largest immunoglobulin (900,000) and also functions to activate complement.

IgA

IgA has the same molecular weight as IgG and comprises about 10–15% of the total immunoglobulins. While IgA can also function to activate complement in serum, IgA is probably more important because it is present in many other body fluids, such as sweat, saliva, and gastrointestinal and bronchial secretions.

Clinical Significance

Normal immunoglobulin synthesis results in a variety of molecules directed toward different foreign antigens (called a polyclonal response). Abnormalities of immunoglobulin production can result in decreased, increased, or absent synthesis (called immunodeficiency). Increased synthesis may be directed toward the host's own antigens (autoimmune). Examples of autoimmune diseases include rheumatoid arthritis and systemic lupus erythematosus. Increased synthesis can also be the hallmark of certain malignant conditions in which a single clone of plasma cells proliferates and produces an abundance of one IgG molecule (called a monoclonal response). Generally this malignant process is multiple myeloma, although some other tumors (such as lymphomas or carcinomas) can also be associated with a monoclonal response.

Monoclonal Proteins

Since a number of malignant conditions can manifest a monoclonal response, detection and classification of monoclonal proteins are extremely important activities in a clinical laboratory. Toward these ends, each laboratory must emphasize techniques such as electrophoresis, immunofixation, immunoelectrophoresis, and light-scattering techniques for identification and quantification of serum and urine monoclonal proteins. These determinations are used by the clinician for diagnosis, along with other laboratory, radiographic, and clinical data. In addition, patients' therapy is monitored by following the increase or decrease in the monoclonal protein as a function of tumor burden. Technical details are discussed elsewhere in this chapter.

Interpretation

The diagnosis of malignant conditions associated with monoclonal proteins is in the province of the clinician; however, the laboratory can assist the clinician by being aware of the diagnostic laboratory criteria. Associated with the monoclonal proliferation characteristic of plasma cells in the bone marrow of patients with multiple myeloma is an increase of the serum concentration of a particular class of immunoglobulins. Most common is IgG (70%), followed by IgA (15%), and the overproduction of light chains (15%). Infrequently, IgD, IgE, and the over-production of heavy chains without attached light chains (heavy-chain disease) are observed. In these cases, the clonal proliferation leads to concomitant decreases in the serum level of the complementary immunoglobulins. For example, an IgG myeloma is most frequently associated with elevated serum levels of IgG *and* decreased levels of IgA and IgM, representing the decreased bone marrow source of IgA and IgM producing plasma cells.

In malignant conditions such as lymphoma, which originate outside the bone marrow, the clonal proliferation does not occur in the bone marrow; thus complementary immunoglobulin levels are not decreased. A specific example is Waldenstrom's macroglobulinemia, in which a clone of mature B lymphocytes is the source of monoclonal IgM. Since this is an extramedullary process, corresponding levels of IgG and IgA are unaffected.

Frequently, monoclonal proteins are observed in which there is no apparent underlying malignant process. These are called "monoclonal proteins of unknown significance" and are most commonly benign. This condition is associated with serum levels of the specific monoclonal protein that are only moderately elevated (if at all) and no decrease in the complementary immunoglobulins. As many as 50% of monoclonal bands observed on routine serum protein electrophoresis fall into this category.

CLINICAL SIGNIFICANCE OF PROTEINS IN CEREBROSPINAL FLUID

Cerebrospinal fluid (CSF) is formed principally by ultrafiltration and active transport mechanisms in the choroid plexus. The average total volume of CSF in humans is nearly constant at about 150 mL; however, fresh CSF is formed at a rate of 0.35 mL/min or about 500 mL/day. To accommodate the nearly 14% hourly turnover in CSF necessary to maintain constant volume, the arachnoid granulations provide a low resistance, pressure-dependent mechanism for absorption of CSF into blood across the blood–CSF barrier.

More than 80% of the total protein content of CSF originates in the serum. Serum proteins enter the CSF compartment predominantly by passive diffusion through the capillaries of the choroid plexus and meninges. As a result, the composition of proteins found in CSF are determined largely by molecular size and concentration in serum.

Concentrations of individual or total protein(s) in CSF can be increased or diminished because of three general processes:

1. disruption in the blood–CSF barrier (i.e. increased permeability of blood–CSF barrier structures),
2. intrathecal production of protein within the central nervous system (CNS), and
3. reduction in CSF flow to the serum compartment.

Because protein passage across the blood–CSF barrier is governed largely by passive diffusion, serum increases in specific proteins and specific protein fractions can profoundly affect those corresponding in CSF. Disturbances in the blood–CSF barrier or improper sample collection can also affect CSF proteins dramatically. For these reasons, interpretation of CSF proteins is difficult or impossible without knowledge of the integrity of the blood–CSF barrier and quantitations of the same proteins in the serum at the time of sampling.

CSF Total Protein

Versions of the Coomassie Brilliant Blue G-250 dye binding method are popular in the clinical laboratory for the determination of CSF total protein. This dye (CBB) binds to protonated amine groups of amino acid residues in the polypeptide chain and the change in absorbance from 465 to 595 nm is measured. This method requires a smaller volume of sample ($\leq 25 \mu L$) than turbidimetric procedures. The reaction underestimates the amount of globulins in the fluid; however, this is not a serious problem, since albumin is the predominant protein in CSF. Reagents and standards for this method are available commercially from several suppliers and are adaptable to a spectrophotometer or a centrifugal analyzer. CBB was originally described for CSF (12) and has subsequently been adapted to urine (13).

Determination of CSF total protein concentration is clinically useful in diagnosing and monitoring a variety of infectious, neoplastic, traumatic, and neurological disease processes. The most striking elevations in CSF protein are observed in bacterial meningitis, spinal cord tumors, and various inflammatory diseases. Specific conditions associated with increased CSF total protein and the levels these disorders attain are listed in Table 2. Fractionation of proteins in various CNS disorders shows that these proteins can arise from serum, through disruption of the blood–CSF barrier, or from intrathecal protein synthesis (i.e., the immunoglobulins). Most commonly, CSF protein increases are associated with a combined effect in which immunoglobulin synthesis is accompanied by increased permeability of the blood–CSF barrier. Decreases in CSF total protein are seen in a relatively few clinical conditions, including water intoxication, CSF rhinorrhea, CSF otorrhea, and hyperthyroidism.

The presence of fresh blood in a CSF specimen (traumatic tap) will invalidate the total protein determination. Centrifugation of the traumatic tap specimen usually yields a clear supernatant, provided samples are delivered to the laboratory expeditiously. Supernatants which are pigmented after centrifugation generally indicate subarachnoid hemorrhage because lysis of erythrocytes occurs *in vivo* if these cells reside in the CSF compartment for more than a few hours.

Specific Protein Indices

Quantitation of most specific CSF proteins is done by immunochemical techniques including immunonephelometry, immunoturbidity, RID, and radioimmunoassay. Because concentrations of most CSF proteins are normally 150- to 200-fold less than in serum, appropriately dilute analytical standards (compared with corresponding assays in serum) must be used for meaningful protein measurement. Interpretation of specific CSF proteins usually requires measurement of the protein in simultaneously collected

Table 2. Cerebrospinal Fluid Total Protein in Various Diseases

Clinical Condition	Appearance and Cells ($\times 10^6$/L)	Total Protein (mg/dL)
Normal	Clear, colorless; 0–5 lymphocytes	15–45[a]
Increased Admixture of Proteins from Blood		
Increased capillary permeability		
Bacterial meningitis	Turbid, opalescent, purulent, usually > 500 polymorphs	80–500
Cryptococcal meningitis	Clear or turbid; 50–150 polymorphs or lymphocytes	25–200
Leptospiral meningitis	Clear to slight haze; polymorphs early, then 5–100 lymphocytes	50–100
Viral meningitis	Clear or slight haze, colorless; usually up to 500 lymphocytes	30–100
Encephalitis	Clear or slight haze, colorless; usually up to 500 lymphocytes	15–100
Poliomyelitis	Clear, colorless; up to 500 lymphocytes	10–300
Brain tumor	Usually clear; 0–80 lymphocytes	15–200 (usually normal)
Mechanical obstruction spinal cord tumor[b]	Clear, colorless, or yellow	100–2000
Hemorrhage: cerebral hemorrahage	Colorless, yellow, or bloody; blood cells	30–150

Table 2. (Continued)

Clinical Condition	Appearance and Cells ($\times 10^6$/L)	Total Protein (mg/dL)
Local Immunoglobulin Production		
Neurosyphilis	Clear, colorless; 10–100 lymphocytes	50–150
Multiple sclerosis	Clear, colorless; 0–10 lymphocytes	25–50
Both Increased Capillary Permeability and Local Immunoglobulin Production		
Tuberculous meningitis	Colorless, fibrin clot, or slightly turbid; 50–500 lymphocytes	50–300 (occasional up to 1000)
Brain abscess	Clear or slightly turbid	20–120
After Myelography (inflammatory reaction)		
		Slight increase

[a] Premature infant: up to 400 mg/dL; children: 30–100 mg/dL, old age: up to 60 mg/dL.
[b] Froin's syndrome lumbar fluid values are much higher than cisternal fluid values.

serum, since even slight disturbances in the blood–CSF barrier can result in substantial increases in all fractions of CSF protein.

Specific protein assays in CSF and serum are useful for assessing the integrity of the blood–CSF barrier. The most rewarding indicator for this purpose involves calculating a ratio for quantitative values of albumin in CSF and serum (*14*). This ratio, termed the CSF/serum albumin index, quotient of albumin, or Q-albumin, is defined thus:

$$\text{CSF/serum albumin index} = \frac{\text{albumin}_{\text{CSF}}\,(\text{mg/dL})}{\text{albumin}_{\text{serum}}\,(\text{mg/dL})} \times 1000$$

Note that the CSF/serum albumin index is unitless, since the quantitative values for CSF and serum albumin are both expressed milligrams per deciliter; the term 1000 is used to give the ratio an integer value. Results of less than 9 for the CSF/serum albumin index indicate an intact blood–CSF barrier. Values for this index of 9 to 14 signify a slight disturbance; results in the 14–30 and 30–100 ranges indicate moderate and severe blood–CSF barrier disturbances. Values for the CSF/serum albumin index that exceed 100 indicate breakdown of the blood–CSF barrier. Disease states documented to show increases in the CSF/serum albumin index include diabetes mellitus, polyneuropathy, intracranial space-occupying lesions, Guillain–Barré syndrome, vascular disease, and CNS degenerative disorders (14).

At the present time, the most clinically important protein synthesized within the central nervous system is immunoglobulin G. Abnormalities in CSF IgG have been demonstrated by a number of algorithms and ratios based on quantitative protein determinations. Some of these algorithms include the CSF IgG/CSF total protein ratio, CSF IgG/CSF albumin ratio, IgG index (15), and IgG synthesis rate (16). Of the various modes for indicating greater-than-normal intrathecal IgG synthesis, the most rewarding is the IgG index (17), calculated as shown.

$$\text{IgG index} = \frac{\text{IgG}_{\text{CSF}}\,(\text{mg/dL})/\text{IgG}_{\text{serum}}\,(\text{mg/dL})}{\text{albumin}_{\text{CSF}}\,(\text{mg/dL})/\text{albumin}_{\text{serum}}\,(\text{mg/dL})}$$

The normal reference interval for the IgG index is up to 0.7; patient values for IgG index exceeding 0.7 indicate abnormal IgG synthesis within the CNS.

Approximately 70% of patients having the demyelinating disease multiple sclerosis (MS) and a large proportion of patients with optic neuritis show an increase (> 0.7) for the IgG index. In addition to MS, Guillain–Barré syndrome, chronic myelopathy of unknown cause, aseptic meningoencephalitis, systemic lupus erythematosus, and some other neurological diseases (18) also may show increases in the IgG index.

Cerebrospinal Fluid Electrophoresis

Electrophoresis of CSF in the clinical laboratory is generally done to evaluate the presence or absence of oligoclonal bands. By definition, oligoclonal bands represent immunoglobulins which show restricted electrophoretic mobility in an agarose matrix. Because immunoglobulins, and therefore immunoglobulin bands, traverse the blood–CSF barrier, electrophoresis of simultaneously collected patient serum is necessary to confirm the CSF origin for these bands. Although many analytical methods for oligoclonal banding assessment have been proposed, conventional agarose electrophoresis (pH 8.6) and agarose isoelectric focusing electrophoresis have been the most successful (18,19) and popular for clinical use.

CLINICAL SIGNIFICANCE OF PROTEINS IN URINE

The process of urine formation is carried out in the kidneys by tubelike functional units called nephrons. Each kidney contains about 2 million nephrons, each one consisting of a glomerulus at the proximal end followed structurally by the proximal convoluted tubule, the loop of Henle, and the distal convoluted tubule. Specialized membranes within the glomerulus function as ultrafiltration devices, restricting passage of most proteins larger than 40,000 daltons, roughly in proportion to their size and plasma concentration. Collectively, the glomeruli filter a volume of 170–200 L of fluid per day. Small proteins ($< 40,000$) pass through the glomerulus but are nearly completely resorbed and metabolized by specialized renal tubular mechanisms, which provide for efficient conservation of water and various solutes.

Urine excretion of up to 150 mg/day of protein is considered to be normal. About two-thirds of the urinary protein normally excreted includes albumin, immunoglobulin fragments, and low molecular weight species. The rest consists mostly of uromucoid or Tamm–Horsfall protein constituting urinary casts.

Urine Total Protein

Screening for excessive amounts of protein in random urine specimens is easily done by various "dipstick" methods. Most of the qualitative methods use dyes such as Tetrabromphenol Blue, which have a high affinity for proteins, especially albumin. Patients showing the presence of excessive protein in a random urine (usually accepted as > 25 mg/dL) should collect a timed urine specimen for quantitative protein determination. Quantitative urine protein can be determined by a modification of the CBB procedure for CSF, described earlier in this chapter.

Even under carefully controlled conditions, accurately timed urine collections are often difficult to obtain. To verify the time period of urine collection, laboratories normalize timed urines to creatinine excretion, since this substance is excreted in urine at a relatively constant rate over time. Although urine creatinine excretion decreases with age and can vary with diet, about 14–26 mg/kg/day of creatinine is excreted by adult males and 11–20 mg/kg/day by adult females.

There are four basic mechanisms leading to increased quantities of protein in urine, or proteinuria: glomerular proteinuria, tubular proteinuria, overload proteinuria, and postrenal proteinuria. Next we discuss each of these mechanisms in detail.

Glomerular Proteinuria

Glomerular proteinuria is the most common and severe form of abnormal protein excretion. Disturbances of this sort result from various injuries which impair the sieving functions of the glomerular membrane system, causing greater-than-normal excretion of protein in urine.

Glomerular proteinuria can be conveniently classified into two types—
selective, in which glomerular injury results in a selective leakage of relatively
lower molecular weight proteins into urine, and *nonselective*, which refers to
progressively severe glomerular injury resulting in leakage of all proteins
regardless of size. Upon urine protein electrophoresis, a pattern showing a
predominance of albumin, the α_1 proteins, and transferrin is consistent with a
selective glomerular proteinuria. In nonselective proteinuria, urine protein
electrophoresis shows a pattern similar to that seen in serum, where proteins
are increased, roughly in proportion to their plasma concentration. In end-
stage renal disease and subsequent renal failure, the number of glomeruli
progressively diminishes, causing a decrease in proteinuria and loss of renal
function. The urine protein electrophoresis pattern for renal failure shows an
absence of most protein fractions.

Table 3 displays conditions associated with glomerular proteinuria. In
systemic lupus erythematosus, poststreptococcal glomerulonephritis, and
membranous glomerulonephritis, there is heavy proteinuria due to an
underlying immune process causing a substantial increase in glomerular
permeability. On kidney biopsies from individuals with these and other
autoimmune disorders, immunoglobulins and components of the complement system can be demonstrated as granular deposits in the glomeruli.
These deposits contribute, along with cell-mediated inflammatory responses,
to increased glomerular permeability.

Benign or functional proteinuria is a class of glomerular proteinuria usually
found in younger individuals. Benign proteinuria involves excretion of
excessive amounts of albumin (usually > 1 g/day) and probably results from
variations in renal blood flow through the glomeruli. Stresses such as
prolonged exposure to cold, severe exercise, and pyrexia can cause functional
proteinuria. Prolonged standing can cause a syndrome termed *postural* or
orthostatic proteinuria. Although postural proteinuria is considered to be a
benign condition, patients exhibiting this phenomenon should be subjected to
follow-up studies, since persistent orthostatic proteinuria may indicate underlying renal disease. Pregnancy often increases urine protein excretion up to
three-fold the upper limit of normal. Proteinuria associated with pregnancy is
transitory and returns to normal after parturition. This benign condition is in
marked contrast to preeclampsia (toxemia of pregnancy) where proteinuria
may exceed 3 g/day.

Tubular Proteinuria

Tubular proteinuria results from defects in, or injury to, the specialized
resorption mechanisms of the proximal convoluted tubules of the kidney; it is
characterized by urinary excretion of these relatively small ($< 40,000$ daltons)

Table 3. Ranges of Protein Excretion Rates in Renal Disorders*

Disorder	Range (mg/day)[b]				
	50	100	1000	3000	> 3000
Exercise proteinuria	····	····			
Febrile proteinuria	····	···			
Postural proteinuria	····	····	∗∗∗∗∗∗		
Bence Jones proteinuria	····	····	····	····	····
Arteriosclerotic renovascular diseases	∗∗∗∗∗∗	∗∗∗∗∗∗			
Hypertension, arterial	∗∗∗∗∗∗	∗∗∗∗∗∗			
Congestive heart failure	····	····	∗∗∗∗∗∗		
Interstitial nephritis	····	····	∗∗∗∗∗∗		
Pyelonephritis	····	····	∗∗∗∗∗∗		
Polycystic kidney disease	····	····	∗∗∗∗∗∗		
Medullary cystic disease	····	····			
Acute glomerulonephritis[c]	····	····	····	····	····
Membranous glomerulonephritis			····	····	····
Membranoproliferative glomerulonephritis			····	····	····
Nephrotic syndrome[d]					····
Kimmelstiehl–Wilson syndrome (diabetic glomerulopathy)			····	····	····
Systemic lupus erythematosus	····	····	····	····	····
Polyarteritis nodosa	····	····	∗∗∗∗∗∗	∗∗∗∗∗∗	
Goodpasture's syndrome	····	····	····	····	····
Systemic sclerosis	····	····	∗∗∗∗∗∗	∗∗∗∗∗∗	
Multiple myeloma[e]	····	····	····	····	····
Nephrotoxins (e.g., Hg, CCl_4)	····	····	····		

[a] The divisions are to be considered approximations rather than the absolute limits of protein excretion rates. Some of the disease categories in which rates of > 3000 mg/day are reached may in fact have excretion rates that exceed 15,000 mg/day.
[b] Dots indicate common, asterisks rare (< 10%) occurrences. Note that scale is logarithmic.
[c] Approximately 10% of cases show rates > 3000 mg/day.
[d] By definitions > 3 g/day.
[e] Refers to generalized disease rather than to light chain (Bence Jones) disease.

proteins. On urine protein electrophoresis, a pattern showing an increase in the α_2, β, and post-γ regions is characteristic of tubular proteinuria.

Tubular proteinuria may be classified into two types: *acute*, which usually resolves totally, and *chronic*, which is usually irreversible. Acute tubular proteinuria is seen in association with burns, acute pancreatitis, and use of renotoxic drugs such as tobramycin or gentamicin. Chronic tubular proteinuria is found in hereditary conditions such as Fanconi's syndrome, with cirrhosis of the liver, or sarcoidosis, and after exposure to renal toxins such as phenacetin and cadmium.

Most commonly, tubular proteinuria occurs in association with glomerular proteinuria. To differentiate a combined tubular and glomerular process, calculation of a *protein–creatinine clearance* is often useful. For calculation of the urinary clearance of individual proteins, the following relationship is applied:

$$\text{protein clearance (mL/min)} = \frac{U \times V}{P}$$

where U and P are the concentration of the protein in urine and plasma and V is the volume of urine excreted per minute. Above-normal protein clearance values imply a loss of selectivity for that protein. In assessing glomerular selectivity, the protein clearance for a relatively small protein (e.g., albumin) and a larger protein (e.g., IgG) are often compared. Although not as reliable as 24-hour collections, random urine samples are often useful for calculation of protein–creatinine indices. For calculation of these indices, a quantitative ratio between the specific protein of interest and creatinine is calculated:

$$\text{protein–creatinine index} = \frac{[\text{specific protein}]}{[\text{creatinine}]}$$

Both the protein–creatinine index and the ratio of protein clearances using random and timed urines, respectively, are useful for evaluation of tubular proteinuria and glomerular selectivity.

Overload Proteinuria

High serum levels of low molecular weight proteins, normally absent or found in low concentration in blood, can saturate or overload the normal resorptive and metabolic capabilities of the kidneys. This condition results in excess urine protein excretion and is termed overload proteinuria. Pathological conditions leading to overload proteinuria include severe muscle breakdown and subsequent urine excretion of myoglobin, hemolysis with release of hemoglobin, and multiple myeloma, which can cause marked increases in urinary excretion of κ and λ immunoglobulin light chains.

Postrenal Proteinuria

Postrenal proteinuria describes abnormal urine protein excretion attributable to inflammatory and degenerative lesions of the urinary tract. Examination of urine sediment from patients with postrenal disease includes microscopic features such as pus or casts containing pus, malignant cells, and casts containing erythrocytes. Because inflammatory exudates are rich in protein, proteinuria always accompanies urine sediment microscopic findings indicative of postrenal disease. In women, possible contamination by vaginal secretions and discharges must be carefully considered and excluded when evaluating proteinuria.

REFERENCES

1. Tiselius A. A new apparatus for electrophoresis: Analysis of colloidal mixtures. *Trans Faraday Soc* 1937;33:524–529.

2. Lubahn DB, Silverman LM. A rapid silver-stain procedure for use with routine electrophoresis of cerebrospinal fluid on agarose gels. *Clin Chem* 1984;30:1689–1691.

3. Alper CA, Johnson AM. Immunofixation electrophoresis: A technique for the study of protein polymorphism. *Vox Sang* 1969;17:445.

4. Ritchie RF, Smith R. Immunofixation. III. Application to the study of monoclonal proteins. *Clin Chem* 1976;22:1982–1985.

5. Mancini G, Carbonara AO, Heremans JF. Immunochemical quantitation of antigens by single radial immunodiffusion. *Immunochemistry* 1965;2:235–254.

6. Fahey JL, McKelvey EM. Quantitative determination of serum immunoglobulins in antibody agar plates. *J Immunol* 1965;94:84–90.

7. Silverman LM, LeGrys VA. The acute phase response and clinically significant proteins. *J. Med Technol* 1987;4:4,154–157.

8. Duff G. Many roles for interleukin-1. *Nature* 1985;313:352–353.

9. Dinarello CA. Interleukin-1. *Rev Infect Dis* 1984;6:51–95.

10. Ramadori G, Sipe JD, Dinarello CA, Mizel SB, Colten HR. Pretranslational modulation of acute phase hepatic protein synthesis by murine recombinant interleukin-1 (IL-1) and purified human IL-1. *J Exp Med* 1985;162:930–942.

11. Dinarello CA. Interleukin-1 and the pathogenesis of the acute phase response. *New Engl J Med* 1984;311:1413–1418.

12. Johnson A, Lott JA. Standardization of the Coomassie Brilliant Blue method for cerebrospinal fluid proteins. *Clin Chem* 1978;24:1931–1933.

13. Lott JA, Stephan VA, Pritchard KA. Evaluation of the Coomassie Brilliant Blue G-250 method for urinary protein. *Clin Chem* 1983;29:1946–1950.

14. Schliep G, Felgenhauer K. Serum–CSF protein gradients, the blood–CSF barrier and the local immune response. *J Neurol* 1978;218:77–96.

15. Tibbling G, Link H, Ohman S. Principles of albumin and IgG analyses in neurologic disorders. I. Establishment of reference values. *Scand J Clin Lab Invest* 1977;37:385–390.

16. Tourtellotte WW, Ma BI. Multiple sclerosis: The blood–brain barrier and the measurement of de novo central nervous system IgG synthesis. *Neurology* (Minneap) 1978;28(2):76–83.

17. Hershey LA, Trotter JL. The use and abuse of the cerebrospinal fluid IgG profile in the adult: A practical evaluation. *Ann Neurol* 1980;8:426–434.

18. Link H, Kostular V. Utility of isoelectric focusing of cerebrospinal fluid and serum on agarose evaluated for neurologic patients. *Clin Chem* 1983;29:810–815.

19. Christenson RH, Russell ME, Gubar KT, et al. Oligoclonal banding in cerebrospinal fluid assessed by electrophoresis on agarose after centrifugal sample concentration through a microconcentrator membrane. *Clin Chem* 1985;32:1734–1736.

CHAPTER 6

ENZYME ANALYSIS

ROBERT H. CHRISTENSON

Durham Veterans Administration Medical Center
Durham, North Carolina

LAWRENCE M. SILVERMAN

North Carolina Memorial Hospital
Chapel Hill, North Carolina

INTRODUCTION

Enzymes are specialized naturally occurring proteins with the ability to catalyze biological reactions. Enzymes are true catalysts because they facilitate formation of key reaction intermediates, but are not themselves consumed or altered during the course of the biochemical reaction. Since all enzymes are proteins, they consist of amino acids joined together by peptide bonds to form polymers, or chains, of various lengths. A prototypical amino acid–peptide bond, formed by the hydrolysis linking reaction between the amine ($-NH_2$) end of amino acid 1 and the carboxylic acid ($-COOH$) end of amino acid 2, is shown in Eq. (1).

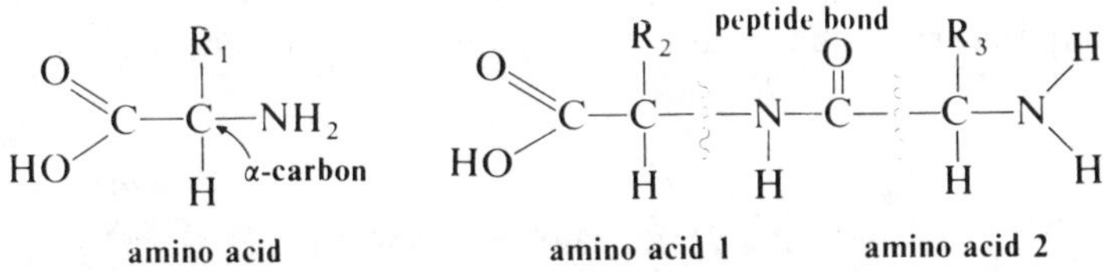

$$\tag{1}$$

Here R_1, R_2, and R_3 may represent any of the 20 chemical groups found on amino acids.

Enzymes of clinical interest are relatively large molecules consisting of between 100 and 4000 amino acid units, having molecular weights between 15,000 and 600,000 daltons. The order sequence of constituent amino acids defines the enzyme's *primary* structure. Since the physicochemical properties of the 20 amino acids commonly found in proteins vary greatly, the overall physical properties of an enzyme represent a composite of the sequence, chemistry, number, and ratio of constituent amino acids.

Unlike fibrous proteins such as α-keratin, which perform structural functions, the one-dimensional arrangement, or *secondary* structure, of enzymes is not predominantly regular and repetitive. Rather, enzymes exist in complex bent and folded globular shapes dictated by the amino acid sequence of their primary structure. Bending and folding result largely from the behavior of integral amino acids in the aqueous pH 7.4 environment. Polar, or hydrophilic, amino acid groups are oriented outward toward the aqueous environment; the nonpolar, or hydrophobic, amino acid groups congregate inward away from the relatively charged aqueous environment. A separate molecular interaction, termed hydrogen bonding, also is operative between amino acids having R groups (see above) containing the elements nitrogen, oxygen, and hydrogen. Hydrogen bonding may occur between these amino acids themselves, or between any of them and the aqueous media. All the various forces, both inter- and intramolecular, and environmental, contribute to the overall three-dimensional shape of enzymes, referred to as *tertiary* structure.

Many enzymes consist of two or more distinct polypeptide chains, each with its own tertiary structure, associated covalently and/or by noncovalent hydrophobic, hydrophilic, and hydrogen bonding forces. In clinical enzymology, each individual polypeptide chain is referred to as a *subunit*. For an individual enzyme, subunits may be identical, similar, or dissimilar based on size and amino acid sequence. When an enzyme has more than one type of subunit, and association of two or more of the subunits is necessary for biological function, the enzyme can exist in multiple forms called *isoenzymes* or *isozymes*. Different isoenzyme forms may vary from each other chemically, physically, and immunologically. For example, creatine kinase, an enzyme useful for the diagnosis of myocardial infarction, may exist in three different forms, MM, MB, and BB, arising from dimeric combinations of the characteristic types of subunits designated M and B. The three-dimensional relationship between subunits is termed *quaternary structure*.

ENZYME NOMENCLATURE

Historically, enzymes were named by adding the suffix ase to the substrate(s) of the catalyzed reaction. Amylase exemplifies this system, since this enzyme was so named because it catalyzes the hydrolysis of amylum, or starch. This rather arbitrary nomenclature system quickly became impractical and cumbersome as the number of enzymes increased and the study of enzymology advanced.

A concise and definitive system for naming enzymes has been developed by the Enzyme Commission (EC) of the International Union of Biochemistry. In the EC system, each enzyme is specified by three designations: (1) a recommended name suitable for everyday use, (2) a systematic name clearly identifying the reaction catalyzed, and (3) a unique numerical code consisting of four integers, separated by periods, preceded by the letters "EC." This standard nomenclature system can be illustrated by creatinine kinase (CK), the *recommended* name for the enzyme catalyzing the reaction

$$\text{ATP} + \text{creatine} \xrightleftharpoons{\text{CK}} \text{ADP} + \text{phosphocreatine}$$

For this CK-catalyzed reaction, ATP: creatine phosphotransferase is the *systematic*, name since this designation summarizes the substrates, products, and type of reaction. The *numerical* designation for creatine kinase is "EC 2.7.3.2" where EC represents Enzyme Commission, 2 indicates the class of the enzyme (a transferase), 7 indicates the subclass (phosphotransferase), 3 designates the sub-subclass for the enzyme, and the fourth number, 2, is a specific serial number for CK within the sub-subclass.

In addition to the standardized system, two or three capital-letter abbreviations have been proposed for several enzymes of clinical interest. Initials and enzymes included in this proposed system are LD for lactate dehydrogenase, CK for creatine kinase, ALT (formerly SGPT) for alanine aminotransferase, and AST (formerly SGOT) for aspartate aminotransferase.

QUANTIFYING ENZYMES

Since enzymes are proteins, development of antibody preparations for use in sensitive and specific immunological assays is possible by standard techniques. Immunochemical methods have found widest application in the area of isoenzyme analysis, although immunoassays for some enzymes (e.g., acid phosphatase) have received considerable acceptance. The majority of enzyme measurements performed in clinical laboratories quantify the amount of *functional enzyme* in patient samples. Therefore, we focus on techniques for quantifying enzyme activity.

Activity Requirements for Enzymes

In addition to the proper polypeptide structural relationships, fundamental factors need to be considered for optimal measurements of enzyme activity.

Some of these important and individualized factors are inclusion of appropriate coenzymes, optimization of reaction pH, assuring the presence (or absence) of various metal ions, and proper reaction temperature control. All these factors *must* be carefully defined and controlled to meaningfully assess and interpret enzymatic activity.

Coenzymes

To achieve maximum catalytic activity, many enzymes, including many of clinical interest, require association with nonprotein substances termed coenzymes. The polypeptide portion of any enzyme requiring a coenzyme is referred to as an *apoenzyme*. When the coenzyme and apoenzyme associate, they form a apoenzyme–coenzyme complex termed the *holoenzyme*. For individual enzyme systems, coenzymes and apoenzymes associate with differing affinity. Some coenzymes bind to apoenzymes so tightly that separation of the coenzyme–apoenzyme complex by equilibrium dialysis is not possible. Such tightly bound coenzymes are called *prosthetic groups*.

For analysis of clinically important enzymes, supplementation of necessary coenzymes into reagent preparations is essential, since blood from some patient groups may have diminished amounts of these substances from the effects of disease or therapeutic intervention.

Assessment in patients undergoing renal dialysis of the activity of the transaminases AST (SGOT) and ALT (SGPT) exemplifies the importance of coenzyme supplementation. During treatment, pyridoxyl-5-phosphate (PLP) is removed from the patient's blood along with other small molecular weight substances such as urea and creatinine. Because PLP is a coenzyme required by AST and ALT for maximum activity, depletion of this coenzyme can lead to incorrectly low assessment of AST/ALT activity. Since monitoring transaminase activity is relied on by clinicians for the diagnosis and monitoring of hepatitis, failure to appropriately supplement PLP into analytical reagents for ALT and AST determination can lead to a missed diagnosis and delayed treatment.

Optimum pH

Enzyme-catalyzed reactions generally show a considerable dependence on pH. Maximum activity for many enzymes of clinical interest is in the pH 7–8 range; however, some enzymes are optimized at higher or lower pH levels. Alkaline phosphatase, for example, shows optimum activity at about pH 10. Acid phosphatase, on the other hand, shows optimum activity at pH 4. Often, the forward and reverse reactions catalyzed by the same enzyme will show different pH maxima. The activity of most enzymes diminishes markedly at pH above or below the optimum resembling a bell-shaped curve; however, some enzymes show maximum activity over a wide pH range. The optimum pH values for all enzymes do not correspond exactly to the intracellular or extracellular environment where they are characteristically located. This factor suggests that pH changes in the intracellular environment play an important role in regulating the functions performed by enzymes.

Temperature Effects

Increasing reaction temperature enhances the probability for molecular interaction. It is therefore not surprising that each 10°C rise in temperature doubles the reaction rate for most enzymes. On the other hand, most enzymes are relatively fragile proteins, susceptible to denaturation and loss of activity by temperatures higher than 55°C. The tradeoff between increased molecular interaction and thermal denaturation results in the different temperatures for optimum activity shown by various enzymes. After thermal deactivation, some enzymes are able to regain their activity upon cooling to moderate thermal levels.

Enzyme assays in the clinical laboratory are usually carried out at 30 or 37°C, since most show high activity and acceptable stability at these temperatures. Although each of these analysis temperatures appears to have distinct advantages, the most important consideration is precise isothermal control, within ±0.1°C, during the entire reaction course.

Factors Governing Reaction Rates

Four factors govern the overall rate of any chemical reaction: the energy required for activation, the concentrations of reactants and reaction inter-mediates, the rate of intermolecular collision, and the orientation of reactant molecules on collision. To examine how protein catalysts affect biochemical reactions, consider a prototypical enzyme reaction:

$$\text{enzyme (E)} + \text{substrate (S)} \qquad (2a)$$

$$\searrow$$

$$\text{enzyme–substrate (E–S) complex} \qquad (2b)$$

$$\searrow$$

$$\text{product (P)} + \text{enzyme (E)} \qquad (2c)$$

Enzymes are generally considered to facilitate biochemical reactions in two ways, both involving rapid formation of the enzyme–substrate (E–S) complex shown in Eq. (2b). The first is because formation of E–S lowers the amount of energy required to achieve the transition state; that is, enzymes diminish the *activation* energy necessary to achieve reaction. Second, binding of substrate (S) to enzyme (E) favorably affects the molecular orientation of the substrate, enhancing formation of products (P).

Quantitative Description of Enzyme Reactions

To describe the measurement of enzymatic activity, it is first necessary to define terms called rate constants, represented as k_i. Use of rate constants allows mathematical description of equilibrium molar concentration ratios of reactants, intermediates, and products at each step of enzymatic (and other) reactions. Stated differently, rate constants allow expression of the "products/reactants" for each step of the reaction. In the equations, brackets [ ] indicate that the species enclosed are in terms of molar concentration. Let us rewrite Eq. (2) in linear form:

$$k_1 = \frac{[\text{E–S}]}{[\text{E}][\text{S}]}$$

$$\text{E} + \text{S} \underset{k_2}{\overset{k_1}{\rightleftharpoons}} \text{E–S} \overset{k_3}{\rightarrow} \text{P} + \text{E} \qquad k_2 = \frac{[\text{E}][\text{S}]}{[\text{E–S}]} \qquad (3)$$

$$k_3 = \frac{[\text{P}][\text{E}]}{[\text{E–S}]}$$

In expression 3, rate constant k_1 describes the rate of formation of the E–S complex by E and S; k_2 describes the reverse reaction involving breakdown of E–S to form E and S. The rate of formation of P from the E–S complex, with simultaneous release of free enzyme (E), is described by k_3. Ideally, the rate of formation of E–S is very rapid (i.e., k_1 is large compared with k_2). This scenario favors fast formation of E–S with slow decomposition of this complex to reactants E and S. Also in the ideal case, k_3 is large compared with k_2, but smaller in magnitude than k_1. The rate-limiting step for the reaction then, is formation of product (P) and release of E from the E–S complex.

Using the rate expression for the prototype enzyme reaction in Eq. (3), the rate of substrate depletion V_{sd} can be described quantitatively as

$$V_{sd} = k_1[\text{S}][\text{E}] - k_2[\text{E–S}] \qquad (4)$$

Similarly, an equation can be written to describe the rate of product formation V_{pf}:

$$V_{pf} = k_3[\text{E–S}] \qquad (5)$$

Michaelis–Menten Kinetics

Analysis of enzymatic activity in the clinical laboratory is contingent upon monitoring either the formation of reaction products or the depletion of reaction substrate by direct or indirect means, or by coupling the enzymatic reaction of interest with secondary reaction(s) producing compounds which are easily measured. To understand the principles behind the analysis of enzymatic activity, it is necessary to become familiar with *Michaelis–Menten* reaction kinetics.

Michaelis–Menten kinetics are described graphically in Figure 1 for an enzyme system like that shown in Eq. (3), containing a constant amount of enzyme, to which is added increasing amounts of reaction substrate. As illustrated, the reaction velocity (y-axis) shows a hyperbolic dependence on substrate (x-axis) as substrate concentration is increased from zero. The maximum velocity of the reaction (V_m in Figure 1) is achieved when sufficient substrate has been added to bind all free enzyme available in the reaction. As shown in Figure 1, the Michaelis–Menten constant K_m corresponds to the substrate concentration at $\frac{1}{2}V_m$.

In the ideal case where $k_1 \gg k_2$ and k_3 is rate limiting, once V_m has been achieved, any enzyme (E) liberated by conversion of E–S to product (P) immediately reacts with readily available substrate to form more of the E–S complex. Under these conditions, both the concentration of E–S and the rate of P formation remain constant, or at *steady state*, when V_m is attained. The steady-state condition can be attained *only* when sufficient substrate has been

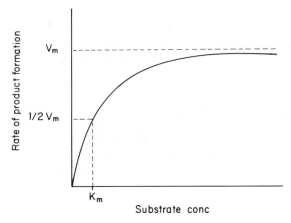

Figure 1. Reaction rate versus substrate plot, representing Michaelis–Menten kinetics. V_m = maximum reaction rate (velocity); K_m = substrate concentration corresponding to half the maximum rate (V_m).

added to the reaction to bind all available enzyme and achieve V_m. In steady state, the term "*zero order*" describes the kinetics of enzymatic reactions, since product formation, once V_m has been reached, is independent of reactant concentration. Analysis of enzyme activity in the clinical laboratory is possible only under the steady-state conditions conducive to zero-order reaction kinetics; analytical reagents are prepared with substrate concentrations 10- to 20-fold greater than the K_m for the amount of enzyme normally found, to assure that steady-state conditions are maintained.

Michaelis–Menten kinetics can be used to describe enzymatic reactions only when the concentration of the enzyme–substrate complex (E–S in Eq. 3) remains constant (i.e., in the steady state). Examination of Eq. (3) shows that to maintain the steady-state condition, the rates of substrate depletion V_{sd} and product formation V_{pf} must be equivalent. When the stipulations of steady state are met, the terms for V_{sd} and V_{pf} in Eqs. (4) and (5) are equal as shown in Eqs. (6) and (7).

$$k_1[S][E] - k_2[E–S] = k_3[E–S] \tag{6}$$

or

$$k_1[S][E] = (k_2 + k_3)[E–S]$$

or

$$\frac{[E]}{[E–S]} = \frac{K_m}{[S]}, \quad \text{where} \quad K_m = \frac{k_2 + k_3}{k_1} \tag{7}$$

As shown, the expression for steady state in Eqs. (6) and (7) leads to an alternate definition of the Michaelis–Menten constant K_m, described graphically in Figure 1.

Further development of the steady-state equation is possible because the total concentration of enzyme, represented here as $[E_t]$, is equivalent to the concentration of free $[E]$ plus the amount of enzyme bound in the $[E–S]$ complex:

$$[E_t] = [E] + [E–S]$$

Substitution into Eq. (7) for $[E]$ and then $[E–S]$, both expressed in terms of $[E_t]$, yields the following useful expressions for $[E–S]$ and $[E]$:

$$[E–S] = \frac{[E_t][S]}{K_m + S} \tag{8a}$$

$$[E] = \frac{[E_t]K_m}{K_m + [S]} \tag{8b}$$

To justify measurement of enzymatic activity by monitoring the rate of product formation V_{pf}, recall again Eq. (5).

$$V_{pf} = k_3 [E-S]$$

By substituting the expression for [E–S] from Eq. (8a), we see

$$V_{pf} = \frac{k_3 [E_t][S]}{K_m + [S]} \tag{9}$$

Simplifying the expression for V_{pf} in Eq. (9) is possible with the following assumptions, valid under the reaction conditions specified for zero-order kinetics. As stated previously, to assure the steady-state condition, substrate concentration in analytical reagents is designed to be 10- to 20-fold greater than that corresponding to K_m. Under these conditions, the substrate concentrations corresponding to K_m become negligible compared with the available [S], and the denominator of Eq. (9), $K_m + [S]$, becomes approximately equal to [S]. Since the denominator is now equal to [S], the [S] terms in the numerator and denominator of Eq. (9) cancel, resulting in Eq. (10).

$$V_{pf} = k_3 [E_t] \tag{10}$$

Inspection of Eq. (10) reveals that when the amount of substrate is great relative to the K_m for the enzyme reaction, the formation of product is directly proportional to the amount of total enzyme present. Equation (10) thus provides a basis for quantitative measurement of enzyme activity.

With similar logical assumptions, monitoring the rate of substrate depletion can also be shown to be a valid means for determining enzymatic activity, as long as steady-state conditions are achieved and maintained. From Eq. (4), the rate of substrate depletion V_{sd} is described by

$$V_{sd} = k_1 [S][E] - k_2 [E-S] \tag{4}$$

Substitution for [E] and [E–S], from Eqs. (8) yields

$$V_{sd} = \frac{k_1 K_m [S][E_t]}{[S] + K_m} - \frac{k_2 [S][E_t]}{[S] + K_m}$$

or

$$V_{sd} = \frac{[S][E_t]/(k_1 K_m - k_2)}{[S] + K_m}$$

and

$$V_{sd} = \frac{K'[S][E_t]}{[S]+K_m} \quad \text{where} \quad K' = k_1 K_m - k_2 \qquad (11)$$

According to Eq. (11), under analytical conditions where the concentration of S is 10- to 20-fold greater than K_m (zero-order kinetic conditions), the denominator ($[S]+K_m$) approximately equals $[S]$. The $[S]$ terms in the numerator and denominator cancel, simplifying the expression to

$$V_{sd} = K'[E_t] \qquad (12)$$

Since Eq. (12) shows that V_{sd} is directly proportional to the total amount of total enzyme $[E_t]$ in the reaction, monitoring the V_{sd} also provides a basis for quantitative activity assessment.

Provided the substrate concentration is high compared with the K_m for the reaction, enzymatic activity can be quantified by measurement of product formation, as shown in Eq. (10), or by substrate depletion as shown in Eq. (12).

Plots other than that shown in Figure 1 have been developed to describe Michaelis–Menten reaction kinetics. The most popular of these is the *Lineweaver–Burk* double-reciprocal plot (Figure 2). For the Lineweaver–Burk plot, $1/v$ represents the ordinate and $1/[S]$ the abscissa. In the absence of inhibitor, the y-intercept of this plot is $1/V_{max}$; the x-intercept represents $-1/K_m$, and the slope equals K_m/V_{max} as shown. Lineweaver–Burk plots are most useful for characterizing various enzyme inhibitors.

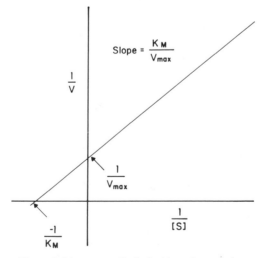

Figure 2. Lineweaver–Burk double-reciprocal plot.

MEASUREMENT OF ENZYME ACTIVITY

Units for Expressing Enzyme Activity

Since measurements of most enzymes in the clinical laboratory are *functional* assays, results for these tests are expressed in terms of catalytic activity. As such, units for reporting enzyme activity represent the quantity of product formed or substrate consumed over a specified time in a measured amount or volume of specimen. Because catalytic activity is dependent on many factors (including pH, ionic strength, temperature, structure of substrate, and presence of various activators), these conditions and concentrations must be specified for each enzyme analyzed.

Recently, use of the international unit (U), as proposed by the Enzyme Commission of the International Union of Biochemists, has become well accepted as the standard measure for quantifying enzymes. For this system, U is defined as the quantity of enzyme able to catalyze one micromole (10^{-6} mole) of substrate to products per minute. Results are usually reported as the concentration of enzyme activity per liter of sample, stated as U/L, or mU/L when more appropriate.

In an effort to be consistent with the Système International (SI), an alternate means for specifying catalytic activity has been proposed using the *katal* as the standard unit. One katal is defined as the number of moles of substrate converted to product per second. With the SI scheme, catalytic concentration is stated per liter of sample, as is the EC system. Conversion of international units to katals is possible with the following equation:

$$16.7 \times 10^9 \text{ katals/L} = 1 \text{ U/L; or } 1.67n \text{ ket} = 1 \text{ U/L}$$

Monitoring Enzyme Activity

Consider the plot of product formation versus time shown in Figure 3. At time zero, analytical reagent containing sufficient substrate for induction of zero-order kinetics, all necessary activators, and appropriate buffers to maintain optimum pH, are mixed with a measured volume of patient sample. After mixture of reagent and sample, represented by point 1 in Figure 3, the reaction is initiated. During the time that enzyme and substrate bind to form the E–S complex (see Eq. 3), a *lag phase* is observed before zero-order kinetics predominate. When .zero-order kinetics prevail (points 3–7), the rate of product formation V_{pf} for the reaction is constant and proportional to total enzyme activity as shown in Eq. (10). As the reaction proceeds to infinity, substrate is eventually depleted until zero-order reaction conditions are no longer met; that is, substrate is no longer 10- to 20-fold higher than K_m. From

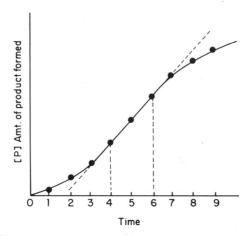

Figure 3. Plot of product formation rate versus time showing the lag phase (points 1–3), region of zero-order kinetics (3–7) and substrate exhaustion (7–9).

this point, represented by points 7–9 in Figure 3, quantifying enzymatic activity by monitoring the rate of product formation or substrate depletion is not valid, since the assumptions used to develop Eqs. (10) and (12) no longer hold true.

Conventional measurement of enzyme activity is possible with two analytical approaches, either by fixed-time measurement or by continuous monitoring. Fixed-time analysis usually refers to enzyme quantitation in which an initial measurement is taken shortly after induction of zero-order kinetics (e.g., at point 4 in Figure 3). At some later time, but still while zero-order kinetics prevail, a final measurement is taken, perhaps at point 6. The total activity in the sample will be reflected by the amount of substrate depleted, or product formed in the reaction over the *fixed time* interval between points 4 and 6. For *continuous monitoring* analysis, frequent measurements are taken during the course of the reaction to approximate a continuum. For the reaction plot in Figure 3, continuous monitoring measurements would be taken at points 1 through 9. The initial mixing, lag phase, induction of zero-order kinetics, and substrate exhaustion portions of the enzyme reaction can be identified with the continuous technique.

Continuous monitoring, rather than fixed-time measurement, is the preferred method for determining enzyme activity. The major problem with fixed-time measurement is that the same final reading may result from a variety of reaction complications, as shown in Figure 4. In one of these possible complications, reactions show a high initial slope; these reactions become substrate depleted, causing spuriously low results. Another problem, also

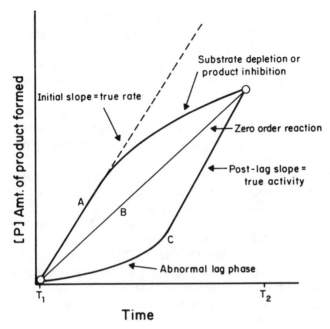

Figure 4. Pitfalls of fixed-time enzyme measurement. A, true rate; B, zero-order reaction; C, post-lag slope.

shown in Figure 4, results from reactions which show an abnormally long lag phase, again causing low enzyme results. For valid enzyme quantification by the fixed-time analysis, the zero-order condition must be maintained throughout the fixed time interval and the enzyme reaction must be subject to few interferences. In contrast, for continuous monitoring analysis, the zero-order condition needs to be maintained for a relatively short period of time—in most cases, four or five consecutive measurements. For example, points 4 through 7 in Figure 3 are sufficient for enzyme quantification by continuous monitoring. Overall, the range of analytical linearity for fixed-time activity measurement is restricted and is subject to more errors from intersample variations compared with continuous monitoring.

Techniques for Monitoring Enzyme Activity

Most enzyme activity measurements are accomplished by monitoring spectrophotometric absorbance changes during the course of the reaction. For absorbance monitoring to reflect the activity of the enzyme, the molecular species actually measured must be altered in proportion with the progress of the reaction. Proportional absorbance changes are possible by three general techniques. The first (Figure 5a) is *direct measurement*, where reactants or products involved in the enzyme reactions absorb light themselves, allowing product formation and substrate consumption to be monitored directly. The second, termed *indirect measurement*, involves quantifying substrate or products with an indicator forming a measurable colored product as shown in Figure 5b. The third (Figure 5c) is termed *enzyme coupling*. Here, product formed in the reaction of interest is linked to secondary enzyme reaction(s) to produce more easily measured products in direct proportion to the activity of the primary enzyme.

The most commonly used and significant chemical substance for monitoring enzyme reactions is the nicotinamide adenine dinucleotide oxidation–reduction couple represented as $NAD^+ + 2H^+ \rightarrow NADH + H^+$. As shown in Figure 6, the reduced form of the couple, NADH, strongly absorbs light at 340 nm while the oxidized form, NAD^+, absorbs light at this wavelength to a far lesser extent. The $NAD^+/NADH$ couple has become widely used for clinical laboratory applications because it is directly involved in, or easily coupled to, many enzyme reactions of clinical interest. Another oxidation–reduction reaction widely used in clinical chemistry is the nicotinamide adenine dinucleotide phosphate oxidation–reduction couple,

Direct measurement

$$S_1 + S_2 + E \rightleftharpoons E - S_1 - S_2 \rightarrow P_1 + P_2 + E$$

Measure depletion of $[S_1]$ or $[S_2]$.
Measure formation of $[P_1]$ or $[P_2]$.

(a)

Indirect measurement

1. Enzymatic reaction

$$S + E \rightleftharpoons E - S \rightarrow P + E$$

2. Indicator reaction

$$S + R \rightarrow colored\ product$$

or

$$S + R_1 \rightarrow colored\ product$$

Measure colored product.

(b)

Coupled reaction

Primary enzyme reaction: $S_1 + E_1 \rightleftharpoons S{-}E_1 \rightarrow P_1 + E_1$

Secondary coupled reaction: $P_1 + S_2 \xrightarrow{E_2} P_2 + P_3 + E_2$

Measure $[P_2]$ or $[P_3]$.

(c)

Figure 5. Schematic diagrams showing various reaction-monitoring techniques.

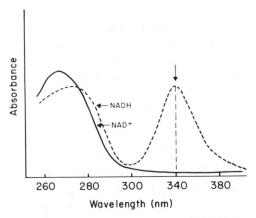

Figure 6. Absorbance versus wavelength plot for the NADH/NAD$^+$ oxidation–reduction couple. Substrate depletion: $X + NADH + H^+ \rightarrow XH_2 + NAD^+$. Product formation: $YH_2 + NAD^+ \rightarrow Y + NADH + H^+$

abbreviated NADP$^+$/NADPH. The absorbance spectra for the NADP$^+$/NADPH couple correspond very closely with spectra for NAD$^+$ and NADH.

The preferred method for enzyme determination is direct measurement. When direct measurement is not practical, enzyme-coupled systems are recommended. Since for most clinically important enzymes, direct measurement and enzyme-coupled methods are available, indirect measurement is used for very few applications in the clinical laboratory.

DIAGNOSTIC ENZYMOLOGY

The enzymes of clinical interest are produced and normally found on the inside of cells, separated from blood by the plasma membrane. For this reason, serum and plasma levels of clinically relevant enzymes are relatively low in healthy subjects. Greater-than-normal enzyme activity in blood can be caused by three general processes: (1) leakage of the enzyme to the extra-cellular compartment, (2) increased intracellular synthesis of enzymes, leading to increased cellular excretion, and (3) increased proliferation of enzyme-producing cells. Enzyme levels found in blood from healthy individuals result from normal cell turnover or from slight leakage of these molecules through the plasma membrane.

Changes in the external environment resulting from deprivation of oxygen, ingestion of organic chemicals, or invasion by viruses can alter the plasma membrane, causing leakage of cellular contents into blood. Increased membrane permeability initially results in leakage of small molecules, followed successively by escape of larger molecules, and finally release of the entire cellular contents during necrosis. Cells of the liver are particularly sensitive to cellular leakage caused by oxygen tension changes, viruses, and various chemical toxins. Other tissues such as skeletal muscle also release enzymes following trauma, hypothermia, or poor perfusion. Because intracellular enzymes are normally found in low amounts in blood, leakage and release of cellular contents cause greatly increased enzyme activity, providing a sensitive indicator for assessment of disease.

Some genetic conditions increase the permeability of the plasma membrane, causing it to offer little resistance to the release of enzymes and resulting in greatly increased activity in the blood of affected individuals. Blood samples from patients with Duchenne's muscular dystrophy, a disease affecting skeletal muscle, often show creatine kinase activity which is several hundred-fold greater than normal, presumably due to increased permeability of muscle cell membranes.

Variation in the serum or plasma activity of some enzymes is also dependent on age. Alkaline phosphatase (ALP) activity in serum from children under age 16 is normally threefold higher than in blood from adults. This difference is due primarily to the increased activity in the bone isoenzyme of ALP in the younger group. Certain drugs can also affect the activity of selected enzymes in blood, through induction of intracellular enzyme systems. For example, ethanol, phenobarbital, and phenytoin induce increased cellular production of γ-glutamyltransferase, resulting in increased serum activity of this enzyme.

Proliferation of tissue, normal and abnormal, can also increase serum and plasma enzyme activity. Serum from men with prostate cancer often shows increased acid phosphatase activity, roughly in proportion to the extent of their disease. This increased activity presumably originates from the abnormal growth of cancerous tissue.

Although the clearance of enzymes from circulation is a poorly understood process, renal excretion is not the primary mechanism, since most enzymes are too large to pass through the glomeruli of the kidney. A preliminary step in enzyme clearance probably involves inactivation and degradation of peptide bonds by intracellular and extracellular proteases.

Diagnostic Use of Enzymes

Selection of enzyme tests for the assessment of clinical disease is based on knowledge of the distribution and per-weight activity of enzymes in various tissues. While the activities of enzymes in blood do not directly reflect the mass of damaged or malfunctioning organ, increases in serum or plasma activity are semiquantitatively related to the extent of tissue involvement. The intracellular locations of enzymes can also provide diagnostic information about the extent of tissue damage. Cytosolic enzymes, for example, indicate less extensive injury than do mitochondrial enzymes. Table 1 lists some clinically important enzymes along with their cellular locations and diagnostic uses.

It is important to note that serum and plasma represent only 5 to 10% of total body water. As such, constituents in blood represent a useful, albeit limited, view of the patient's overall well-being. Interpretation of enzyme activity, and indeed all clinical tests, must be done only in light of the patient's illness and other clinical findings.

Selected Enzymes

Acid Phosphatase (ACP)

The preferred specimen for ACP determination is serum, separated expeditiously from blood collected in a red-top tube. ACP is an extremely labile enzyme and must be quantified immediately or stored, at $4°C$, buffered at pH4-5 by addition of disodium citrate (10 mg/mL). Specimens for ACP determination must be free from hemolysis, since erythrocytes have high ACP activity.

Immunological methods for ACP include counterimmunoelectrophoresis, enzyme immunoassay, and radioimmunoassay; all are based on antisera specific for the prostatic fraction. Immunochemical methods offer only slight advantages over chemical means and are substantially more costly.

Chemical methods for ACP measurement also attempt to fractionate the prostatic fraction. The most popular methods use thymolphthalein monophosphate (TMP) and α-naphthylphosphate as substrates because both ostensibly react specifically with prostatic ACP. Since the prostatic fraction of ACP is sensitive to inhibition by tartrate, nonspecific substrates such as 4-nitrophenyl phosphate can be used to derive the prostatic fraction by subtracting from the total ACP activity that activity remaining after tartrate inhibition. Use of the substrate TMP is probably the most specific chemical method; tartrate inhibition is thought to be the least specific.

In the two-step TMP substrate reaction shown below, hydroxide is used to halt the reaction with measurement of thymolphthalein anion at 600 nm.

$$\text{thymolphthalein monophosphate} \xrightarrow[\text{pH 5.6}]{\text{ACP}} \text{thymolphthalein} + \text{inorganic}$$

phosphate

$$\text{thymolphthalein} \xrightarrow[\text{pH 12}]{\text{OH}^-} \text{thymolphthalein anion}$$

Table 1. Some Clinically Important Enzymes

Enzyme (abbreviation)	Enzyme Commission Number	Storage Stability at 0–4°C	Preferred Method of Analysis (reference)	Normal Reference Interval	Tissue Source	Principal Clinical Application
Acid phosphatase (ACP)	EC 3.1.3.2	3 days at pH 3–4	At pH 5.4, thymolphthalein monophosphate is hydrolyzed to thymolphthalein, which is measurable, in basic solution at 595 nm.	0.0–0.80 U/L at 37°C	Prostate, erythrocytes	Monitoring carcinoma of prostate
Alanine aminotransferase (ALT; SGPT)	EC 2.6.1.2	5 days	Primary reaction: L-alanine + α-oxoglutarate → pyruvate + L-glutamate, in presence of pyridoxyl-5-phosphate as activator. Pyruvate formation is coupled to lactate production by LDH: concurrent oxidation of NADH to NAD⁺ allows measurement at 340 nm.	5–35 U/L at 30°C	Liver, skeletal muscle, heart	Hepatic parenchymal disease

126

Enzyme	EC number	Stability	Method / Reaction	Reference range	Tissue source	Clinical associations
Aspartate aminotransferase (AST; SGOT)	EC 2.6.1.1	1 week	Primary reaction: L-aspartate + α-ketoglutarate $\rightarrow$ oxaloacetate + L-glutamate, in presence of pyridoxyl-5-phosphate as activator. Production of oxaloacetate is coupled to formation of L-malate by MDH; concurrent oxidation of $NADH \rightarrow NAD^+$ allows measurement at 340 nm.	5–35 U/L at 30°C	Liver, skeletal muscle, heart, kidney, erythrocytes	Hepatic parenchymal disease, myocardial infarction, muscle disease
Alkaline phosphatase (AP)	EC 3.1.3.1	2–3 days	Substrate, 4-nitrophenyl phosphate, is hydrolyzed at pH 10.3; AMP serves as both an alkaline buffer and a phosphate acceptor. Formed 4-nitrophenoxide is measured at 405 nm.	Males: 35–94 U/L Females: 25–80 U/L Children: < 350 U/L at 30°C	Liver, bone, intestinal mucosa, placenta, kidney	Bone disease, hepatobiliary disease
α-Amylase (AMS)	EC 3.2.1.1	7 months	(a) Saccarogenic assays: measurement of formed sugars and dextrins (rarely used) (b) Amyloclastic assays: measurement of decreases in starch substrate	25–125 U/L 15–37°C by Beckman DS assay	Salivary glands, pancreas, ovaries	Pancreatic diseases

Table 1. (Continued)

Enzyme (abbreviation)	Enzyme Commission Number	Storage Stability at 0–4°C	Preferred Method of Analysis (reference)	Normal Reference Interval	Tissue Source	Principal Clinical Application
			(c) Chromolytic analyses: dye-labeled amylase substrates produce measurable dyes when attached by amylase			
			(d) Specific substrates: amylopectin and maltopentaose			
Creatine kinase (CK).	EC 2.7.3.2	1 week	Primary reaction: phosphocreatine + ADP → creatine + ATP at pH 6.8 in presence of N-acetylcysteine (NAC) as activator. Coupling production of ATP ultimately with conversion of NADP → NADPH allows measurement at 340 nm.	20–120 U/L at 30°C	Skeletal muscle, brain, heart, smooth muscle	Myocardial infarction, muscle diseases

128

Enzyme	EC number	Stability	Method	Reference range	Tissue source	Clinical significance
γ-Glutamyltransferase (GGT)	EC 2.3.2.2	1 week	Substrate, L-γ-glutamyl-3-carboxyl-4-nitroanalide donates a glutamyl group to glycylglycine. Formation of p-nitroaniline is monitored at 405 nm.	5–30 U/L	Liver, kidney	Hepatobiliary disease, alcoholism
Lactate dehydrogenase (LD)	EC 1.1.1.27	± 1 week	Either forward or reverse of the following reaction: L-lactate + NAD $\underset{\text{pH } 7.4-7.8}{\overset{\text{pH } 8.8-9.8}{\rightleftharpoons}}$ pyruvate + NADH. Each is acceptable, and each is monitored at 340 nm.	95–200 U/L (P→L) at 30°C; 35–88 U/L (L→P) at 30°C	Heart, liver, skeletal muscle, erythrocytes, platelets, lymph nodes	Myocardial infarction, hepatic parenchymal diseases
5'-Nucleotidase (5'-ND)	EC 3.1.3.5	1 week	Substrate, adenosine 5'-monophosphate, is hydrolyzed to adenosine, which is converted to ammonia and inosine. Production of ammonia is coupled to conversion of NAD⁺ → NADH with measurement at 340 nm.	5–13 U/L	Hepatobiliary tract	Hepatobiliary disease

TMP is used as substrate to quantify ACP activity on the du Pont aca. Although fixed-time measurement is used in the aca, this means of analysis is successful because ACP is subject to relatively few inhibitors and the analytical conditions in this instrument are carefully maintained.

Serum acid phosphatase determination should not'be used as a screening test for prostatic adenocarcinoma since this enzyme, including the prostatic fraction, also is increased in prostatic infarct and hyperplasia. In conjunction with other parameters, however, ACP is useful in staging carcinoma of the prostate and for indicating when malignant disease has extended beyond the capsule. This enzyme is also of use for monitoring patient response to treatment following therapy for prostatic carcinoma.

Above-normal ACP activity has been associated with Paget's disease, hyperparathyroidism, and metastasis to bone by cancer. Goucher's disease, some hematological disorders, and Nieman–Pick disease all show ACP increases of nonprostatic origin. Forensic investigations of rape and similar crimes use ACP measurements because semen contains very high activity of this enzyme.

Alkaline Phosphatase (ALP)

For ALP determination, serum from blood collected in a red-top tube is the preferred specimen. Since increases in ALP activity occur between 2 and 4 hours after a fatty meal, fasting specimens are necessary. From childhood to puberty, ALP levels are two- to threefold higher than the upper normal limit for adults. Pregnant women also show increased activity compared with normal.

For analysis of ALP, the International Federation for Clinical Chemistry recommends use of 4-nitrophenyl phosphate as substrate and 2-amino-2-methyl-1-propanol (AMP) as both an alkaline buffer and a phosphate acceptor in the reaction

$$\text{4-nitrophenyl phosphate} + H_2O \xrightarrow[Mg^{2+},\ pH\ 10.3]{ALP} \text{phosphate} + \text{nitrophenoxide}$$

Because Zn^{2+} and Mg^{2+} inhibit ALP when present in excess, the chelating agent N-hydroxyethyl ethylenediaminetriacetic acid (EDTA) is added to reagent preparations. For quantification of ALP activity, formation of nitrophenoxide can be continuously monitored at 502 nm.

There are four major isoenzymes of ALP: intestine, liver, bone, and placenta, named according to tissue where each is found in high activity. Two of the four, the liver and bone isoenzymes, are normally found in serum. Increases in

ALP activity seen in pregnancy are due to the placental isoenzyme. Interestingly, a fifth form of ALP, termed the Regan isoenzyme, is found in serum from some patients with malignant cancer. The Regan isoenzyme is reportedly identical to that found in the placenta.

Biliary obstruction induces increased synthesis of ALP in hepatocytes adjacent to the biliary canaliculi. Obstructions located within the liver (intrahepatic) due to hepatic cancer or to drugs (e.g., chlorpromazine) result in a two- to threefold increase in ALP above normal. Extrahepatic obstructions, caused by gallbladder stones or cancer in the head of the pancreas, result in ALP increases greater than threefold above normal. In general, hepatitis B infections result in only moderate increases in serum ALP activity, although there may be individual differences.

Above-normal ALP activity may also result from bone disease. Paget's disease (osteitis deformans), may cause a 10- to 20-fold increase in ALP. Two- to four-fold increases in serum ALP are often seen in association with rickets and during the healing of bone fractures. ALP increases are also seen with osteogenic bone cancer and Fanconi's syndrome.

Alanine Aminotransferase (ALT; SGPT; GPT)

The recommended specimen for ALT determination is serum, free from excess hemolysis, separated from blood collected in a red-top tube. ALT is stable at room temperature for 2–3 days and refrigerated, at 4°C, for 1 week.

The reaction catalyzed by ALT is the transfer of an amino group ($—NH_2$) from L-alanine to α-oxoglutarate according to the reaction

$$\text{L-alanine} + \alpha\text{-oxoglutarate} \underset{\text{PLP, pH 7.8}}{\overset{\text{ALT}}{\rightleftharpoons}} \text{pyruvate} + \text{L-glutamate}$$

Supplementation of analytical reagent with pyridoxyl-5-phosphate (PLP) is critical to optimize and standardize ALT measurement, since some patient samples may be deficient in this coenzyme. Directly monitoring the ALT-catalyzed reaction is not feasible. The most popular method involves coupling pyruvate production (see above) to lactate formation with concurrent oxidation of NADH, catalyzed by lactate dehydrogenase (LDH):

$$\text{pyruvate} + \text{NADH} \xrightarrow{\text{LDH}} \text{lactate} + \text{NAD}^+$$

The rate of decreasing absorbance due to conversion of NADH to NAD^+ can be monitored continuously, at 340 nm, and is proportional to ALT activity.

ALT activity is usually used clinically in conjunction with aspartate aminotransferase (AST) to monitor and diagnose parenchymal liver dysfunction. Although ALT activity is more specific and sensitive for indicating liver illness, AST is usually more elevated in alcoholic liver disease. In carcinoma of the liver, ALT levels may be increased five- to ten-fold above normal. Drugs such as opiates, salicylate, and ampicillin may be associated with moderate ALT increases. Although cardiac muscle is low in ALT activity, this enzyme may be increased following myocardial infarction due to secondary hypoperfusion of the liver. Slight elevations in ALT activity can occur from nonhepatic disorders such as various muscle diseases, dermatomyosidis, trauma, and gangrene.

Aspartate Aminotransferase (AST; SGOT; GOT)

Serum from blood collected in a red-top tube is preferred for AST determination. AST retains 90% of initial activity when stored at room temperature for 3 days, or refrigerated at 4°C for one week.

AST catalyzes the transfer of an amino ($-NH_2$) group from L-aspartate to α-oxoglutarate according to the reaction

$$\text{L-aspartate} + \alpha\text{-oxoglutarate} \underset{\text{PLP, pH 7.8}}{\overset{\text{AST}}{\rightleftharpoons}} \text{oxaloacetate} + \text{L-glutamate}$$

As with ALT, directly measuring the depletion of reactants or formation of products is not facile. For AST determination, formation of oxaloacetate is coupled, using malate dehydrogenase (MDH), for oxidation of NADH via the reaction

$$\text{oxaloacetate} + \text{NADH} \xrightarrow{\text{MDH}} \text{NAD}^+ + \text{L-malate}$$

Oxidation of NADH is monitored continuously at 340 nm to derive AST activity. As with ALT, supplementing AST analytical reagent with pyridoxyl-5-phosphate (PLP) is critical, since this coenzyme is required for maximum activity.

Clinically, AST and ALT are used to monitor and diagnose liver disease, particularly conditions involving the parenchyma. AST increases after myocardial infarction (MI), since heart tissue contains substantial activity of this enzyme. The rise and fall in AST after MI parallels that of CK. Acute pancreatitis, hemolytic disease, and diseases affecting striated muscle, dermatomyositis, gangrene, and trauma can increase serum AST activity from two- to ten-fold above the upper limit of normal.

L-*Amylase (AML)*

Serum for AML determinations should be from blood collected in a red-top tube, although heparinized plasma is acceptable. AML is stable, when refrigerated, for several months. Urine for AML determination should be collected without a preservative, over a timed interval.

Two groups of AML isoenzymes are present in human serum, one mainly from the salivary glands, coined the S type, and the other mainly from the pancreas, termed the P type. Because AML has a molecular weight between 40,000 and 50,000 daltons, this enzyme readily passes through the glomeruli of the kidney. AML is not absorbed by the renal tubules and therefore is one of the only enzymes normally present in urine. In addition to the S-type and P-type amylases, there is a third AML formed by complexation of ordinary serum AML (usually the S type) with either IgG or IgA. This larger form, appropriately termed macroamylase, is enzymatically active but is not excreted in urine because of its large molecular weight ($> 200,000$ daltons). No known clinical symptoms are associated with macroamylasemia.

Until recently, three general methodologies have been available for AML determination: (1) saccharogenic methods, where AML activity is measured by monitoring formation of reducing substances, (2) amyloclastic methods, whereby AML is quantified by following the decrease in starch substrate, and (3) chromolytic assays, where AML activity is assessed by colorimetric measurement of dyes liberated by α_{1-4}-bond cleavage. In the past decade, more clearly defined substrates such as maltopentaose, amylopectin, malto-tetraose, and 4-NP-(glucose)$_7$ have become increasingly popular, especially for adaptation of AML determination to automated high volume instruments.

Measurements of AML activity with the Beckman Astra are done by monitoring the rate of decrease in sample turbidity. For this method, amylopectin serves as substrate; conversion of this substrate to maltose, according to the following reaction, is followed at 520 nm.

$$\text{amylopectin} \xrightarrow{\text{AML}} \text{dextrin fragments}$$

$$\text{dextrin fragments} \xrightarrow{\text{AML}} \text{maltose}$$

Although this method has good specificity for AML and may be done rapidly, optically turbid, lipemic, or hemolyzed samples can yield depressed results.

Another well-accepted method, available with the du Pont aca instrument, uses maltopentaose as substrate in the following coupled system.

$$\text{maltopentaose} \xrightarrow{\text{AML}} \text{maltotriose} + \text{maltose}$$

$$\text{maltotriose} + \text{maltose} \xrightarrow{\text{L-glucosidase}} \text{5-glucose}$$

$$\text{glucose} + \text{ATP} \xrightarrow{\text{hexokinase}} \text{glucose-6-phosphate} + \text{ADP}$$

$$\text{glucose-6-phosphate} + \text{NAD}^+ \xrightarrow{\text{G-6-P}} \text{6-phospho-gluconolactone} + \text{NADH} + \text{H}^+$$

The absorbance increase due to conversion of $\text{NAD}^+ \rightarrow \text{NADH}$ is monitored at 340 nm for AML quantification. High blank interference from short-chain oligosaccharides, present in some patient samples, is successfully avoided because of the well-controlled preincubation and measurement conditions of the aca. Usually in acute pancreatitis AML activity begins increasing 2–12 hours after the attack, reaching maximum activity after 12–48 hours at levels four- to six-fold greater than normal. In uncomplicated cases AML activity returns to normal after 3–4 days.

A useful calculation for assessing amylase release and excretion is the amylase creatinine clearance ratio (ACCR):

$$\text{ACCR}(\%) = \frac{\text{urine amylase (U/L)} \times \text{serum creatinine (mg/L)}}{\text{serum amylase (U/L)} \times \text{urine creatinine (mg/L)}} \times 100\%$$

Use of the ACCR allows short (2–4 hours) urine collections and relates renal clearance by comparing AML excretion to that of creatinine. The normal value for the ACCR is 2–5%; usually the ACCR is more than 8% in acute pancreatitis. Results must be interpreted cautiously; however, since keto-acidosis, burns, multiple myeloma, orthostatic hemoglobulinuria, and other conditions can also cause elevations in the ACCR.

In chronic pancreatitis, serum AML is often normal; therefore, a urine determination of AML and calculation of the ACCR are particularly useful. Substantial elevations in serum and urine AML may occur with pelvic inflammatory disease, salivary gland lesions, biliary tract disease, cholecystitis, and mumps.

Creatine Kinase (CK)

Although heparinized plasma is acceptable for CK analysis, the preferred specimen is serum from blood collected in a red-top tube. CK measurements should be performed expeditiously, since this enzyme shows diminished activity after 4 hours at room temperature, 8–12 hours at 4°C, or 2–3 days when frozen. Structurally CK is a dimer consisting of two subunits, each of which may be of two types, either M (for muscle) or B (for brain). A hybrid form of CK, the MB isoenzyme, is found in high activity in cardiac tissue.

The most popular method for assessing total CK activity is the coupled enzyme system outlined as follows:

(a) $\qquad$ phosphocreatine + ADP $\underset{}{\overset{CK\ Mg^{2+},\ pH\ 9.6}{\rightleftharpoons}}$ creatine + ATP

(b) $\qquad$ ATP + glucose $\xrightarrow{hexokinase}$ glucose-6-phosphate + ADP

(c) $\quad$ glucose-6-phosphate + NADP$^+$ $\xrightarrow{GPD}$ 6-phosphogluconate

$$+ NADPH + H^+$$

For CK measurement with this coupled system, increasing absorbance due to the reduction of NADP$^+$, catalyzed by glucose-6-phosphate dehydrogenase (GPD), is monitored at 340 nm. The pH optimum for this exothermic reaction system is 6.8–6.9. Although erythrocytes do not contain substantial CK activity, grossly hemolyzed specimens are not suitable for analysis. This is because these cells contain adenylate kinase, an enzyme which facilitates conversion of 2 ATP molecules to 1 AMP and 1 ATP, thus interfering with reaction (b) above.

While CK is relatively unstable in serum, it is possible to preserve and restore some activity by fortifying reagent preparations with any of various sulfhydryl compounds. The best accepted of these restorative sulfhydryl compounds is N-accetylcysteine (NAC), because of its low expense, stability, and odorlessness.

As with some other enzymes, metal ions such as Mg^{2+} (which is activating in low concentrations), Zn^{2+}, Cu^{2+}, and Ca^{2+} inhibit CK. The chelating reagent EDTA is thus added to reagent preparations to eliminate this potential interference.

Measurement of total CK activity is clinically useful for diagnosis and monitoring of various diseases involving skeletal muscle and the central nervous system. Polymyositis, alcoholic rhabdomyalysis, and Duchenne's muscular dystrophy are all conditions which increase serum CK activity 20- to 200-fold above normal. Potential victims of malignant hyperthermia may also show increased baseline levels of CK activity. Neurogenic causes for elevations in CK activity include acute cerebrovascular disease and Reye's syndrome, which may increase CK up to 10-fold above normal. Non-pathological elevations in CK activity may be seen after intramuscular injections or exercise. Assessment of the MB isoenzyme of CK has shown to be particularly valuable in the diagnosis of myocardial infarction, as discussed in the section on isoenzymes.

Lactate Dehydrogenase (LDH; LD)

Serum from blood collected in a red-top tube is acceptable for LDH determination, as is heparinized plasma. Since erythrocytes contain LD activity which is 150-fold higher than normally found in serum, hemolyzed specimens are not suitable for analysis. For some time, the stability of LDH and its five isoenzymes has been a source of considerable discussion. The consensus is that isoenzymes LD-4 and LD-5 are labile upon freezing, and therefore specimens for determination of LDH and its isoenzymes should be kept at room temperature if analysis is to be done in 3–5 days, and 4°C for extended storage.

Direct monitoring of LDH is possible at 340 nm, since the catalyzed reaction involves the $NAD^+/NADH$ couple:

$$\text{lactate} + NAD + \underset{\text{pH } 7.4-7.8}{\overset{\overset{\text{LDH}}{\text{pH } 8.8-9.8}}{\rightleftharpoons}} + NADH + H^+ + \text{pyruvate}$$

Reagent formulations for both the forward lactate →pyruvate (L→P) and reverse pyruvate→lactate (P→L) reactions are available, since assessing LDH activity in either direction offers benefits

Monitoring the forward reaction involving reduction of NAD^+, the L→P direction, offers three analytical advantages: (1) lactate, present in excess as substrate in reagent formulations for the forward reaction, inhibits LDH less than does the pyruvate present in excess for quantification in the reverse direction, (2) the L→P reaction is linear to higher LDH activity, and (3) there are apparently fewer LDH inhibitors present in commercial preparations of NAD^+ than in preparations of NADH. LDH measurement in the reverse P→L direction, on the other hand, requires less expensive reagents and, analytically, the reverse reaction is more precise, since the absorbance change is greater in this direction. The forward L→P and reverse P→L reactions for LDH determination are about equally popular in clinical laboratories.

The cellular location of LDH in all human tissues is the cytoplasm. Although the tissue distribution of LDH is almost ubiquitous, the liver, heart, skeletal muscle, and kidney contain especially high activities, nearly 500-fold greater than normally found in serum. Fractionation of the LDH isoenzymes may be useful in interpreting above-normal serum LDH activity. In liver and skeletal muscle, isoenzymes LD-4 and LD-5 predominate; in cardiac and kidney tissue LD-1 and LD-2 predominate.

Diseases of the liver are usually associated with increased serum LDH activity. Because of the lack of specificity for LDH increases, suspected hepatic disease should be followed with more specific tests including AST, ALT, ALK, and bilirubin. Hypoxic cardiorespiratory disease results in two-to five fold increases in serum LDH activity, ostensibly from leakage or release of the enzyme from numerous sources, including cardiac tissue, the liver (secondary to liver congestion), and other tissues affected by resulting ischemia and oxygen deprevation. Neoplastic states, the hemolytic anemias, megaloblastic anemias, renal infarct, and acute pancreatitis are all associated with substantial increases in serum LDH activity.

γ-Glutamyltransferase (GGT)

The preferred specimen for GGT analysis is serum, free from hemolysis, collected in a red-top tube. Although heparinized plasma interfers with popular GGT methodology, EDTA plasma is acceptable for analysis. Presumably because the prostate contains substantial GGT activity, normal reference intervals for men are approximately 50% higher than for women.

The function of GGT is the specific transfer of terminal γ-glutamyl groups containing 5- or γ-carboxyl residues from a peptide, or peptide-like compound, to an acceptor. The molecule accepting the γ-glutamyl group may be a different portion of the same molecule, a different molecule, or even water. The conventional method for GGT measurement entails direct monitoring of GGT transferase function with substrate containing the chromophore p-nitroanaline, as in the following scheme.

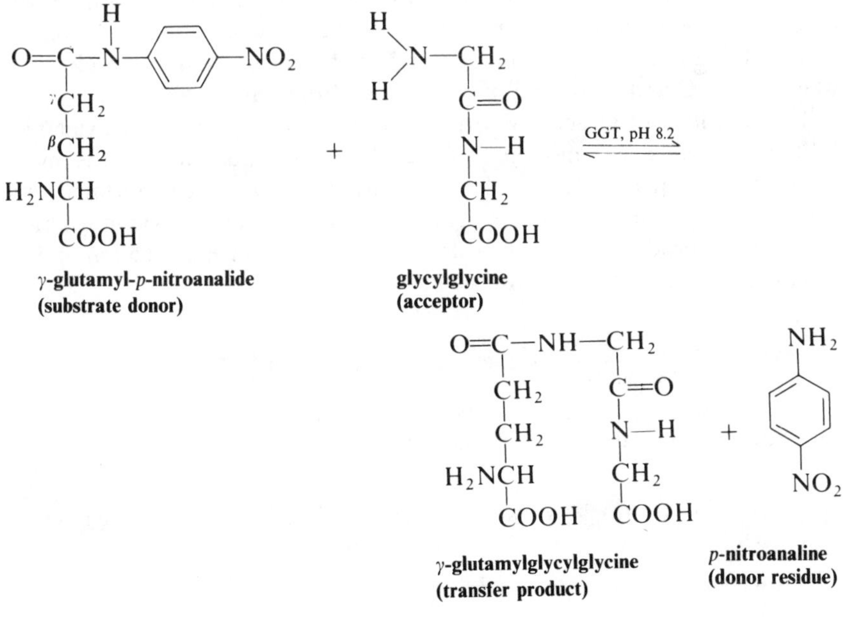

γ-glutamyl-p-nitroanalide
(substrate donor)

glycylglycine
(acceptor)

γ-glutamylglycylglycine
(transfer product)

p-nitroanaline
(donor residue)

As the reaction progresses, the release of p-nitroanaline, proportional to GGT activity, is continuously monitored at 405 nm.

Besides the γ-glutamyl-p-nitroanaline substrate shown, other substrates are available to quantify GGT which offer better solubility and enhanced reaction activity with the enzyme. Use of one such alternate substrate, γ-glutamyl-3-carboxy-nitroanilide, has been proposed by the International Federation for Clinical Chemistry (IFCC). In their recommended method, the IFCC retains glycylglycine as the γ-glutamyl acceptor.

GGT activity measurement is the most sensitive enzyme test for indicating the presence of liver disease, since a normal value for this enzyme is almost never observed when there is hepatic damage. Obtaining a GGT determination is useful for establishing a hepatic origin for ALK elevations in pregnant women, in children, and in skeletal disease. However, GGT activity measurements are of little help for discriminating the specific type of liver disease. The highest elevations in GGT activity, 5- to 30-fold above normal, are seen in association with intrahepatic or posthepatic obstruction. Moderate GGT elevations are seen with hepatitis or in patients ingesting certain drugs (e.g., phenytoin or phenobarbitol); heavy users of ethanol also show moderate increases in GGT activity. Increases in GGT, from two- to five-fold above normal, are seen in association with pancreatitis and pancreatic malignancy.

5'-Nucleotidase (5'-ND)

Although plasma samples collected with heparin, EDTA, or oxalate are acceptable, the preferred specimen for 5'-ND analysis is serum from blood collected in a red-top tube. Samples for 5'-ND measurement are stable for 1 week at 0–4°C and for several months when frozen at −40°C.

To quantify 5'-ND activity, two coupled-enzyme systems are available; both use adenosine 5-monophosphate (AMP) as substrate. In the most popular 5'-ND quantitation method, adenosine formation (reaction (a) below) is coupled to inosine production using adenosine deaminase (AD in reaction (b)). Inosine production causes a decrease in absorbance at 265 nm and is usually measured after a fixed time interval.

(a) $\quad \text{AMP} + \text{H}_2\text{O} \xrightarrow[\text{pH } 6.6-7.0]{5'\text{-ND}} \text{adenosine} + \text{P (inorganic)}$

(b) $\quad \text{adenosine} + \text{H}_2\text{O} \xrightarrow{\text{AD}} \text{inosine} + \text{NH}_4^+$

(c) $\quad \text{NH}_4^+ + 2\text{-oxoglutarate} + \text{NADH} + \text{H}^+ \xrightarrow{\text{GLDH}} \text{L-glutamate} + \text{NAD}^+ + \text{H}_2\text{O}$

In the second method for 5'-ND determination, reactions (a) and (b) are used. In this method, ammonium (NH_4^+) production from reaction (b) is coupled by L-glutamic dehydrogenase (GLDH) to conversion of NADH to NAD^+ as shown in reaction (c). Continuous monitoring of NADH oxidation at 340 nm is usually used with the three-step procedure, rather than fixed-time measurement.

A two- to six-fold increase above normal in 5'-ND activity is very specific for hepatobiliary disease, since this enzyme is not usually increased in skeletal disease, in childhood, or with pregnancy. Assessing 5'-ND activity is useful for differentiating hepatobiliary versus skeletal elevations in ALT.

METHODS OF ISOENZYME ANALYSIS

There is no single method for analyzing all the clinically useful isoenzyme families. While each of the following methods has enjoyed some historic popularity, newer techniques involving biotechnology (e.g., monoclonal antibodies, recombinant DNA) may in the future supplant these older methods and allow isoenzyme analyses to be automated and, perhaps, performed in a random access manner, rather than with the batch techniques of today.

Electrophoresis is the most popular technique for isoenzyme separation and analysis, particularly when agarose is the support medium. Many isoenzyme families can be separated rapidly, based on charge differences and subsequently stained using specific substrate mixtures. Scanning densitometry can then be used to estimate the relative amount of activity residing in each separated isoenzyme fraction. For CK and LD isoenzyme fractionation, electrophoresis represents the best compromise of sensitivity, cost-effectiveness, and turnaround time. However, the major limitations of electrophoresis reside in the nature of electrophoretic procedures; that is, they are batch

Table 2. Methods of Isoenzyme Analysis

Method	Examples	Disadvantages
Electrophoresis	LD, CK	Labor intensive
Chromatography	Acid phosphatase CK, LD	Difficult to automate
Selective inhibition	Alkaline phosphatase	Difficulties with more than 2 isoenzymes
Antibody techniques	CK, LD, acid phosphatase	Some methods are not cost effective

techniques, which are relatively inflexible. While there has been controversy over the relative sensitivities of electrophoresis and antibody techniques, for most clinical situations involving CK and LD, electrophoresis is adequate.

Chromatographic techniques, usually involving ion-exchange resins, are primarily used in research settings today. Historically, these methods have been very important techniques which bridged the period of time before the commercial availability of procedures involving electrophoresis and antibodies. Currently, chromatographic techniques are useful only for very small volume situations or for a reference method employed for comparison studies.

Selective inhibition is again rarely used but does provide some historical interest. These techniques are based on research involving inhibitors which are selective for one particular isoenzyme over another. Thus, tartrate has been used for measuring acid phosphatase of prostatic origin; pyruvate, heat, and lactate for discriminating LD coming from liver or muscle; and heat, urea, phenylalanine, and homoarginine for discriminating alkaline phosphatase isoenzymes. These techniques are less useful, however, when more than two isoenzymes exist and need to be differentiated. Currently, only acid phosphatase and occasionally alkaline phosphatase are measured using selective inhibition, although antibody techniques for prostatic acid phosphatase are available and growing in popularity.

Antibody techniques hold much of the promise in this field. Isoenzymes which are the product of different gene loci can be detected by specific antibodies, either polyclonal or monoclonal. Depending on the epitope (antigen recognition site) and the design of the assay, these techniques can be based on inhibition of one or more isoenzyme, precipitation of one or more isoenzyme, or a combination of both approaches. The advantages of this approach are many, the most obvious being the ability to use automated, random access analyzers. As more antibody products appear, the cost of reagents will decrease, eliminating the major disadvantage of current products. Presently, there are antibody techniques available for most of the clinically important isoenzymes, with the exception of the bone and liver isoenzymes of alkaline phosphatase, which appear to be the product of a single gene locus, thus not amenable to this technique.

INTERPRETATION OF ISOENZYMES

The interpretation of isoenzymes can be grouped into two classifications: (1) isoenzyme analyses that can be completed on the basis of the test results, and (2) those analyses in which the appropriate interpretation depends on additional data. In the first group we can include alkaline and acid phosphatase isoenzymes; the latter group includes lactate dehydrogenase and creatine kinase isoenzymes.

Acid phosphatase isoenzymes are primarily ordered in patients in which prostatic cancer is known or highly suspected. Whether the methods are immunological or involve selective inhibition, a high prostatic acid fraction is consistent with prostatic cancer. However, there are other sources of this isoenzyme, which may occur in hematological malignancies, such as leukemia. One way to rule out this source is to check the white blood cell count, since elevated levels of this isoenzyme are seen with severe leukocytosis (WBC > 50,000).

Alkaline phosphatase isoenzymes may be ordered for a variety of reasons; however, the most common clinical situation involves discriminating liver from the heat labile bone fraction. Other situations in which alkaline phosphatase isoenzymes are clinically useful include

1. amniotic fluid analysis to detect cystic fibrosis (low levels of the intestinal isoenzymes are seen),
2. certain malignancies associated with a placental-like isoenzyme, and
3. discrimination of certain types of biliary and intestinal disturbance based on biliary and intestinal isoenzymes.

Nevertheless, these situations are relatively uncommon compared with the more routine request to differentiate bone from liver disease. As mentioned above, since both these isoenzymes appear to have the same primary protein structure but differ in sialic acid content, differentiating bone from liver disease solely on the basis of alkaline phosphatase isoenzyme values is not recommended. Frequently, γ-glutamyltransferase, a relatively specific marker of liver involvement, is used as an aid in interpreting alkaline phosphatase isoenzyme results.

The second group of isoenzymes, which often require additional data for adequate interpretation, includes creatine kinase and lactate dehydrogenase. Rather than describe specific cases, I have developed algorithms to aid in interpretation. The material, however, is designed for adult patients who have not had cardiac surgery.

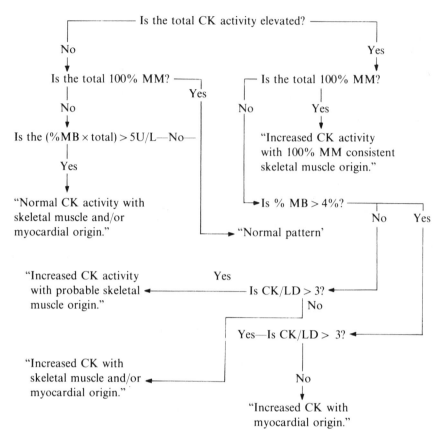

Algorithm for CK isoenzyme interpretation

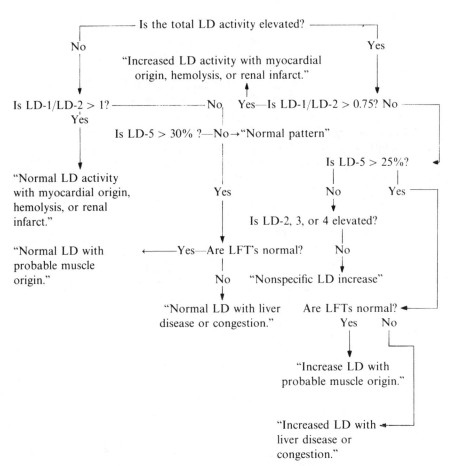

Algorithm for LD isoenzyme interpretation: LFT = liver function test. *Note:* Increased LD activity with multisystem diseases or malignancies can present as elevations in several fractions, such as LD-2, 3, and 4. Also, patients with myocardial involvement can present with increased LD activity with both LD-1/LD-2 > 0.75 and LD-5 > 25% if there is concomitant liver involvement.

REFERENCES

1. Lehninger AL, *Biochemistry: The Molecular Basis of Cell Structure and Function,* 2nd ed. New York: Worth, 19

2. Moss DW, Henderson AR, Kachmar JF. Enzymes, in Tietz NW (ed): *Fundamentals of Clinical Chemistry.* Philadelphia: Saunders, 1987, pp 346–417.

3. Moss DW, Henderson AR, Kachmar JF. Enzymes, in Tietz NW (ed): *Textbook of Clinical Chemistry.* Philadelphia: Saunders, 1986, pp 619–762.

4. Hohnadel DC. Enzymes, in Kaplan LA, Pesce AJ (eds): *Clinical Chemistry: Theory, Analysis, and Correlation.* St. Louis: Mosby, 1984, pp 927–961.

CHAPTER 7

HORMONE IMMUNOASSAYS

RONALD J. WHITLEY

University of Kentucky, Lexington, Kentucky

INTRODUCTION

Biochemical evaluation of endocrine function is tremendously dependent on the availability of sensitive and accurate laboratory procedures for measuring plasma levels of hormones or urinary excretion of hormones or metabolites. Assay methods for hormones and their metabolites can be divided into three main groups: bioassays, physical–chemical assays, and binding assays.

Bioassays

At one time, hormones were almost always measured using biological assays. Bioassays, however, depend on the physiological response of a living organism and tend to be expensive and difficult to perform. Also, they are relatively insensitive and may lack specificity (i.e., nonhormonal substances present in serum or urine may modulate the response). At present, bioassays are occasionally used to evaluate biological activities of purified hormone preparations.

Physical–Chemical Assays

Physical and chemical assays were initially developed for nonprotein, low molecular weight hormones such as steroids and catecholamines. These methods were generally faster and easier than bioassays, more reproducible, and more suited for use in the hospital laboratory. In contrast, chemical and physical assays for protein and polypeptide hormones were much more difficult to develop. Consequently, bioassays continued to be used to assay large molecular weight hormones such as FSH and LH until binding assays were developed in the 1960s. Today, binding assays have been applied to the determination of virtually every known hormone of physiological importance.

145

Binding Assays

Hormone binding assays embrace a variety of *in vitro* analytical methods that depend on the reaction between a hormone and a specific binding protein. Such assays can be divided into immunoassays (in which the binding protein is a specific antibody), receptor binding assays (in which the binding protein is a biological receptor protein obtained from the target tissue of the hormone), and competitive protein binding assays (in which the binding agent is a naturally occurring protein found in blood).

Several years ago, competitive protein binding assays were the most sensitive methods for hormone determination, particularly steroids. For example, corticosteroid binding globulin was widely used for the measurements of cortisol, progesterone, and other corticosteroids. Naturally occurring binding proteins have advantages in that they are stable, easy to prepare, and relatively inexpensive; however, they may not be specific for a particular hormone. Moreover, competitive protein binding assays are available for only a limited number of compounds. Receptor assays also have limited applications, partly because of their unstable nature and partly because of the complexity of their preparation and purification.

Immunoassays employing specific antibodies are the most common hormone binding assays in use today for several reasons: (1) antibodies can be produced that are capable of discriminating a particular hormone antigen from structurally similar compounds, (2) picomolar concentrations of hormones can be measured as a result of the high affinity with which the antibody binds the hormone antigen, and (3) antibodies can be produced that are capable of binding a wide variety of natural and synthetic hormones.

Antibodies used in binding assays are usually produced by immunizing animals with a suitable preparation of the hormone of interest. Some hormones, such as steroids, are not immunogenic in themselves but can become immunogenic when covalently conjugated to carrier proteins before injection. In recent years, antibodies have also been produced using hybridomas obtained by fusing antibody-forming spleen cells with myeloma tumor cells.

ANTIBODY–ANTIGEN REACTION

The binding of a hormone ligand to an antibody is an equilibrium reaction involving noncovalent bonds (electrostatic, hydrogen bonding, and van der Waals interactions). In many assay systems, the initial combination of antibody and antigen is followed by growth of the immune complex to form aggregates. Depending on the relative concentrations of antigen and antibody, these aggregates may cross-link and form precipitable complexes. Some of the methods discussed in this chapter examine the formation of these large immune complexes as an index of antigen–antibody reaction. A few examine other secondary effects such as agglutination. Most, however, are concerned with the primary combination of hormone antigen and antibody.

The initial or primary reaction between antigen and antibody is often described by the law of mass action:

$$Ab + H \underset{k_{-1}}{\overset{k_1}{\rightleftharpoons}} Ab:H$$

$$K_a = \frac{k_1}{k_{-1}} = \frac{[Ab:H]}{[Ab][H]}$$

Here Ab denotes the antibody, H the hormone antigen, and Ab:H the antibody–antigen complex; k_1 and k_{-1} are the rate constants for the association and dissociation reactions, respectively; K_a is defined as an association constant for the overall binding reaction and is expressed in liters per mole (L/mol).

K_a is also referred to as the affinity or avidity constant. The former is an expression of the binding strength of a single antibody combining site for the hormone ligand, whereas the latter refers to the sum of the binding affinities of all the individual combining sites. For steroid–antibody binding, K_a is about 10^6–10^{10} L/mol, but for protein hormones the upper limit is about 10^{12} L/mol. K_a is particularly important to the sensitivity of an immunoassay (i.e., the minimal detectable concentration). Thus, largely because of the multivalent nature of the protein antigen, immunoassays for protein hormones are generally more sensitive than those for steroids.

In addition to their avidity, antibodies are characterized by specificity. The specificity of an antibody for a particular hormone is measured by its capacity to bind the hormone of interest and not other structurally related compounds. If cross-reacting compounds are present, they may bind to the antibody with the same affinity, causing an overestimation of hormone concentration. The specificity of antibodies raised against high molecular weight hormone antigens is rather unpredictable, whereas it is generally possible to obtain well-defined antisera for steroids. Generally speaking, steroid antisera tend to be specific for the part of the molecule farthest removed from the site of carrier protein conjugation. Figure 1 illustrates the specificity of antisera raised

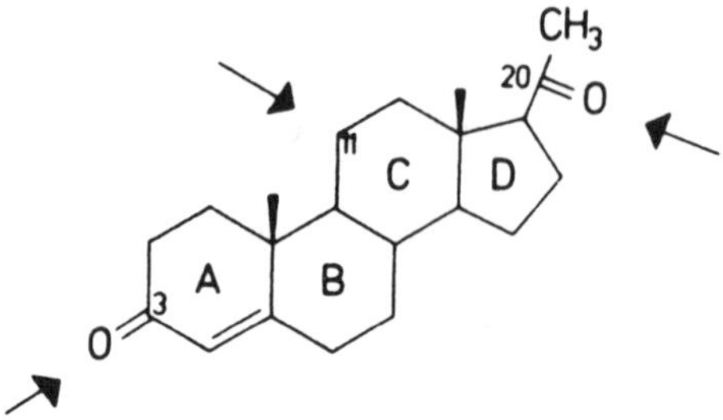

Steroid	Cross-reaction		
	P-20	P-3	P-11
Progesterone	100	100	100
Pregnenolone	1.1	13	0.5
17α-hydroxyprogesterone	98	4.6	1.2
Testosterone	95	0.05	0.04
11α-hydroxyprogesterone	7.1	13	34.5

Figure 1. Sites of conjugation of progesterone for generation of antisera, and specificity of antisera. [From Riad-Fahmy D, et al. Steroid immunoassays in endocrinology, in Voller A, et al (eds): *Immunoassays for the 80's,* 1981, p. 206. Reproduced with permission of MTP Press Ltd., Lancaster].

against progesterone coupled to the 20, 3, and 11 positions. Regardless of the size of the hormone antigen, it is important to determine antibody specificity for each assay system, preferably by testing patient samples directly for possible cross-reacting compounds.

Until recently, most antisera were heterogeneous (i.e., polyclonal) mixtures of different populations of antibodies. Not surprisingly, polyclonal antibodies often bind the hormone antigen as well as structurally related compounds. In contrast, monoclonal antibodies offer the potential for selecting antibodies that have essentially no cross-reactivity with other compounds (*1*). Table 1 illustrates the case of six antibodies obtained for hCG. It should be noted, however, that monoclonal antibodies are not always better than polyclonal antisera, and in some assay systems monoclonal antibodies have yet to achieve the high avidity of polyclonal antisera.

An alternative approach to the achievement of assay specificity in hormone immunoassays is to purify the sample before performing the immuno-reaction—for example, by means of solvent extraction or chromatography. Even with nonspecific antisera, preassay purification procedures usually provide accurate results; however, such techniques are generally too time-consuming. In fact, one of the major advances in hormone immunoassays in

Table 1. Cross-Reactivity of Six Antibodies for hCG

Antibody	Relative Affinity (%)				
	hCG	β-hCG	LH	TSH	FSH
1	30	100	10	<1	7
2	<1	100	<1	<1	<1
3	100	1600	2	<1	<1
4	100	<1	5	1	<1
5	100	<1	40	3	4
6	100	120	1	<1	<1

Source: Modified from Siddle K. Properties and applications of monoclonal antibodies, in Collins WP (ed): *Alternative Immunoassays*. New York: Wiley, 1985, p 24. Reprinted with permission of John Wiley & Sons, Ltd.

recent years has been the development of direct assay methods that avoid these preliminary steps.

CLASSIFICATION OF IMMUNOASSAYS

Immunoassays for hormone detection and measurement can be classified according to the technique used to demonstrate that an antigen–antibody reaction has taken place.

Labeled Antigen

When an atom or molecule capable of generating a signal for monitoring the binding reaction is attached to the hormone antigen, the labeled antigen serves as a tracer to follow the distribution of hormone between the unbound and antibody-bound fractions.

Labeled antigens have found wide applications in competitive binding assays. Typically, a sample containing unlabeled hormone is incubated simultaneously with labeled hormone and specific antibody. During this incubation step, the labeled and unlabeled ligands compete for a limited number of antibody binding sites, usually until equilibrium is achieved. Competitive binding assays of this type are also referred to as "saturation analysis," to indicate that labeled and unlabeled hormones are in excess of the antibody. Since these assays obey the law of mass action, less labeled hormone is bound as the quantity of unlabeled hormone increases. By plotting the percentage of labeled hormone bound as a function of the concentration of unlabeled hormone standards, a calibration curve (dose–response curve) can

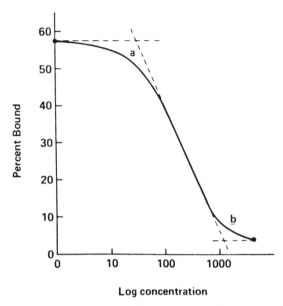

Figure 2. Dose–response curve for a typical radioimmunoassay. The useful portion of the curve is bracketed by points *a* and *b*. [From Buffone G. Principles of immunochemical techniques, in Tietz NW (ed): *Textbook of Clinical Chemistry*. Philadelphia: Saunders, 1986, p 226. Reproduced with permission.]

be constructed. As shown in Figure 2, the amount of tracer bound to antibody is inversely proportional to the concentration of hormone in the sample.

Immunoassays employing labeled antigens can also be performed before binding has reached equilibrium. In the nonequilibrium or sequential approach, unlabeled hormone is incubated with excess antibody before the tracer is added.

$$Ab + H \rightleftharpoons Ab:H + Ab \overset{H^*}{\rightleftharpoons} Ab:H + Ab:H^*$$

When this sequential approach is used, more unlabeled hormone can be bound by the antibody than in the corresponding competitive binding assay, thus providing an increase in assay sensitivity.

Labeled Antibody

Immunoassays employing labeled antibody are also known as immunometric assays. Although competitive binding techniques using labeled antibodies were once widely employed, most procedures now use excess labeled antibodies in noncompetitive formats (i.e., "reagent-excess methods"). In general, noncompetitive immunometric assays offer several important analytical advantages over competitive antigen-labeled methods. For example, labeled antibodies are more stable and easier to prepare. Furthermore, excess labeled antibody systems are capable of providing faster reaction times, improved assay sensitivity, expanded working ranges, improved precision, and higher specificity for the hormone of interest. Until recently, inadequate amounts of pure antibody severely restricted the development of immunometric assays. With the availability of monoclonal antibodies, abundant supplies are now assured (2).

In the original form of the immunometric assay, the test sample was reacted with excess labeled antibody. The unreacted labeled antibody was then separated by use of antigen coupled to a solid phase (3). The amount of bound label in the supernate provided a direct measure of antigen concentration. In subsequent developments, "two-site sandwich" immunometric assays were introduced for measuring hormone molecules with more than one antigenic determinant (e.g., FSH, LH, prolactin). In a typical assay, the test sample is first incubated with excess unlabeled antibody linked to an insoluble support. Unlabeled hormone antigen, if present, attaches to the bound antibody. After incubation and washing, a labeled second antibody directed against a different part of the hormone antigen is added. This antibody also binds to the hormone, creating an antigen "sandwich" between the two antibodies.

$$\text{\Large\}—Ab_1 + H \rightarrow \text{\Large\}—Ab_1 : H$$

$$\text{\Large\}—Ab_1 : H + Ab_2^* \rightarrow \text{\Large\}—Ab_1 : H : Ab_2^*$$

Because the immune complex is anchored to a solid phase, the remaining free label is conveniently removed by washing. The amount of label present in the bound fraction is directly related to the amount of antigen added (Figure 3).

If the hormone antigen has two similar binding sites, a single polyclonal antibody can be used for labeling as well as for coupling to the solid phase. If the hormone has antigenic sites of differing specificities, different monoclonal antibodies often can be produced. For use in sandwich assays, monoclonal antibodies are almost always preferred. In many cases the test sample and the labeled antibody can be added simultaneously to the solid phase antibody, thus eliminating one incubation step and one washing step.

To improve assay sensitivity, variations of this two-site sandwich protocol are available. For example, both antibodies can be added together, or the

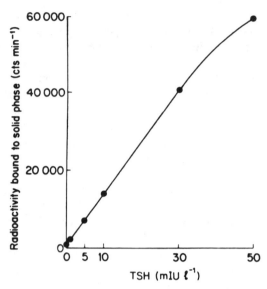

Figure 3. Dose–response curve for a typical immunoradiometric assay. [From Siddle K. Properties and applications of monoclonal antibodies, in Collins WP (ed): *Alternative Immunoassays*. New York: Wiley, 1985, p 30. Reprinted with permission of John Wiley & Sons, Ltd.]

hormone antigen can be reacted with the labeled antibody before addition of the solid phase antibody. To develop assay systems common for a large variety of analytes, a number of "three-site" sandwich immunoassays also have been developed. For example, a labeled second-antibody format has been used in which antibodies A and B, react with the antigen, and a third labeled antibody (C) reacts with antibody B.

$$\text{\Large\}\!\!-Ab_A : Ag : Ab_B : Ab_C^*$$

Antibody A is anchored to a solid phase. One important advantage of this assay format is that the same labeled antibody can be used for several different antigens, provided antibodies A and B are produced in different animals.

With the widespread availability of monoclonal antibodies, three-site assays have been modified to include two monoclonal antibodies that recognize different binding sites of the hormone antigen. For example, one antibody can be labeled with fluorescein isothiocyanate (FITC) and the other with an enzyme label (*4*). The immune sandwich that forms when hormone is present is captured by anti-FITC antibodies covalently immobilized on solid phase particles.

$$\text{\textexclamdown}{-}Ab + FITC\text{-}Ab_1 + Ag + Ab_2^* \rightarrow \text{\textexclamdown}{-}Ab : FITC\text{-}Ab_1 : Ag : Ab_2^*$$

This "common capture" format eliminates the need to optimize antibody–solid phase coupling conditions for each individual antibody and also permits the convenience of running several immunometric assays simultaneously.

Nonlabels

Some hormone immunoassays do not use labeled antigens or antibodies to monitor the changes associated with antibody binding. For many years, light-scattering techniques have been used to follow the growth of antigen–antibody complexes. Other nonlabel techniques such as immuno-electrophoresis and radial immunodiffusion are also available for following the formation of a precipitin band or ring when a hormone antigen combines with its specific antibody. Although nonlabeled immunoassays are relatively simple to perform, they are usually applied only to large molecular weight hormones that are present in relatively high concentrations.

A number of different materials have been used to label antigens or antibodies (Table 2). Some are employed in heterogeneous assays in which a separation step is required. Others are used in homogeneous protocols that do not require separation of bound and free label. A few of these heterogeneous and homogeneous immunoassay systems are discussed in the sections that follow.

Table 2. Labels Used in Hormone Immunoassays

Radioisotopes
Enzymes; coenzymes; enzyme substrates, prosthetic groups, inhibitors, or activators
Fluorescent and phosphorescent molecules
Chemiluminescent and bioluminescent molecules
Proteins
Particles: erythrocytes, latex, sols
Metals
Bacteriophages
Free radicals
Immunoreactive liposomes
Immunoselective electrodes

RADIOACTIVE LABELS

Radioctive atoms have been widely employed as immunoassay labels. Of all immunoassay procedures, those employing radioactive labels have been used most often for the quantitation of hormones. Since development of the technique about 25 years ago, radioimmunoassay determinations have increased from 52 million worldwide in 1975 to more than 400 million in 1985 (5). As a consequence of the phenomenal impact RIA has had on medicine, particularly endocrinology, a Nobel Prize was awarded in 1977 to three of its pioneers.

Choice of Radioactive Label

Radioactive labels fall into two groups: β-emitting isotopes such as tritium, and γ-emitting isotopes such as ^{125}I. For many years, steroid immunoassays used tritium-labeled ligands. Tritiated steroids behave very much like unlabeled steroids and are often stable over a 6-month period. Other advantages of tritium labels include long half-life and the ease with which they can be attached to most steroids. Tritium labels have several disadvantages, though, including the quenching of light emission, the high cost of scintillation fluids and β counters, and the difficulty and expense of automation. Moreover, immunoassays based on the use of tritiated reagents are time-consuming, particularly if single-channel instruments are used for counting. Most laboratories prefer to use γ-emitting isotopes such as ^{125}I for several reasons: (1) assay tubes can be counted directly without the need for scintillation fluid, (2) corrections for quenching are not necessary, (3) shorter counting times are possible because of the higher specific activities of iodine-labeled hormones, and (4) γ-counters are available in multichannel form.

Many procedures have been used to introduce radioactive iodine into hormone antigens or antibodies. For peptides or proteins containing tyrosine and/or histidine, chloramine T methods can be easily used (6). Other techniques include lactoperoxidase (7) and the introduction of iodinated acyl groups (8). The latter may be used to label compounds that do not contain tyrosine groups. Except for phenolic estrogens, direct radioiodination of steroid hormones usually is not possible. For this reason, steroids often are conjugated to bridge structures that can be radioiodinated (9). Regardless of the nature of the radioactive tracer or bridge structure, if either is coupled to important antigenic sites on the hormone or antibody, assay sensitivity will be significantly decreased.

Choice of Separation System

For radiolabeled immunoassays, the distribution of hormone between the free and antibody-bound fractions is determined by measuring the radioactivity of either fraction after physical separation of the two components. An ideal separation technique would not disturb the antigen–antibody equilibrium reaction. Moreover, it would quantitatively separate bound and free fractions, and it would be rapid, simple, and inexpensive to perform.

A variety of separation systems are available (Table 3). In general, methods based on differential migration of bound and free fractions (e.g., electrophoresis, gel filtration) are not practical for routine clinical applications. In contrast, systems that adsorb the free fraction onto an insoluble matrix (e.g., dextran-coated charcoal) or use protein precipitation to convert the bound fraction into an insoluble form have enjoyed wider acceptance. In these instances, centrifugation is usually chosen to achieve phase separation, although filtration methods have also been described. Adsorption and protein precipitation procedures, however, are not as popular as they once were, largely because considerable effort is required to carefully optimize each assay.

Table 3. Methods of Separating Free and Bound Label

Adsorption
    Dextran-coated charcoal
    Silicates (Florisil, talc)
Ion-exchange resins
Gel filtration
Antigen–antibody affinity columns
Electrophoresis
Protein precipitation: ethanol, dioxane, $(NH_4)_2SO_4$, polyethylene glycol
Immunological precipitation: double (second) antibody
Solid phase supports
    Plastic surfaces (polystyrene–polypropylene coated tubes, microtiter plates, dipsticks, polystyrene beads or balls, polyacrylamide beads, etc.)
    Microcrystalline cellulose
    Glass
    Magnetic particles
    Sepharose, Sephadex, Sephacryl
    Suspendable microbeads
Sucrose layering
Radial partition

Immunological precipitation techniques continue to be used for many competitive RIAs. In the double-antibody system, for example, the antibody-bound antigen is precipitated immunologically by using a second antibody. To achieve complete precipitation, however, prolonged incubation times are frequently required; moreover, refrigerated centrifuges are sometimes needed. To overcome some of these problems, accelerated liquid phase second-antibody (e.g., a mixture of PEG and second antibody) or solid phase second-antibody techniques have been used.

The current trend in separation systems is toward the use of solid phases to insolubilize either the bound or free ligand. For example, whole antibody (or the purified IgG fraction) can be covalently or noncovalently attached to such solid supports as test tubes and microparticles. In addition to reducing incubation times, solid phase supports are simple to use, and assay precision is noticeably improved compared with other separation systems. Solid phase materials have other advantages, as well. For example, some solid phase particles (e.g., microcrystalline cellulose) stay suspended during incubation, thus exposing a large surface area for antibody–antigen binding and avoiding the need for mixing. Others, such as antibody-coated tubes, beads, or magnetic particles, avoid the need for centrifugation. Still others facilitate automated separation techniques, such as sucrose layering or internal sample attenuation. The latter uses bismuth oxide, a radiation-absorbing material, to shield the radiation from either the bound or free radioligand (10). For further discussions of the advantages and disadvantages of separation techniques, the interested reader is referred to recent workshop proceedings (11).

Applications of Radiolabeled Immunoassays

From an operational standpoint, radiolabeled immunoassays may be divided into two categories: those in which antigen is labeled with a radioisotope (radioimmunoassay, RIA) and those in which antibody is labeled (immuno-radiometric assay, IRMA). The former are employed as competitive or sequential procedures, whereas the latter are developed as noncompetitive techniques. In principle, radiolabeled assays can be used for the quantitative determination of almost any substance that is available in pure form and to which an antibody can be produced. In recent years, complete commercial kits as well as individual components have become available for nearly every known hormone. We do not attempt to review the vast number of radio-labeled procedures developed for specific hormones [current textbooks, journals, or product guides may be consulted for further information (12,13)]. Instead, a general discussion of current and future trends in radiolabeled immunoassays follows.

A number of developments in radioisotope-labeled immunoassays have been aimed at simplifying assay procedures while retaining or even increasing their high sensitivity for the measurement of very low concentrations of hormone analytes.

1. *Direct Assays.* Most polypeptide and protein hormones can be analyzed without prior extraction and concentration of hormone from the serum or urine sample. An increasing number of steroid immunoassays are also being adapted for direct measurement. Previously, steroid hormones required lengthy solvent extraction or column separation procedures to displace binding proteins or to remove interfering lipids and cross-reacting substances.

2. *Extended Sensitivity.* In a number of instances, improvements in the sensitivity of present assay methods would be clinically beneficial. For example, most radioimmunoassays for TSH have been characterized by inadequate sensitivity in the normal and subnormal range. The availability of highly sensitive immunoradiometric assays for TSH has already begun to provide clinicians with enhanced diagnostic capabilities, especially in the hyperthyroid range (*14*). Over the next few years, the need for enhanced sensitivity may also include the measurement of free or non-protein-bound hormones. In this regard, it is quite likely that labeled antibody procedures will continue to replace a significant number of competitive RIAs.

3. *Automation.* The development of fully automated radiolabeled assay systems has been hampered by the need to physically separate free from bound label. Nevertheless, the wish to increase sample throughput has encouraged a number of different approaches to solve this problem. Both discrete and continuous-flow instruments are commercially available, and new developments can be expected (*15*).

4. *Dual Labels.* A rapidly developing area of RIA technology is the ability to measure two hormones in the same reaction mixture by using two radioactive labels having nonoverlapping emission spectra. Dual-label assays for hormones such as LH and FSH have already been developed (*16*). In these cases, ^{57}Co and ^{125}I were used as radioisotopes.

NONISOTOPIC LABELS

In recent years many efforts have been made to develop alternative immuno-assays that do not rely on the use of radiolabels. A number of disadvantages associated with radioisotopes underlie current interest in nonisotopic labels: (1) limited shelf life of radioiodinated reagents, (2) relatively low specific activity of radiolabels, (3) potential dangers of handling radioactive materials, (4) licensing requirements, (5) radiation damage to sensitive ligands, and

(6) automation difficulties encountered because radiolabels do not lend themselves to fully automated, separation-free assays. Some of the reasons offered against radioisotope methods are debatable. Nevertheless, important advantages would result if nonisotopic immunoassays could be demonstrated to be superior in their analytical performance (e.g., more precise), practicality (e.g., lower in cost), or diagnostic utility (e.g., enhanced sensitivity).

The sections that follow discuss nonisotopic labels of various types in terms of their role in hormone immunoassays. In many cases the relation between these alternative technologies and established radiolabeled procedures is also considered.

Enzyme Labels

A number of compounds measured via enzymatic processes may be used as immunochemical labels in place of radioactive isotopes: enzymes, coenzymes, enzyme substrates, enzyme inhibitors or activators, enzyme prosthetic groups, and apoenzymes. Enzymes, in particular, appear to be the most sensitive and are undoubtedly the most widely used of all nonisotopic tracers. As biological catalysts, enzyme labels can trigger the formation of large quantities of product molecules, which can then be measured and related to the amount of unlabeled hormone in a test sample. Enzyme activity is chiefly determined by photometry, but fluorescent and chemiluminescent substrates as well as changes in pH or conductivity have also been used to monitor the enzyme reaction.

Enzyme immunoassays (EIA) generally are of two types: heterogeneous and homogeneous. In the heterogeneous system, antigen–antibody binding does not affect enzyme activity; however, a procedure is required for separating the antibody-bound and unbound labeled fractions. In homogeneous systems, antibody binding modulates the activity of the enzyme, usually by increasing or decreasing the signal. In this case, enzyme activity is measured without separating the bound and free fractions. Numerous EIA configurations have been described, and some are available as commercial kits.

Choice of Enzyme Labels

A number of factors govern the selection of a particular enzyme label (*17*). A few of the enzymes that have been successfully used in heterogeneous and homogeneous hormone assays are listed in Table 4.

Heterogeneous EIAs. Most EIAs that require separation of the bound antigen from the unbound fraction are based on principles analogous to

**Table 4. Enzyme Labels Commonly Used in
Enzyme Immunoassays**

Heterogeneous Assays

Horseradish peroxidase
Alkaline phosphatase
β-D-Galactosidase

Homogeneous Assays

Malate dehydrogenase
Glucose-6-phosphate dehydrogenase

conventional radioimmunoassays except that enzyme activity is measured instead of radioactivity. Assays that combine the merits of solid phase technology with those of enzyme-labeled antigen or antibody are often referred to as ELISA (enzyme-linked immunosorbent assay) procedures. Heterogeneous EIAs may be divided into two categories: those in which antigen is labeled with enzyme, and those in which antibody is labeled.

Labeled Antigen. Heterogeneous EIAs using labeled antigens are usually employed as competitive procedures similar to antigen-labeled RIAs. In the reaction that follows, enzyme-labeled hormone (H–E) and unlabeled hormone (H) compete for a limited amount of solid phase antibodies.

$$H + H\text{-}E + \text{\textbf{\}}\text{—}Ab \rightleftarrows \text{\textbf{\}}\text{—}Ab : H + \text{\textbf{\}}\text{—}Ab : H\text{-}E \subset \begin{smallmatrix} S \\ P \end{smallmatrix}$$
(free)   **(bound)**

After a short incubation period, the unbound or free fraction is washed away, and the antibody-bound fraction is assayed using a suitable enzyme substrate(s). Enzyme activity is thus inversely related to the concentration of hormone in the sample. In many cases very small quantities of hormones can be measured. For example, the sensitivity of a competitive EIA for progesterone was found to be 4 pg per tube (*18*). In this case, horseradish peroxidase was used as the enzyme label and microcrystalline cellulose was used as the solid phase matrix. Sensitive and specific EIAs for nearly all naturally occurring steroids of clinical value have now been developed. In addition to steroids, competitive EIAs have been reported for other small hormones such as thyroxine (T_4). In one commercial T_4 assay system adapted for automation, serum is incubated with peroxidase-labeled T_4 in a test tube coated with T_4

antibody; endogenous T_4 present in the sample competes with enzyme-labeled T_4 for binding sites on the antibody. Recently, a common capture immunoassay using enzyme-labeled T_4 as the tracer was reported. This competitive EIA was shown to be both sensitive and rapid.

Another approach to heterogeneous enzyme immunoassays, termed steric hindrance enzyme immunoassay (SHEIA), has been applied to measurements of thyroxine and human placental lactogen (19a). In this assay system, β-D-galactosidase is used to label the hormone antigen. Following competition of unlabeled hormone and enzyme-labeled hormone for a limited amount of antibody, a pseudosubstrate inhibitor P is added.

$$H + H\text{-}E + Ab \rightleftarrows Ab:H + Ab:H\text{-}E$$
$$\textbf{(soluble)}$$

$$H\text{-}E + \text{\textexclamdown}\!\!-\!P \rightleftarrows \text{\textexclamdown}\!\!-\!P\text{-}E\text{-}H$$
$$\textbf{(insoluble)}$$

$$Ab:H\text{-}E + \text{\textexclamdown}\!\!-\!P \rightarrow NR$$

The free enzyme-labeled hormone (H–E) reversibly binds to the inhibitor, whereas the enzyme-labeled hormone–antibody complex (Ab : H–E) does not, probably because of steric hindrance. The enzyme activity of the soluble fraction is usually measured.

Most heterogeneous enzyme immunoassays depend on interactions between antigens and antibodies. Several years ago, a novel approach to these assays was described in which the enzyme label was linked to the antigen of interest as well as a tag molecule such as biotin (19b). Immunoassays based on this procedure are known as antibody masking, enzyme tagged immunoassays (AMETIA). Free antigen and the antigen–enzyme–tag conjugate compete for available antibody binding sites.

$$Ag + Ag\text{-}E\text{-}T + Ab \rightleftarrows Ab:Ag + Ab:Ag\text{-}E\text{-}T$$

$$\text{\textexclamdown}\!\!-\!R + Ab:Ag\text{-}E\text{-}T \rightarrow NR$$
$$\textbf{(masked)}$$

$$\text{\textexclamdown}\!\!-\!R + Ag\text{-}E\text{-}T \rightarrow \text{\textexclamdown}\!\!-\!R\text{-}T\text{-}E\text{-}Ag$$

If the antigen–enzyme–tag conjugate is bound to antibody, the tag molecule becomes masked and will not bind to its receptor (such as avidin) immobilized on a solid support. Enzyme activity in the solid phase complex is found to increase in proportion to antigen concentration.

Labeled Antibody. Enzyme immunoassays involving the use of labeled antibody are generally performed as solid phase competitive techniques or as noncompetitive sandwich type-assays. One example of a competitive EIA using labeled antibody, often referred to as inhibition enzyme immunoassay, is based on the competition of unlabeled antigen and solid phase antigen for a limited amount of enzyme-labeled antibody (Ab-E).

$$\dashv\!\!\!\!\dashv\text{—Ag} + \text{Ag} + \text{Ab-E} \rightleftarrows \text{Ag}:\text{Ab-E} + \dashv\!\!\!\!\dashv\text{—Ag}:\text{Ab-E}\overset{S}{\underset{P}{\subset}}$$

$$\qquad\qquad\qquad\qquad\qquad\text{(free)}\qquad\qquad\text{(bound)}$$

Enzyme activity in the solid phase complex is inversely proportional to the concentration of sample antigen. A modification of this inhibition enzyme immunoassay, called competitive enzyme-linked immunoassay (CELIA), has been used for the detection of hCG (20) and testosterone (21). In this method, a specific antibody (Ab_1) competitively binds free and solid phase antigen.

$$\dashv\!\!\!\!\dashv\text{—Ag} + \text{Ag} + \text{Ab}_1 \rightleftarrows \dashv\!\!\!\!\dashv\text{—Ag}:\text{Ab}_1 + \text{Ag}:\text{Ab}_1$$

$$\dashv\!\!\!\!\dashv\text{—Ag}:\text{Ab}_1 + \text{Ab}_2 \rightarrow \dashv\!\!\!\!\dashv\text{—Ag}:\text{Ab}_1:\text{Ab}_2$$

$$\dashv\!\!\!\!\dashv\text{—Ag}:\text{Ab}_1:\text{Ab}_2 + \text{Ab}_3:\text{E} \rightarrow \dashv\!\!\!\!\dashv\text{—Ag}:\text{Ab}_1:\text{Ab}_2:\text{Ab}_3:\text{E}\overset{S}{\underset{P}{\subset}}$$

In a subsequent step an anti-immunoglobulin antibody (Ab_2) is added. After washing, a soluble peroxidase–antiperoxidase immune complex ($\text{Ab}_3:\text{E}$) is also added. The amount of bound enzyme is inversely related to the amount of hormone in the sample.

Over the past few years there has been a move toward using immunoen-zymometric assays (IEMAs) based on excess labeled antibodies. Several configurations are possible. In one format similar to the original form of the IRMA, unlabeled sample hormone is reacted with excess enzyme-labeled antibody; the remaining unreacted labeled antibody is separated by using excess solid phase antigen. Enzyme activity of the supernate increases in proportion to antigen concentration.

$$\text{H} + \text{Ab-E} \rightarrow \text{Ab-E} + \text{H}:\text{Ab-E}$$

$$\qquad\qquad\qquad\qquad\text{(soluble)}$$

$$\dashv\!\!\!\!\dashv\text{—H} + \text{Ab-E} \rightarrow \dashv\!\!\!\!\dashv\text{—H}:\text{Ab-E}$$

$$\qquad\qquad\qquad\qquad\text{(bound)}$$

This approach seems to work quite well with hormone antigens having single antigenic determinants.

A double-antibody IEMA for determination of hapten hormones has also been described (22). This method uses a two-antibody complex in which an antigen-specific first antibody is indirectly labeled with an enzyme-labeled second antibody. In a typical assay, unlabeled sample hormone is reacted with an excess of the double-antibody complex. The remaining unreacted antibody complex is then separated by means of a solid phase coupled antigen. An important advantage of this indirect labeling method is that one enzyme-labeled antibody can be used to measure several different hormone antigens.

There is a two-site immunoenzymometric assay analogous to the two-site sandwich IRMA technique. This noncompetitive method requires a separation step and is usually used with polypeptide–protein hormones having multiple antigenic sites. Typically, standard or sample is incubated with an excess of a capture antibody anchored to a solid phase support.

$$\text{—Ab}_1 + \text{H} \rightarrow \text{—Ab}_1 : \text{H}$$

$$\text{—Ab}_1 : \text{H} + \text{Ab}_2\text{-E} \rightarrow \text{—Ab}_1 : \text{H} : \text{Ab}_2\text{-E} \underset{\searrow \text{P}}{\overset{\text{S}}{\subset}}$$

Hormone, if present, attaches to the bound antibody. After incubation and washing, excess enzyme-labeled antibody is added, which also binds to the antigen. After further washing, the enzyme activity present in the bound fraction is found to be directly proportional to the amount of hormone in the test sample. Sandwich assays are probably the most popular of all the EIAs in use today. In terms of sensitivity and simplicity, these assays offer results that are comparable to or even exceed those using radioisotopes as labels. Sandwich IEMAs have been developed for a number of hormones such as hCG, LH, TSH, prolactin, and insulin; only a few representative examples from the recent literature are noted here (4,23–29). Some are available as commercial kits. Others, such as urinary hCG and LH, have also been developed as dipsticks (30,31).

Enzyme-Amplified Immunoassays. Originally it was thought that enzyme-based immunoassays would provide greater sensitivity than that offered by RIA or IRMA procedures. Unfortunately, this expected benefit is not always obtained. To enhance the sensitivity of enzyme immunoassays, alternative approaches can be used such as enzyme amplification.

An enzyme-amplified immunoassay for TSH has been reported and can be used to illustrate the principles involved (32). This immunoenzymometric assay uses two TSH monoclonal antibodies: one is immobilized to a

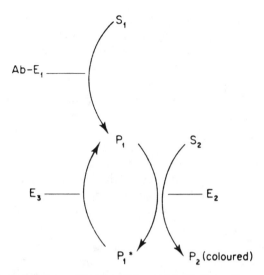

Figure 4. Principle of enzyme amplification. [From Siddle K. Properties and applications of monoclonal antibodies, in Collins WP (ed): *Alternative Immunoassays*. New York: Wiley, 1985, p 31. Reprinted with permission of John Wiley & Sons, Ltd.]

polystyrene surface, and the other is linked to alkaline phosphatase. Samples are first reacted with both antibodies for 2 hours. After excess reagents have been removed by washing, the bound enzyme is measured using a redox amplification system. As illustrated in Figure 4, antibody-bound E_1 catalyzes the conversion of S_1 to P_1 in a primary reaction. The P_1 that is generated is then used as the trigger for a secondary reaction in which S_2 is converted to P_2. A third enzyme E_3 regenerates P_1, thereby allowing recycling of P_1. Compared to conventional enzyme assays, this amplified procedure results in a 100-fold increase in colored product (P_2). For TSH, a detection limit of 0.037 mIU/L and a working range of 0.13–24.0 mIU/L were obtained.

Radial Partition Enzyme Immunoassay. In radial partition enzyme immunoassay, radial chromatography is used to separate the free and bound labeled analyte. The entire immunoassay is conducted on glass fiber filter paper coated with specific antibody. Although a variety of labels can be used (e.g., fluorophores and radioisotopes), enzymes are used most often and are discussed here. Both low and high molecular weight hormones such as hCG, cortisol, and thyroxine can be measured on automated instruments, usually in 10 minutes or less (*33–35*).

There are three different types of radial partition enzyme immunoassay: competitive, sequential, and sandwich. Enzyme-labeled antigens as well as enzyme-labeled antibodies may be used. For example, measurement of total intact hCG in serum or plasma is based on the two-site sandwich technique (34). In this procedure, two monoclonal hCG antibodies are used: one is linked to the glass fiber filter paper, and the other (directed against a different hCG antigenic site) is linked to alkaline phosphatase. The patient sample is applied to the filter paper, and after a short incubation, an excess of the enzyme-labeled antibody is added. After a suitable incubation, unbound labeled antibody is washed from the filter paper by radial elution. This wash solution also contains the substrate for the enzyme reaction, 4-methylumbelliferyl phosphate. Enzyme activity in the filter paper is measured by front-surface fluorometry, and the increase in fluorescence is directly proportional to the concentration of hCG in the test sample.

Homogeneous EIAs. Homogeneous enzyme immunoassays have been reported for several important hormones, particularly low molecular weight ones such as cortisol and thyroxine. At present, homogeneous enzyme immunoassays are less sensitive but more rapid, simpler to use, and easier to adapt to automation than heterogeneous EIAs. Compounds of various types have been used as labels in homogeneous enzyme immunoassays. Only a few examples are described here to illustrate some of the configurations available.

Enzyme as Label. One of the first separation-free EIAs applied widely in the endocrine laboratory used enzymes to label the antigens of interest. In this assay procedure, commonly known as the enzyme multiplied immunoassay technique (EMIT), binding of antibody to enzyme-labeled hormone so alters the enzyme activity that physical separation of antibody-bound and unbound labeled hormone is not required. Two enzymes are frequently used in EMIT assay systems for small hormones: glucose-6-phosphate dehydrogenase and malate dehydrogenase. In the EMIT cortisol assay, conjugation of glucose-6-phosphate dehydrogenase to the steroid hormone does not inhibit enzyme activity (36). However, binding of cortisol-specific antibody to the enzyme-labeled hormone does reduce enzyme activity, perhaps as a result of steric or allosteric inhibition.

$$H + H\text{-}E \underset{\longleftarrow}{\overset{Ab}{\longrightarrow}} Ab\text{:}H + Ab\text{:}H\text{-}E$$
$$\text{(active)} \qquad\qquad \text{(inactive)}$$

When unlabeled hormone is added, there is competition with enzyme-labeled cortisol for a limited number of antibody binding sites. As the concentration of unlabeled cortisol increases, less enzyme-labeled steroid is bound by the antibody. As a result, the catalytic activity of the free enzyme-labeled hormone increases in direct proportion to the amount of cortisol in the sample.

The homogeneous EMIT assay for thyroxine uses a malate dehydrogenase enzyme chemically bound to T_4 as the tracer (37). This T_4–enzyme conjugate is enzymatically inactive, perhaps due to T_4 blocking the enzyme active site. Binding of specific T_4 antibodies to the T_4–enzyme conjugate results in an increase in enzyme activity. As the concentration of unlabeled T_4 increases, less antibody is available for binding to the T_4–enzyme conjugate, and enzyme activity decreases.

Homogeneous EIAs using enzyme-labeled antibodies have also been developed for a few large molecular weight hormone antigens (38). One configuration uses a signal amplification system based on principles of enzyme channeling (39). In enzyme channelling, two enzymes are used to catalyze consecutive reactions such that the product of the first enzyme serves as substrate for the second.

$$S \xrightarrow{E_1} P_1 \xrightarrow{E_2} P_2$$

When both enzymes are brought close together, such as during an antibody–antigen binding reaction, catalytic formation of product is maximized. Adaptation of this technique to a qualitative test strip immunoassay for urinary hCG has been described (40). In this assay, the surface of the test strip consists of an enzyme (glucose oxidase) and a specific antibody to the α subunit of hCG coimmobilized onto a cellulose support. Pretreatment of the urine sample with a horseradish peroxidase (HRP) conjugate of anti-βhCG is necessary before the test strip is added. After incubation in a sonicator, the test strip is transferred to a solution containing glucose (S_1) and chloronaphthol (S_2) substrates.

$$hCG + Ab_\beta\text{-HRP} \rightarrow hCG:Ab_\beta\text{-HRP}$$

The hydrogen peroxidase produced in the first reaction (P_1) reacts with chloronaphthol in the second reaction to generate a color in proportion to the amount of hormone in the sample. A unique aspect of this assay is the use of ultrasonic energy to accelerate hormone binding to immobilized antibody. The entire assay takes less than 15 minutes to perform, and good correlation was obtained with a commercial ELISA method.

Substrate Label. An interesting new development in competitive homogeneous EIAs is the labeling of antigens with fluorogenic enzyme substrates (*41*). In the absence of unlabeled antigen, substrate-labeled ligand will bind to antibody and prevent substrate turnover. In the presence of unlabeled antigen, however, substrate-labeled antigen will be unbound and free to react with the enzyme. Substrate-labeled fluorescence immunoassays (SLIAs) do not rely on the amplification properties of the enzymes. Instead, the enzyme is used to measure only the amount of unbound substrate. Not surprisingly, this assay technique has limited sensitivity and has not been extensively applied to hormone measurements.

Enzyme Modulator Label. Another separation-free competitive EIA uses enzyme modulators as labels (*42*). Enzyme modulators may be either reversible or irreversible inhibitors or activators of enzyme activity. For example, a thyroxine assay has been developed using a T_4-labeled cholinesterase inhibitor as the enzyme modulator (*43*). As illustrated in the reactions that follow, unlabeled T_4 and T_4 labeled with the enzyme modulator (H-M) compete for a limited amount of antibody.

$$H + H\text{-}M \underset{}{\overset{Ab}{\rightleftharpoons}} Ab:H + Ab:H\text{-}M$$

$$H\text{-}M + E \rightarrow H\text{-}M:E$$
$$\text{(inactive)}$$

As the concentration of T_4 increases, more H-M is left to complex with the free enzyme, which in this case is acetylcholinesterase. Decreases in enzyme activity are proportional to the concentration of unlabeled T_4.

Coenzymes and Prosthetic Group Labels. Coenzymes and enzyme prosthetic groups have also been used as labels for homogeneous EIAs (*44*). These assays can be illustrated as follows:

$$HL + HL\text{-}NAD + Ab \rightleftharpoons Ab:HL + Ab:HL\text{-}NAD$$

$$HL\text{-}NAD + A\text{-}E \rightarrow HL\text{-}E \begin{smallmatrix} S \\ \curvearrowright \\ P \end{smallmatrix}$$

As the concentration of unlabeled hormone ligand (HL) increases, more of the coenzyme-labeled hormone is left free to combine with an apoenzyme (A-E), thereby forming an enzymatically active holoenzyme. One sensitive homogeneous coenzyme immunoassay for plasma estriol uses an NAD-estriol conjugate and malic–alcoholic dehydrogenases (45). Interferences from endogenous coenzymes in serum or urine, however, tend to limit applications. Prosthetic groups such as flavin adenine dinucleotide (FAD) can also serve as labels, and homogeneous prosthetic group labeled EIAs (PGLEIAs) have been reported for low molecular weight analytes (e.g., theophylline) as well as for high molecular weight analytes (e.g., IgG) (46). Prosthetic group labels, however, have rarely been applied to hormone measurements.

Liposome Immunoassay. Another type of homogeneous enzyme immunoassay is based on the use of immunoreactive liposomes (47,48). Liposomes are artificial membrane vesicles consisting of a lipid bilayer that separates internal and external aqueous compartments. Liposomes can be designed to contain a wide variety of materials such as enzymes, dyes, or ions. Upon lysis of the liposome membrane, these materials can be released and used as markers in immunoassay systems. Liposome immunoassays (LIA) can be divided into two categories: complement dependent and complement independent. The principle of complement dependent LIA can be illustrated with a determination of serum thyroxine (49). In this assay, glucose-6-phosphate dehydrogenase is encapsulated in liposomes that are "sensitized" by attaching a T_4–phosphatidylethanolamine conjugate to the surface membrane. Unlabeled and liposomal-labeled molecules of T_4 compete for binding antibody. In the absence of serum T_4, the liposome-labeled antigen and antibody form a complex that can be lysed by complement, thus allowing entrapped marker enzymes access to substrate molecules. In the presence of T_4, more liposome-labeled antigen is left uncomplexed. Lysis does not occur, and enzyme activity decreases in proportion to the concentration of T_4 in the sample. This homogeneous T_4 assay was developed for use on both continuous-flow and discrete automated analyzers.

Many of the disadvantages associated with complement-dependent assays have been overcome by using cytolytic agents. In the complement-independent system, the antigen is labeled with a cytolysin (H-C), such as bee venom melittin, which is capable of lysing the liposomal membrane. As shown, free antigen and cytolysin-labeled antigen compete for available antibody.

$$H + H\text{-}C + Ab \rightleftarrows Ab{:}H + Ab{:}H\text{-}C$$

As H increases, less H-C is bound to the antibody, leaving more cytolysin-labeled antigen free to lyse the liposome.

$$H\text{-}C + E \rightarrow lysis \rightarrow E\underset{\rightarrow P}{\overset{S}{\diagdown}}$$

Release of the enzyme markers can then be measured spectrophotometrically using conventional substrates or potentiometrically using immunoselective electrodes.

Fluorescent Labels

Fluorescent labels are gaining increasing interest as alternatives to radioisotopes (50–53). To a great extent, initial development of fluorescence-based immunoassays was hampered by the decreased sensitivity caused by the high background fluorescence present in the measurement. However, recent improvements in fluorometers, fluorescent labels, and solid phase separation systems have significantly reduced the background noise such that fluorescence immunoassays now rival RIA methods for situations calling for high sensitivity.

Basis of Fluorescence Measurement

Luminescent molecules have the property of being able to absorb light at one wavelength and emit light at a longer wavelength. As shown in Figure 5, upon absorption of appropriate excitation energy, a luminescent molecule will emit light as fluorescence, as the molecule moves from the singlet (S_1) to the ground state (S_0), or as phosphorescence, as the molecule relaxes from the triplet (T_1) to the ground state. The energy that is lost in luminescence can be seen as the difference between the excitation and emission energy (wavelengths). This

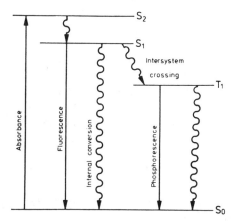

Figure 5. A Jablonski diagram illustrating the electronic energy levels and transitions in fluorescence and phosphorescence. [Reprinted with permission from the AACC from *Clinical Chemistry*. Volume 31 (1985), pg. 360, Figure 1. Copyright American Association for Clinical Chemistry, Inc.]

difference is referred to as the Stokes shift. Fluorescence usually has a small Stokes shift (30–50 nm), a relatively short lifetime (nanoseconds), and a high quantum yield (defined as the ratio of the number of emitted photons to the number of exciting photons). By contrast, phosphorescence has a lower quantum yield, a longer lifetime (milliseconds), and a larger Stokes shift.

Fluorescence measurements can be very sensitive. However, sensitivity may be limited because of high background problems resulting from light scattering, intrinsic background fluorescent signals, or quenching. High concentrations of proteins, lipids, or other large complexes are examples of major light-scattering interferences in serum. In these cases, scattering of excitation light occurs either from dissolved molecules (i.e., Rayleigh scattering) or from colloidal particles (i.e., Tyndall scattering). Since Rayleigh and Tyndall scattering have the same wavelength as the excitation light, it is often helpful if the excitation and emission wavelengths of fluorescent labels are well separated (i.e., large Stokes shifts); this prevents light scattering from contributing to the fluorescence seen at emission wavelengths.

High background fluorescent signals can also be caused by fluorescent compounds inherent in serum samples (e.g., bilirubin, NADH). Various procedures have been used to reduce this intrinsic background fluorescence: chemically pretreating the sample with peracetic or persulfuric acid, using blank measurements, or using fluorescent labels that have excitation and emission wavelengths far removed from the background noise.

Fluorescent signals can be quenched (decreased) as well as enhanced (increased) by a number of factors. For example, binding of fluorescent labels to serum proteins, or the presence of heavy atoms like iodine can impair fluorescence. Self-quenching can also occur, particularly if several fluorescent groups are relatively close together.

Choice of Fluorescent Labels

Fluorescent labels have requirements similar to radio- or enzyme labels in that they should be attached to hormone antigens or antibodies without significant loss of immunoreactivity. For optimal assay sensitivity, a fluorescent label should also have a high molar absorptivity and quantum yield. Moreover, the fluorescence emission should be distinguishable from background noise, and binding of the label to the immunoreactant should not quench the label's original fluorescence. Table 5 lists examples of fluorophores used as labels for hormone immunoassays. Of these, fluoroscein is currently the most popular for several reasons: (1) it has a high fluorescent intensity, (2) its fluorescence can be excited by several common light sources, (3) labeling techniques are simple, and (4) the shelf life of labeled antigen or antibody is

Table 5. Fluorescent Labels Commonly Used in FIA

Fluorophore	Excitation Wavelength (nm)	Emission Wavelength (nm)	Molar Absorptivity, ε (L/mol)	Decay Time (ns)
Fluorescein	492	520	70,000	4.5
Rhodamines	550	580	50,000	3.0
Umbelliferones	380	450	20,000	
Europium chelates	340	613	30,000	500,000

practically indefinite. Fluoroscein, however, has a small Stokes shift, and light scattering can be a problem. More importantly, serum bilirubin may contribute to the fluorescence background.

Among the interesting molecules that have been advocated recently for use in FIA are chelates of lanthanide rare earth ions, such as europium and terbium, and the polycyclic hydrocarbons, such as pyrene. These fluorescent probes are particularly attractive because of their extraordinarily large Stokes shifts. For example, the sharp emission peak of europium (613 nm) can be easily separated from scattering caused by the excitation light (340 nm) or from interfering substances in serum (400–600 nm). Another characteristic of these highly fluorescent lanthanide chelates is their very long fluorescent decay time (10^3–10^6 ns) compared to the fluorescence decay time of the background (1–20 ns) or other fluorophores such as fluorescein (4.5 ns) (54). Using time-resolved fluorometers, emission fluorescence is easily measured after a certain time has elapsed from the moment of excitation (Figure 6). For most applications, lanthanide ions are attached to specific antisera using polycarboxylic acids such as EDTA. Since, however, these labeled antibodies are essentially nonfluorescent, the lanthanide ion must be dissociated after the antigen–antibody reaction has taken place and then coupled to another chelating agent, such as a β-diketone, to produce intense fluorescence.

Heterogeneous FIAs. Heterogeneous FIAs involve a necessary separation of free and antibody-bound fractions for measurement. Separation techniques such as PEG or double-antibody precipitations are not used frequently. Instead, most assay systems make extensive use of solid phase separations. Solid phases permit convenient separation of free and bound fractions as well as removal of endogenous fluorophores or other interfering substances. In this way, most background problems can be directly avoided and assay sensitivity increased. A number of solid phase materials are widely used, including polyacrylamide beads, magnetizable cellulose particles, and cellulose

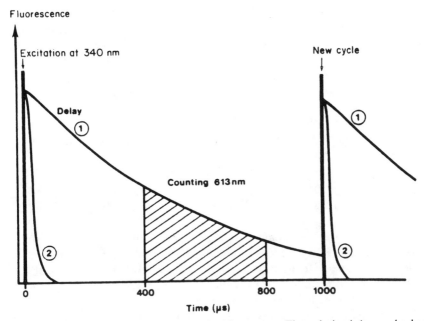

Figure 6. Measurement principle of time-resolved fluorescence. The cycle time is 1 ms and pulsed excitation less than 1 µs occurs at the beginning of each cycle. The delay time after the pulsed excitation is 400 µs, and the actual counting time within the cycle has the same duration. The total measurement time is 1 s. Curve 1 represents the fluorescence of an europium chelate and curve 2 the background fluorescence (actual decay time less than 1 µs). [From Lovgren L, et al. Time-resolved fluorometry in immunoassay, in Collins WP (ed): *Alternative Immunoassays.* New York: Wiley, 1985, p 205. Reprinted with permission of John Wiley & Sons, Ltd.]

acetate–nitrate dipsticks. Coated plastic tubes are generally not used because of optical problems.

Labeled Antigen. Heterogeneous FIAs employing labeled antigen have been developed as competitive or sequential procedures. In one competitive commercial system employed for measuring T_4 and cortisol, unlabeled hormone in the sample competes with fluorescein–labeled hormone for a limited amount of primary antibody (55). To separate the bound fluorescent tracer from the free label, a second-antibody precipitation technique is used. After incubation, the tubes are removed from the analyzer and centrifuged, and the supernatant containing the free fraction and other interfering factors is decanted. The tubes are then returned to the analyzer where the precipitate is automatically dissolved and the fluorescence of the resulting solution measured. As in competitive RIA, the fluorescent signal is inversely proportional to the amount of antigen present. A number of heterogeneous FIAs using antisera attached to polyacrylamide beads or magnetizable particles have been established for steroids such as cortisol, progesterone, and estriol, as well as T_3 and T_4 (*56–59*). The use of magnetizable particles is particularly convenient and eliminates the need for centrifugation.

Another development in separation FIAs has been the use of the sequential reagent addition technique in which addition of the label is delayed. In a sequential FIA for T_4 (*60*), serum is incubated with an excess of antibody covalently linked to magnetizable cellulose particles.

$$\begin{array}{l}{-}Ab\\{-}Ab\end{array} + H \rightleftarrows \begin{array}{l}{-}Ab\\{-}Ab:H\end{array} \xrightleftharpoons{\text{H-F}} \begin{array}{l}{-}Ab:H\text{-}F\\{-}Ab:H\end{array} + H\text{-}F$$

The bound antigen is separated by applying a magnetic field, and the supernatant containing endogenous fluorophores or other interfering compounds is aspirated to waste. Excess fluorescein-labeled T_4 is then added. Some become bound to the unoccupied antibody binding sites, and the remainder is left in the supernatant. The fluorescence of the labeled antigen remaining in the supernatant is measured and directly related to the amount of T_4 in the sample. Results correlate very closely with those using RIA techniques.

Labeled Antibody. Fluoroimmunoassays involving the use of labeled antibody are performed as sandwich-type assays or as solid phase competitive techniques. The same solid phases employed for labeled antigens can be used for labeled-antibody methods, thus providing easy washing and separation as well as reducing fluorescence background and light-scattering problems. One example of a solid phase, labeled-antibody competitive technique is the measurement of 17-β-estradiol (*61*). In this assay, immobilized estradiol competes with endogenous steroid in the sample for known amounts of antisera labeled with 4-methylumbelliferone. Following incubation, assay tubes are centrifuged, and aliquots of the supernatant are used for fluorescence measurement of the free labeled antibody. Sensitivity was only slightly less than RIA.

Recently, a competitive immunofluorometric assay (IFMA) was described for serum cortisol based on the time-resolved fluorescence technique (*62*). In this direct assay, cortisol present in serum samples competes with cortisol immobilized on the surface of microtiter strips for a limited amount of europium-labeled antibody. After washing, Eu^{3+} is released from the bound complex and a highly fluorescent europium chelate is formed. The fluorescent signal is inversely proportional to the amount of cortisol in the sample. The entire assay is carried out in 2 hours at room temperature. A similar competitive time-resolved immunofluorometric assay (TR-FIA) technique has been applied to the analysis of serum testosterone (63).

TR-FIAs of larger antigens such as TSH, PRL, hCG, and insulin are usually performed as sandwich-type assays. In a recent procedure for insulin (64), two different monoclonal antibodies were used. The first was immobilized on the surface of microtiter strips, and the other was labeled with Eu^{3+}. Standards or serum samples were first incubated at room temperature for 2 hours in the antibody-coated wells with europium-labeled antibody. The bound europium label was then dissociated from the solid surface with enhancement solution and the resulting fluorescence measured with a time-resolved fluorometer. The fluorescent signal was directly proportional to the concentration of insulin in the serum sample.

Some TR-FIAs are available as commercial kits under the trade name DELFIA (dissociation-enhanced lanthanide fluoroimmunoassay). For example, the TSH DELFIA is a two-site, solid phase immunofluorometric assay using microtiter strips as the solid phase (65). In this assay, two monoclonal antibodies are used: one is attached to the solid phase and directed against the β subunit of the TSH molecule, and the other is labeled with europium and directed against an antigenic determinant that overlaps both α and β subunits. Because of low cross-reactivity (hCG < 0.1%, hLH < 0.4%), the serum sample and the tracer could be added simultaneously to the assay wells. Only one incubation step was required, and assay time was less than 4 hours. Even so, the high sensitivity of the assay (0.03 μIU/mL) allowed TSH to be measured in serum of hyperthyroid patients.

Not all TR-FIAs use microtiter strips as the solid phase. In a recent procedure for prolactin (66), polystyrene tubes coated with monoclonal antibody to prolactin were used as a solid phase. In this case, a pulsed nitrogen laser was used to excite the europium.

Homogeneous FIAs. A variety of homogeneous fluorescence methods have been devised for detecting antigen–antibody reactions without separating the bound and free components. Most are competitive assays in which antigen–antibody binding changes a fluorescent property of the labeled immunoreactant. In general, homogeneous fluorescence assays are simple, requiring only one incubation step and no washing. However, the sensitivity of these assays is often limited by serum interferences.

Direct Quenching FIA. In certain cases, antibody binding decreases (quenches) the fluorescent signal. For example, in a homogeneous fluorescence quenching immunoassay described for cortisol (*67*), binding of fluorescein-labeled cortisol to antibody caused a decrease in the intensity of the fluorescent signal. Competition for antibody binding sites by unlabeled cortisol decreased the amount of fluorescein-labeled hormone, and fluorescence intensity increased. Although direct quenching FIA is simple and rapid, the degree of quenching depends on the nature of the hormone antigen. In general, this method is not applicable to large protein hormones. Another limitation of direct quenching FIAs is the dependence on electron donors near the antibody binding site. To avoid these restrictions, some methods amplify the fluorescence quenching effect by adding a quenching group to the antibody (e.g., fluorescence excitation transfer immunoassays), while others use antibodies directed against the fluorescent label itself (e.g., indirect quenching or fluorescence protection immunoassay).

Fluorescence Excitation Transfer Immunoassay (FETIA). Competitive immunoassays based on the principle of fluorescence excitation transfer are very useful for assaying antigens with multivalent antigenic determinents. Typically, two labels are used: fluorescein as the donor/fluorescer to label the antigen, and rhodamine as the acceptor/quencher to label the specific antibody. Because the emission spectrum of fluorescein overlaps the absorption spectrum of rhodamine, rhodamine is able to absorb the emission from fluorescein. Energy transfer, however, is a function of the donor–acceptor distance. When a fluorescein-labeled antigen binds to a rhodamine-labeled antibody, energy transfer can easily occur. As a result, the fluorescein label is quenched and the fluorescent signal decreases. Competition for antibody binding sites by unlabeled antigen, however, reverses this effect, and the amount of quenching is decreased.

$$H + H\text{-}F + Ab\langle^R_R \rightleftarrows Ab\langle^R_R : H\text{-}F + Ab\langle^R_R : H$$

(quenched)

The measured fluorescence intensity will increase and will be directly proportional to the concentration of unlabeled antigen. Homogeneous immunoassays based on this technique have been applied to both low and high molecular weight hormones such as thyroxine and TBG (*68*). Unlike the case of direct quenching FIA, a number of fluorescence excitation transfer immunoassays have been commercially developed.

Indirect Quenching FIA or Protection FIA. An entirely different approach to amplifying the fluorescence quenching effect employs three reagents: antibodies directed against a hormone antigen (Ab_L), a fluorescent-labeled antigen (H-F), and antibodies directed against the fluorescent label itself (Ab_F). If the sample does not contain free unlabeled antigen, the labeled antigen binds the specific antibody, thus sterically protecting the fluorescent label from binding to the quenching antibody. If unlabeled antigen is present, a competitive reaction occurs.

$$H + H\text{-}F + Ab_L \rightleftarrows Ab : H + Ab_L : H\text{-}F$$

$$H\text{-}F + Ab_F \rightleftarrows Ab_F : H\text{-}F$$
(quenched)

Less labeled antigen binds to Ab_L and more binds to Ab_F, quenching fluorescence. Low molecular weight molecules, such as T_4 (69), as well as macromolecules, have been measured using this method. Indirect quenching FIA, however, has not found wide use in endocrinology.

Fluorescence Enhancement Immunoassay. It is interesting that fluorescence quenching can be turned around with antigens such as T_4 and T_3, and actual enhancement of fluorescence can be produced upon binding of antibody (70). In one study, the fluorescence intensity of a fluorescein–T_4 conjugate was noted to be low, probably because of internal quenching of fluorescein by iodine atoms. When this conjugate was bound to antibody, however, a fourfold increase in fluorescence resulted, presumably due to partial inhibition of the quenching effects of the iodine atoms. This assay can be performed with a conventional fluorometer, and no separation step is required. Practical applications, however, are limited at present.

Fluorescence Polarization Immunoassay (FPIA). A simple but rapid and precise homogeneous FIA is based on the change in fluorescence polarization after an immunological reaction. For example, when a small, freely tumbling molecule such as a fluorescent-labeled antigen is excited with polarized light, the polarization of the emitted light will be low. When the fluorescent-labeled antigen is complexed with antibody, however, the molecule becomes much larger. Consequently,, molecular motion (Brownian rotation) is slowed and the fluorescence polarization is enhanced. When unlabeled antigen is added, the free form of the labeled antigen with its rapid movement is increased, and the fluorescence polarization is decreased. Thus, the degree of polarization varies inversely with the amount of unlabeled antigen added.

FPIAs have been described for a number of hormones, including serum T_4, serum and urine cortisol, insulin, hCG, 17β-estradiol, and estriol (71–75). An instrument for conveniently measuring fluorescence polarization in the clinical laboratory has also been developed and is commercially available. Although FPIA is simple and rapid for small antigens, it is generally not suitable for hormones with molecular weights above 20,000. For large antigens, antigen–antibody binding will not result in a marked increase in effective size, and a change in fluorescence polarization may not be detectable. Because Brownian rotation is influenced by factors such as temperature and viscosity, assay conditions must be strictly controlled. The sensitivity of FPIA is generally limited to the micromolar range, and its linear range is often narrow. Because FPIA is prone to a number of interferences (e.g., hemolysis, bilirubin), sample blanks or correction factors may also be necessary.

Chemiluminescent and Bioluminescent Labels

Chemiluminescence and bioluminescence may be defined as the chemical production of visible light. Here the free energy of a chemical reaction supplies the energy required to produce molecules in an excited state. Visible light is then emitted as these excited molecules return to the ground state. Chemiluminescence and bioluminescence are collectively referred to as luminescence, and instruments for measuring light emission are known as luminometers. Luminescent reactions derived from biological systems are referred to as bioluminescence.

In recent years the feasibility of using chemiluminescent and bioluminescent molecules as labels for hormone immunoassays has been demonstrated (76–81). It is possible to distinguish three different types of luminescent immunoassay. The first category involves the direct labeling of antigens or antibodies with luminescent molecules. The second category involves the labeling of immunoreactants with catalysts or cofactors of luminescent reactions. The third category involves the use of luminescence to analyze the product generated by an enzyme label.

Lumigenic Labels

Both chemiluminescent and bioluminescent compounds have been used to tag the antigen or antibody. In early work, luminol (5-aminophthalhydrazide) was used as the probe, and the amount of free or bound label was determined by initiating the chemiluminescent reaction and measuring the light that was produced. As the scheme illustrates, light is produced when luminol is treated with an oxidizing reagent such as H_2O_2 under basic conditions in the presence of a suitable metal catalyst. The catalyst may vary from transition metal cations like Mn^{2+} and Ni^{2+} to heme-containing compounds like horseradish peroxidase. Currently, one of the most widely used catalysts is microperoxidase, a proteolytic product of cytochrome C. Although the light-emitting reactions of luminol itself are efficient, loss of chemiluminescence often occurs when luminol is attached to antigens or antibodies. For this reason, luminescent labels such as isoluminol (6-aminophthalhydrazide) have been designed. For isoluminol derivatives, coupling to antigen or antibody actually enhances light output.

In recent work, interest in chemiluminescent molecules known as acridinium esters has been increasing. Unlike luminol or isoluminol, aromatic acridinium esters do not require a catalyst for the light-emitting reaction to occur.

The nature of this reaction is such that oxidative cleavage results in an excited product molecule, n-methylacridone, being formed from the parent molecule prior to light emission. This feature minimizes serious quenching when acridinium esters are attached to antigens or antibodies.

The general design of hormone immunoassay systems using lumigenic labels is the same as that used in other immunoassays. Both heterogeneous (separation required) and homogeneous (nonseparation) methods have been described.

Heterogeneous Assays. Separation of bound and free fractions can be achieved using liquid or solid phase methods. Liquid phase methods often include second antibody or dextran-coated charcoal. A variety of solid phase supports have also been used in which the immunoreactant either is absorbed to polystyrene or polypropylene tubes or polystyrene balls, or is covalently linked to polyacrylamide beads, plastic microspheres, magnetic particles, or microcrystalline cellulose. Coated tubes and magnetized particles are particularly convenient, since they eliminate the need for centrifugation.

Labeled Antigen. Almost all labeled antigen assays involve aminobutylethylisoluminol (ABEI) and competitive binding formats. Some use liquid phase separations to measure plasma hormone levels (e.g., progesterone, estradiol, testosterone, cortisol) (*82–84*). Most, however, use solid phase supports. Measurements of progesterone, estradiol, and testosterone in plasma, as well as estriol, estrone, and pregnanediol in urine, are examples of steroid hormones included in this group of solid phase heterogeneous chemiluminescent immunoassays (*85–87*).

One of the most significant advances in hormone (immunoassays has been the development of procedures using unextracted serum or plasma. Recently, methods have been reported for the direct measurement of cortisol, progesterone, and estradiol in plasma using steroid–isoluminol conjugates (*88–90*). In the direct solid phase chemiluminescent assay for serum progesterone, danazol displaced progesterone from endogenous binding proteins, and polyacrylamide beads covalently coupled to progesterone antibody served as the solid phase. Delayed (sequential) addition of the label contributed to the sensitivity of this assay (1.7 pg/tube).

In addition to steroid haptens, competitive binding chemiluminescent assays have also been developed for polypeptide hormones such as hCG and LH (*91,92*). Solid phase separation techniques were used in both cases, and derivatives of isoluminol were used to label the antigens.

In all the chemiluminescent immunoassays discussed so far, the actual light measurement was preceded by incubation with sodium hydroxide at high temperature. This step is necessary because luminol and isoluminol have low quantum yields, and the antigen–antibody complex must be dissociated before the chemiluminescent reaction is initiated, to enhance sensitivity. As noted previously, acridinium esters do not require a dissociation step.

Recently, a progesterone acridinium ester has been synthesized and used as the labeled antigen in a solid phase chemiluminescent immunoassay (93).

Labeled Antibody. Heterogeneous methods for measuring hormones using chemiluminescent-labeled antibodies have also been described. Both competitive and noncompetitive formats are used. An example of the former is the solid phase antigen luminescence technique (SPALT). In this assay unlabeled hormone in the test sample and solid phase coupled antigen compete for antigen-specific antibody. Excess second antibody labeled with isoluminol is used as a "universal" indicator. After washing, the bound fraction is reacted with sodium hydroxide, whereupon chemiluminescence is initiated with microperoxidase and hydrogen peroxide. Immunoassays based on this technique have been developed for hormones such as hCG, LH, FSH, and prolactin (94). To date, wider interest in this approach has been limited by the availability of appropriate solid phase antigens.

Labeled antibody procedures have also been applied to the development of several immunochemiluminometric assays (ICMA) for polypeptide and peptide amine hormones. For example, a two-site sandwich assay for serum TSH was recently developed that employs two TSH monoclonal antibodies (95). One was labeled with an acridinium ester and the other was immobilized onto magnetic particles. After simultaneous incubation of serum with both monoclonal antibodies, separation of bound and free label was effected magnetically. The standard curve was linear between 0.3 and 100 mIU/mL, and detection sensitivity was less than 0.1 μIU/mL. ICMAs for the measurement of hCG and thyroxine have also been developed (91,96).

Homogeneous Assays. Homogeneous luminescent immunoassays do not require the separation of bound from free label before the chemiluminescent reaction is initiated. These homogeneous assays are based on the fact that binding of labeled antigen to its specific antibody actually enhances total light production. This process is inhibited in a competitive manner by addition of unlabeled hormone. Assays based on this principle have been developed for progesterone, cortisol and estriol in serum, and estriol glucuronide in urine (97–100). Assay sensitivity equal to or greater than RIA can be obtained; however, these assays are often affected by interferences present in serum or urine.

Recently, a unique homogeneous chemiluminescent immunoassay was used to measure serum progesterone (101). This assay is based on the observation that isoluminol-labeled antigen bound to fluorescein-labeled antibody transfers its energy to fluorescein and yields green emission. However, if isoluminol-labeled antigen does not bind to fluorescent-labeled antibody, blue chemiluminescent light is produced. The amount of chemi-luminescent label bound to the fluorescent antibody was determined by simultaneously measuring chemiluminescence at two wavelengths.

Catalysts or Cofactor Labels

Catalysts or cofactors of luminescent reactions have often been employed as labels in immunoassays. Of the various compounds used as catalytic labels in reactions involving luminol, only peroxidase has been applied to hormone measurements. The amount of peroxidase-labeled antigen or antibody may be determined by adding excess luminol/H_2O_2 and measuring steady-state chemiluminescence. Such systems are often referred to as "enhanced lumine-scence" assays.

Labeled Antigen. Enhanced luminescent immunoassays have been described for the measurement of T_4, T_3, and T_3 uptake, and cortisol (*102,103*). In the case of the thyroid haptens, the test sample and a hapten–horseradish peroxidase conjugate are reacted with first antibody in microtiter wells coated with second antibody. After one hour, the wells are washed, luminol/H_2O_2 is added, and the luminescence measured.

Labeled Antibody. Quantitative immunometric assays based on enhanced luminescence have also been reported for several glycoprotein hormones, including hCG, LH, and TSH (*104–106*). These heterogeneous assays use microtiter wells coated with primary monoclonal antibody. Test sample is added and incubated, and after washing, second antibody conjugated to horseradish peroxidase is added. Following washing and incubation, a signal reagent is added and the luminescence read.

Cofactors of bioluminescent reactions may also be used as labels. For example, homogeneous assays for urinary estriol and plasma progesterone have been developed using NAD^+ as the cofactor label (*107*). After enzyme reduction, labeled steroids (H-NADH) are quantitated using the bacterial luciferase system.

$$\text{H-NADH} + \text{FMN} \xrightarrow{\text{oxidoreductase}} \text{H-NAD} + \text{FMNH}_2$$

$$\text{FMNH}_2 + \text{RCHO} + \text{O}_2 \xrightarrow[\text{luciferase}]{\text{bacterial}} \text{FMN} + \text{RCO}_2\text{H} + \text{light}$$

The basis of this competitive assay is the reduction (estriol) or enhancement (progesterone) in bioluminescence when the steroid–cofactor conjugate is bound to specific antibody. In the presence of unlabeled hormone, these changes in light yield are reversed. Unfortunately, it is difficult to couple cofactors to hormone antigens or antibodies. This technique also lacks sensitivity and is difficult to apply to serum or urine.

Enzyme Labels

Chemiluminescence and bioluminescence may be used to analyze the product generated by an enzyme label. For example, pyruvate kinase has been used as a label in a bioluminescent assay for insulin (*108*). ADP and phosphoenol pyruvate were chosen as substrates. The ATP produced was then monitored by the firefly reaction:

$$ATP + luciferin + O_2 \xrightarrow[Mg^{2+}]{firefly\ luciferase} oxyluciferin + AMP + PP$$
$$+ CO_2 + light$$

A chemiluminescent enzyme immunoassay for the measurement of 17α-hydroxyprogesterone has also been reported using glucose oxidase as the label (*109*). In this case, the hydrogen peroxide that was formed was detected using an oxalate ester–fluorophore system.

Protein Labels

Most nonlabeled hormone immunoassays are limited to measuring multivalent antigens such as peptides or proteins. High concentrations of these proteins are also needed to increase the size of the immune complex until it becomes able to form a precipitin line or to scatter light. Consequently, sensitivity problems have prevented nonlabeled methods from exerting a major impact on hormone analysis. However, by labeling low molecular weight hormones with large proteins such as bovine serum albumin or ferritin, light-scattering techniques can be made more attractive. For example, a light-scattering immunoassay using a hormone–protein conjugate has been described for progesterone (*110*). In this assay, unlabeled hormone and protein-labeled hormone compete for a limited amount of antibody. As the free hormone increases, immune complex formation decreases. The resulting decrease in light scattering is related to the concentration of free hormone. When nephelometry is used to measure the changes in light scattering, this agglutination assay is referred to as nephelometric inhibition immunoassay (NINIA). Although sensitivity and precision of NINIA for low molecular

Table 6. Particle-Enhanced Light-Scattering Techniques

Direct agglutination
Particle counting
Turbidimetric agglutination inhibition
Quasi-elastic scattering
Anisotropic scattering

weight hormones generally are greater than those of the corresponding direct agglutination assay, applications remain limited to hormones present in relatively high concentrations in serum or urine.

Particle Labels

Agglutination assays have been used for many years for qualitative and quantitative measurements of hormone antigens. Even when large carrier proteins are used as labels, high concentrations of hormone are generally necessary for agglutinated products to become visible or able to scatter light. To increase assay sensitivity, the size of the immune complex can be conveniently increased by labeling the antigen or antibody with various inert particles such as red blood cells, polystyrene (latex) particles, dyes, or sols. Over the years a number of particle-enhanced methods have been developed using agglutination and agglutination inhibition formats. For qualitative work, visual observation of the agglutination process is usually sufficient; for quantitative immunoassays, a wide range of light-scattering techniques has been employed (Table 6).

Erythrocytes and Latex

For several years red blood cells and latex particles have served as labels for a large number of immunoassays involving visible detection of agglutination or agglutination inhibition reactions. These particles can be coated (sensitized) with antigens or antibodies in a variety of ways. RBCs, for example, can be sensitized by direct adsorption of antigen or antibody, by covalent chemical attachment of immunoreactants, or by using cells treated with tannic acid.

Erythrocytes and latex particles have formed the basis for a number of qualitative immunoassays, particularly urinary hCG pregnancy tests (111). These tests are generally rapid, inexpensive, and accurate. Also, they can be conveniently conducted on glass slides or in test tubes. Currently, most slide and tube test assays for urinary hCG use agglutination inhibition procedures.

In the slide test, for example, hCG-coated latex particles are mixed with urine and anti-hCG antibodies. If hCG is not present, the hCG–latex particles combine with the antiserum and cause agglutination (i.e., negative test). If hCG is present, the hormone combines with and neutralizes the antiserum, thereby inhibiting particle agglutination (i.e., positive test). Tube tests, on the other hand, use hCG-coated erythrocytes rather than latex as particle reagents. If hCG is present in the urine, hemagglutination does not occur, and the RBCs settle to the bottom of the tube forming a visible ring (positive test). Unlike slide tests, which require only a couple of minutes to perform, tube tests may take up to 2 hours to complete. Several commercial urinary hCG assays are available. Most, however, are only qualitative, and many do not detect hCG levels below 1000–2000 IU/L; thus, early or abnormal pregnancies may be missed.

Because they can be easily made and are readily available, latex particles have also been used in a number of sensitive quantitative immunoassays (see Table 6). For example, a particle-enhanced direct agglutination assay has been described for hCG (112). In this case, agglutination between the latex-labeled hormone and the corresponding antibody was followed using a light-scattering technique such as turbidity.

Quantitative particle-enhanced procedures based on particle counting (particle counting immunoassay, PACIA) are much more common than direct agglutination assays. In early configurations, latex particles coated with specific antibody were incubated with hormone antigen, and the decrease in the number of particles lost by agglutination was determined using an instrument that counts blood cells. In later work, particle counting assays were developed using agglutination inhibition reactions. For example, in a test for T_4 two particle reagents were used: anti-T_4 attached to latex particles (Ab-L) and T_4 antigen coupled to dextran (T_4-D) (113). In the absence of free hormone, antigen and antibody particles agglutinate; but in the presence of increasing amounts of free T_4, binding sites on the antibody particle are blocked, and agglutination with the dextran-labeled hormone is inhibited. The number of unagglutinated antigen particles is counted and related to the amount of added hormone. Assay sensitivity was 10 μg/L, comparable to RIA. Automated PACIA systems have been reported for other hormones such as hCG and growth hormone (114,115).

Particle-enhanced immunoassays involving turbidimetric measurements have also been described (particle-enhanced turbidimetric agglutination inhibition immunoassay, PETINIA). In a test for T_4, the rate of agglutination between a T_4–Ficoll conjugate and a latex-coupled T_4 antibody in the presence of serum T_4 was measured turbidimetrically at 600 nm; T_4 in the specimen inhibited agglutination competitively. An automated method using this system is available commercially.

A more sophisticated light-scattering method using latex particle reagents has also been described. Known as quasi-elastic light-scattering immunoassy (QLS), this laser light-scattering technique measures the mean diffusion constant of agglutinated particles. This constant is then used to calculate hormone concentration. QLS inhibition immunoassays have been developed for hCG and LH (*116*). Assay sensitivity for both hormones was 1 ng/mL, comparable with RIA methods. By measuring the angular anisotropy of the scattered laser light, sensitivity could be further increased to 0.1 ng/mL.

Sols

Sol particles (sols) are colloidal suspensions of inorganic metals such as gold and silver, or organic compounds such as dyes. Recently, sol particles have been used as labels for quantitative immunoassays (SPIA) in homogeneous agglutination assays as well as in heterogeneous sandwich assays. Sol suspensions are often associated with intense colors that vary with particle size; thus, colorimetry can often be used for detection. Carbon rod atomic absorption spectrophotometry has also been used to detect sols, with sensitivity often equal to that of radioisotopes.

A homogeneous (separation-free) assay for urinary hCG has been described using gold sol particles (*117*). In this assay, gold particles coated with antibody were added to the urine sample and incubated for a fixed time; then the color was assessed either visually (qualitative test) or spectrophotometrically (quantitative test). If hCG is present, the antibody–gold particles agglutinate and the absorbance at 540 nm decreases. A sensitivity of 100 IU/L was reported.

Sol labels have also been applied to heterogeneous sandwich assays. Both colloidal inorganic metals and disperse organic dyes have been used. In a typical sandwich assay the sample is first incubated with excess antibody covalently linked to microtiter plates. After incubation and washing, a second antibody labeled with a gold sol or dye is added and the mixture incubated. After further washing, the label bound to the microtiter wells is redispersed (gold sol) or dissolved (dye) and the absorbance read in a spectrophotometer. Sandwich assays for hCG and human placental lactogen (hPL) have been described (*118*). By labeling anti-hCG with gold sol and anti-hPL with silver sol, both hormones could be determined simultaneously in a single sample using atomic absorption spectrophotometry.

Metal Labels

Metal atoms have been used as labels in heterogeneous assays for steroid hormones such as estrone, estradiol, and estriol (*119*). Some of the metal ions that have been used include iron, mercury, cobalt, and platinum. In these immunoassays, metal-labeled antigen and unlabeled antigen competitively react with antibody. After separation of bound and free fractions, the metal content is measured using emission, absorption, or fluorescence spectrometry, electrochemical methods, or neutron activation. To date, most metal immunoassays lack sensitivity and require complex detection systems. Consequently, these assays have not enjoyed wide acceptance in the endocrine laboratory.

Bacteriophage Labels

Homogeneous immunoassays employing bacteriophage viruses as labels have been developed for several steroid and peptide hormones, such as estradiol, progesterone, aldosterone, and insulin (120,121). If a suitable culture is infected with bacteriophage viruses, the bacterial cells will die, and plaques will form. It is possible, however, to inactivate the plaque-forming activity of the bacteriophages by attaching antigen molecules to the surface of the virus and reacting the product with antigen-specific antibody. Immunoassays based on competitive inactivation of bacteriophage-labeled antigen with antigen-specific antibodies are known as viroimmunoassays. Bacteriophage-labeled hormone, unlabeled hormone, and antibody are incubated and then mixed with E. coli. The mixtures are plated and the plaques counted several hours later. Compared with corresponding RIAs, viroimmunoassays for estradiol and progesterone were three-fold more sensitive. These bacteriophage-labeled procedures, however, are complex and are not widely used as routine clinical assays. Other methods for measuring lysis of host bacteria are available and have been shown to be useful alternatives to these tedious plating assays (122).

Free-Radical Labels

Atoms or compounds containing unpaired electrons (e.g., free radicals or other paramagnetic species) have also been used as labels in homogeneous hormone immunoassays (123). When placed in a magnetic field and irradiated with electromagnetic radiation, free radicals absorb and scatter energy by resonance as the unpaired electrons go from one spin state to another. Immunoassays based on electron spin resonance (ESR) spectrometry take advantage of the fact that antigens labeled with unpaired electrons give a different resonance signal when bound to antibody than when free. Homogeneous immunoassays based on the use of these "spin" labels are also known as spin immunoassays (SIA) and have been described for steroids such as progesterone and testosterone (124,125). Direct measurement of spin-labeled compounds lack sensitivity. To amplify the spin signal, compounds containing unpaired electrons have also been incorporated into liposomes (126).

IMMUNOSELECTIVE ELECTRODES

One of the newest developments in immunoassay technology involves the use of immunoselective electrodes. Earlier in this discussion we noted the development of homogeneous liposome enzyme immunoassays (LIA) using electrodes (see "Enzyme Labels"). Other hormone immunoassays that use electrochemical sensors have also been reported. For example, a competitive enzyme immunoassay using an iodide-selective electrode has been developed for 17β-estradiol (127). In this method, unlabeled hormone in the test sample competed with an estradiol–horseradish peroxidase conjugate for a limited quantity of antibody immobilized on an artificial protein membrane. After incubation, the membrane was placed on the surface of an iodide-sensitive electrode. Enzyme activity was then evaluated in the presence of KI and H_2O_2 substrates. Variations of electrode potentials were recorded as a function of time and noted to be proportional to enzymatic oxidation of iodide.

Potentiometric immunoassay sensors have also been applied to measurements of cortisol and hCG. In the case of cortisol, the unlabeled steroid is first incubated with specific antibody followed by the addition of cortisol labeled with asparaginase, a deaminating enzyme (128). After further incubation, a second antibody immobilized on agarose beads is used to precipitate the immune complex. After washing and centrifugation, an ammonia gas-sensing membrane electrode is immersed into a resuspension of the immune complex. Asparagine is then used to start the enzyme reaction.

For hCG, a direct immunosensor was used in which specific antibody was chemically fixed to a titanium wire. When this electrode was immersed into a solution containing free hCG, there occurred at the probe's tip an antigen–antibody binding reaction, which was converted into an electrical impulse. Steady-state potentials were noted to occur after about 10 minutes. Even with careful control of pH, temperature, and ionic strength, assay sensitivity using this electrode was generally insufficient for clinical use.

CONCLUSION

Immunoassays play a leading role in the routine determination of hormones in biological fluids. Most assay systems continue to use radioisotopes to monitor the immunological reaction, but in recent years a number of nonisotopic procedures have challenged the sensitivity, precision, wide applicability, and overall ruggedness of traditional RIAs. There is little doubt that nonisotopic assays will eventually replace most radioligand assays in the clinical laboratory.

REFERENCES

1. Rock RC, Perlstein MT. Monoclonal antibodies in endocrinology: Principles and selected applications, in Gordon DS (ed): *Monoclonal Antibodies in Clinical Diagnostic Medicine*. New York: Igaku-Shoin, 1985, pp 159–167.
2. Sevier ED, David GS, Martinis J, Desmond WJ, Bartholomew RM, Wang R. Monoclonal antibodies in clinical immunology. *Clin Chem* 1981;27:1797–1806.
3. Miles LEM, Hales CN. *Nature* 1968;219:186–189.
4. Kang J, Kaladas P, Chang C, et al. A highly sensitive immunoenzymometric assay involving "common capture" particles and membrane filtration. *Clin Chem* 1986;32:1682–1686.
5. Dwenger A. Radioimmunoassay: An overview. *J. Clin Chem Clin Biochem* 1984;22:883–894.
6. Greenwood FC, Hunter WM, Glover JS. The preparation of ^{131}I-labeled human growth hormone of high specific activity. *Biochem J* 1963;89:114–123.
7. Marchalonis JJ. An enzymatic method for the trace iodination of immunoglobulins and other proteins. *Biochem J* 1969;113:299–305.
8. Bolton AE, Hunter WM. The labeling of proteins to high specific radioactivities by conjugation to a ^{125}I-containing acylating agent. *Biochem J* 1973;133:529–539.
9. Corrie JET. [125]Iodinated tracers for steroid radioimmunoassay: The problem of bridge recognition, in Hunter WM, Corrie JET (eds): *Immunoassays for Clinical Chemistry*. Edinburgh: Churchill & Livingstone, 1983, pp 353–357.
10. Thorell JI. Internal sample attenuator counting (ISAC). A new technique for separating and measuring bound and free activity in radioimmunoassay. *Clin Chem* 1981;27:1969–1973.
11. Hunter WM, Corrie JET (eds). *Immunoassays for Clinical Chemistry*. Edinburgh: Churchill & Livingstone, 1983.
12. Lane KW (ed). Gold book. Directory and buyer's guide. *Lab Manage* (special issue) 1987;25(2):1–92.
13. Chattoraj SC, Watts NB. Endocrinology, in Tietz NW (ed): *Textbook of Clinical Chemistry*. Philadelphia: Saunders, 1986, pp 997–1171.
14. Klee GC, Hay ID. Assessment of sensitive thyrotropin assays for an expanded role in thyroid function testing: Proposed criteria for analytical performance and clinical utility. *J Clin Endocrinol Methods* 1987;64:461–471.
15. Chen I-W. Commercially available fully automated systems for radioligand assay. Part 1. Overview. *Ligand Rev* 1980;2(2):46–50.

16. Beinlich CJ, Piper JA, O'Neal JC, White OD. Evaluation of dual-label simultaneous assays for lutropin and follitropin in serum. *Clin Chem* 1985;31:2014–2018.

17. Avrameas S. Heterogenous enzyme immunoassays, in Voller A, Bartlett A, Bidwell D (eds): *Immunoassays for the 80s*. Baltimore: University Park Press, 1981, pp 85–90.

18. Riad-Fahmy, Read GF, Joyce BG, Walker RF. Steroid immunoassays in endocrinology, in Voller A, Bartlett A, Bidwell D (eds): *Immunoassays for the 80s*. Baltimore: University Park Press, 1981, pp 205–261.

19a. Castro A, Monji N. Steric hindrance enzyme immunoassay (SHEIA), in Ngo T, Lenhoff H (eds): *Enzyme-Mediated Immunoassays*. New York: Plenum, 1985, pp 291–298.

19b. Ngo TT, Lenhoff HM. Enzyme immunoassays using tagged enzyme-ligand conjugates, in Ngo T, Lenhoff H (eds): *Enzyme-Mediated Immunoassays*. New York: Plenum, 1985, pp 313–323.

20. Yorde DE, Sasse EA, Wang TY, Hussa RO, Garancis JC. Competitive enzyme-linked immunoassay with use of soluble enzyme/antibody immune complexes for labeling. *Clin Chem* 1976;22:1372–1377.

21. Yorde DE, Pluta PE, Sassa EA. Competitive enzyme-linked immunoassay with the use of soluble enzyme/antibody immune complex for labeling, in Pal S (ed): *Proceedings of an International Symposium on Enzyme-Labeled Immunoassay of Hormones and Drugs*. Berlin: Walter de Gruyter, 1978, pp 359ff.

22. Gnemmi E, O'Sullivan MJ, Chieregatti G, Simmons M, Simmonds A, Bridges JW, Mark V. A sensitive immunoenzymometric assay (IEMA) to quantitate hormones and drugs, in Pal S (ed): *Proceedings of an International Symposium on Enzyme Labeled Immunoassays of Hormones and Drugs*. Berlin: Walter de Gruyter, 1978, pp 29–41.

23. Fitzgerald K, Pepin K, Simon F. A simultaneous immunoenzymetric assay (IEMA) for the quantitative/qualitative measurement of hCG in serum. *Clin Chem* 1986;32:1157(A 531).

24. Braunstein GD, Kelley L, Farber S, Sigall ER, Wade ME. Two rapid, sensitive, and specific immunoenzymatic assays of human choriogonadotropin in urine evaluated. *Clin Chem* 1986;32:1413–1414.

25. Parenti L, Vallejo R, Simon F, Yeh S. A simultaneous immunoenzymetric assay (IEMA) for human luteinizing hormone in serum. *Clin Chem* 1986;32:1167 (A 580).

26. Pekary AE, Turner LF, Hershman JM. New immunoenzymatic assay for human thyrotropin compared with two radioimmunoassays. *Clin Chem* 1986;32:511–514.

27. Wada HG, Danisck RJ, Baxter SR, Federici MM, Fraser RC, Brownmiller LJ, Lankford JC. Enzyme immunoassay of glycoprotein tropic hormones—choriogonadotropin, lutropin, thyrotropin—with solid-phase monoclonal antibody for the α-subunit and enzyme-coupled monoclonal antibody specific for the β-subunit. *Clin Chem* 1982;28:1862–1866.

28. DeTuri MP, Coleman PF, Haden B. Solid-phase enzyme immunoassay for the quantitation of prolactin in human serum. *Clin Chem* 1986;32:1156(A 524).

29. Franken N, Haug H, Deeg R, Wahlefeld A. A new one-step enzyme immunoassay for insulin. *Clin Chem* 1986;32:1066(A 082).

30. Baxter SR, Rundle DD, Lankford JC, Wada HG. A dipstick enzyme immunoassay for visual detection of choriogonadotropin. *Clin Chem* 1983;29:1192(A 131).

31. Kasper KC, Rodrick-Highberg G, Wada HG. Dipstick enzyme immunoassay for human luteinizing hormone in urine. *Clin Chem* 1983;29:1192(A 132).

32. Clark PMS, Price CP. Enzyme-amplified immunoassays: A new ultrasensitive assay of thyrotropin evaluated. *Clin Chem* 1986;32:88–92.

33. Giegel JL. Radial partition enzyme immunoassay, in Ngo TT, Lenhoff HF (eds): *Enzyme-Mediated Immunoassay*. New York: Plenum, 1985, pp 343–362.

34. Rugg JA, Rige CT. Leung K, Lamar SL, Welsh M, Le Blanc M, Evans SA. Radial partition immunoassay applied to automated quantification of human choriogonadotropin with use of two monoclonal antibodies. *Clin Chem* 1986;32:1844–1848.

35. Soto A, Morejon C, Delgado J, Chirte J, Gil P, Singh P, Ni WC. Radial partition immunoassay for thyroxin. *Clin Chem* 1986;32:1165(A 573).

36. Crowe CP, Gibbons I, Schneider RS. Recent advances in homogeneous enzyme immunoassays for haptens and proteins, in Nakamura RM, Dito WR, Tucker ES (eds): *Immunoassays: Clinical Laboratory Techniques for the 1980s*. New York: Liss, 1980, pp 89–126.

37. Van Lente F, Galen RS. Determination of thyroxine by enzyme-immunoassay, in Maggio ET (ed): *Enzyme-Immunoassay*. Boca Raton, FL: CRC Press, 1980, pp 135–153.

38. Gibbons I. Nonseparation enzyme immunoassays for macromolecules, in Ngo TT, Lenhoff HF (eds): *Enzyme-Mediated Immunoassays*. New York: Plenum, 1985, pp 121–143.

39. Litman DJ. Test strip enzyme immunoassay, in Ngo TT, Lenhoff HF (eds): *Enzyme-Mediated Immunoassays*. New York: Plenum, 1985, pp 155–190.

40. Chen R, Weng L, Sizto N, Osorio B, Hsu C-J, Rodgers R, Litman D. Ultrasound-accelerated immunoassay, as exemplified by enzyme immunoassay of choriogonadotropin. *Clin Chem* 1984;30:1446–1451.

41. Ngo TT, Wong RC. Fluorogenic substrate labeled separation-free enzyme-mediated immunoassays for haptens and macromolecules, in Ngo TT, Lenhoff HF (eds): *Enzyme-Mediated Immunoassays*. New York: Plenum, 1985, pp 85–110.

42. Ngo TT. Enzyme modulator as label in separation-free immunoassays: Enzyme modulator mediated immunoassay (EMMIA), in Ngo TT, Lenhoff HF (eds): *Enzyme-Mediated Immunoassays*. New York: Plenum, 1985, pp 57–72.

43. Finley PR, Williams RJ, Linchti DA. Evaluation of new homogeneous enzyme inhibitor immunoassay of serum thyroxine with use of bichromatic analyzer. *Clin Chem* 1980;26:1723–1726.

44. Miyai K. Advances in nonisotopic immunoassay. *Adv Clin Chem* 1985;24:61–110.

45. Kohen F, Hollander Z, Yeager FM, Carrico RJ, Boguslaski RC. A homogeneous EIA for oestriol monitored by co-enzymatic cycling reactions, in Pal S (ed):

Proceedings of an International Symposium on Enzyme Labeled Immunoassay of Hormones and Drugs. Berlin: Walter de Gruyter, 1978, pp 67–79.

46. Ngo TT. Prosthetic group labeled enzyme immunoassay, in Ngo TT, Lenhoff HM (eds): *Enzyme-Mediated Immunoassay*. New York: Plenum, 1985, pp 73–84.

47. Monroe D. Liposome immunoassay: A new ultrasensitive analytical method. *Am Clin Prod Rev* 1987;5(12):34–41.

48. Litchfield WJ, Freytag JW. Liposome-entrapped enzyme mediated immunoassays, in Ngo TT, Lenhoff HF (eds): *Enzyme-Mediated Immunoassays*. New York: Plenum, 1985, pp 145–154.

49. Piran U, Uretsky L, Law SJ, Stastny M. Homogeneous liposome immunoassay for thyroxine on automated chemistry analyzers. *Clin Chem* 1986;32:1167 (A 582).

50. Hemmila I. Fluoroimmunoassays and immunofluorometric assays. *Clin Chem* 1985;31:359–370.

51. Nakamura RM. Advances in analytical fluorescence immunoassays: Methods and clinical applications, in Nakamura RM, Dito WR, Tucker ES (eds): *Clinical Laboratory Assays*. New York: Masson, 1983, pp 33–60.

52. Landon J, Kamel RS. Immunoassays employing reactants labeled with fluorophore, in Voller A, Bartlett A, Bidwell D (eds): *Immunoassays for the 80s*. Baltimore: University Park Press, 1981, pp 91–112.

53. Sidki AM, Landon J. Fluoroimmunoassays and phosphoroimmunoassays, in Collins WP (ed): *Alternative Immunoassays*. New York: Wiley, 1985, pp 185–201.

54. Lovgren T, Hemmila I, Petterson K, Halolnen P. Time-resolved fluorometry in immunoassay, in Collins WP (ed): *Alternative Immunoassays*. New York: Wiley, 1985, pp 203–217.

55. Brinkley M. An automated high sensitivity fluorescence immunoassay system. *Am Clin Prod Rev* 1986;5(1):32–35.

56. Curry RE, Heitzman H, Riege DH, Sweet RV, Simonsen MG. A systems approach to fluorescent immunoassay: General principles and representative applications. *Clin Chem* 1979;25:1591–1595.

57. Pourfarzaneh M, White GW, Landon J, Smith DS. Cortisol directly determined in serum by fluoroimmunoassay with magnetizable solid phase. *Clin Chem* 1980;26:730–733.

58. Allma BL, Shot F, James VHT. Fluoroimmunoassay of progesterone in human serum of plasma. *Clin Chem* 1981;27:1176–1179.

59. Ekeke G, Landon J, Edwards CRW, Whie GE, Shridi F. Magnetizable solid-phase separation immunoassay for total estriol in pregnancy serum. *Clin Chim Acta* 1981;109:31–37.

60. Nargessi RD, Ackland J, Hassan M, Forrest GS, Smith DS, Landon J. Magnetizable solid-phase fluoroimmunoassay of thyroxine by sequential addition technique. *Clin Chem* 1980;26:1701–1703.

61. Ekeke GI, Exley D, Abuknesha R. Immunofluorimetric assay of estradiol-17β. *J Steroid Biochem* 1979;11:1597–1600.

62. Eskola JU, Nanto V, Meurling L, Lovgren TNE. Direct solid-phase time-resolved immunofluorometric assay of cortisol in serum. *Clin Chem* 1985;31:1731–1734.

63. Bertoft E, Eskola JU, Nanto V, Lovgren T. Competitive solid-phase immuno-assay of testosterone using time-resolved fluorescence. *FEBS Lett* 984;173:213–216.

64. Toivonen E, Hemmila I, Marniemi J, Jorgensen PN, Lovgren T. Two-site time-resolved immunofluormetric assay of human insulin. *Clin Chem* 1986;32:637–640.

65. Kaihola HL. Irjala K, Vikari J, Nanto V. Determination of thyrotropin in serum by time-resolved fluoroimmunoassay evaluated. *Clin Chem* 1985;31:1706–1709.

66. Dechaud H, Bador R, Claustrat F, Desuzines C. Laser-excited immunofluoro-metric assay of prolactin, with use of antibodies coupled to lanthanide-labeled diethylenetriaminepentaacetic acid. *Clin Chem* 1986;32:1323–1327.

67. Kobayaski Y, Tsubota N, Miyai K, Watanabe F. Fluorescence quenching immunoassay of serum cortisol. *Steroid* 1979;34:829–834.

68. Van Der Werf P, Chang CH. Determination of thyroxine binding globulin (TBG) in human serum by fluorescence excitation transfer immunoassay. *J. Immunol Methods* 1980;36:339–347.

69. Ullman EF. Recent advances in fluorescence immunoassay techniques, in Langan J, Clapp JJ (eds): *Ligand Assay.* New York: Masson, 1981, pp 113–136.

70. Smith DS. Enhancement fluoroimmunoassay of thyroxine. *FEBS Lett* 1977; 77:25–27.

71. Symons RG, Vining RF. An evaluation of a fluorescence polarization immuno-assay of thyroxin and thyroxin-uptake. *Clin Chem* 1985;31:1342–1348.

72. Kobayashi Y, Amitani K, Watanabe F, Miyai K. Fluorescence polarization immunoassay for cortisol. *Clin Chim Acta* 1979;92:241–247.

73. Yamaguchi, Hayashi C, Miyai K. Fluorscence polarization immunoassay for insulin preparations. *Anal Lett* 1982;15:731–737.

74. Urios P, Cittanova N, Jayle M-F. Immunoassay of human chorionic gonado-trophin using fluorescence polarization. *FEBS Lett* 1978;94:54–58.

75. Strarup-Brynes I, Osikowicz G, Vanderbilt AS, Fino J, Shipchandler M. A fluorescence polarization immunoassay quantitating unconjugated (free) estriol in serum. *Clin Chem* 1986;32:1170(A 596).

76. Seitz WR. Immunoassay labels based on chemiluminescence and biolumine-scence. *Clin Biochem* 1984;17:120–125.

77. Olsson T, Thore A. Chemiluminescence and its use in immunoassay, in Voller A, Bartlett A, Bidwell D (eds): *Immunoassays for the 80s.* Baltimore: University Park Press, 1981, pp 113–125.

78. Barnard GJR, Kim JB, William JL. Chemiluminescence immunoassays and immunochemiluminometric assays, in Collins WP (ed): *Alternative Immuno-assays.* New York: Wiley, 1985, pp 123–152.

79. Kohen F, Pazzagli M, Serio M, de Boever J, Vandekerckhoves D. Chemiluminescence and bioluminescence immunoassays, in Collins WP (ed): *Alternative Immunoassays*. New York: Wiley, 1985, pp 103–122.

80. Wood WG. Luminescence immunoassays: Problems and possibilities. *J Clin Chem Biochem* 1984;22:905–918.

81. Metzel PS, Moris N. A new chemiluminescence immunoassay system. *Am Clin Prod Rev* 1986;5(5):32–35.

82. Pazzagli M, Kim JB, Messeri G, Martinazzo G, Kohen F, Francheschetti F, Tomassi A, Salerno R, Serio M. Luminescent immunoassay (LIA) for progesterone in a heterogeneous system. *Clin Chim Acta* 1981;115:287–296.

83. Pazzagli M, Serio M, Munsun P, Rodbard D. A chemiluminescent immunoassay (LIA) for testosterone, in *Radioimmunoassays and Related Procedures in Medicine*. Vienna: Unipub, 1983, pp 747–755.

84. Pazzagli M, Kim JB, Messeri G, Kohen F, Bolelli GF, Tommari A, Salerno R, Serio M. Luminescent immunoassays (LIA) for cortisol. *J Steroid Biochem* 1981; 14:1181–1187.

85. Kohen F, Kim JB, Lindner HR, Collins WP. Development of a solid-phase chemiluminescence immunoassay for plasma progesterone. *Steroids* 1981; 38:73–88.

86. De Boever J, Kohen F, Vanderkerckhove D. A solid phase chemiluminescence immunoassay for plasma estradiol-17β for gonadotropin therapy compared with two different redioimmunoassays. *Clin Chem* 1983;29:2068–2072.

87. Kohen F, Lindner HR, Gilad S. Development of chemiluminescence monitored immunoassays for steroid hormones. *J Steroid Biochem* 1983;19:413–418.

88. Lindstrom L, Meurling, Lovgren T. The measurement of serum cortisol by a solid-phase chemiluminescence immunoassay. *J Steroid Biochem* 1982;16:577–580.

89. De Boever J, Kohen F, Vandekerckhove D, Van Maele G. Solid-phase chemiluminescence immunoassay for progesterone in unextracted serum. *Clin Chem* 1984;30:1637–1641.

90. De Boever J, Kohen F, Usanachitt C, Vandekerckhove D, Leyseele D, Vandewalle L. Direct chemiluminescence immunoassay for estradiol in serum. *Clin Chem* 1986;32:1895–1900.

91. Barnard G, Kim JB, Brockelbank JL, Collins WP, Kohen F, Gaier B. The measurement of choriogonadotropin by chemiluminescence immunoassay and immunochemiluminometric assay. 1. Use of isoluminol derivatives. *Clin Chem* 1984;30:538–541.

92. Brockelbank JL, Barnard G, Kim JB, Collins WP, Kohen F, Gaier B. The measurement of urinary LH by a solid-phase chemiluminescence immunoassay. *Ann Clin Biochem* 1984;21:284–289.

93. Richardson AP, Kim JB, Barnard GJ, Collins WP, McCapra F. Chemiluminescence immunoassay of plasma progesterone with progesterone–acridinum ester used as the labeled antigen. *Clin Chem* 1985;31:1664–1668.

94. Cheng P-J, Hemmila I, Lovgren T. Development of solid-phase immunoassay using chemiluminescent IgG conjugates. *J. Immunol Methods* 1982;48:159–168.

95. Miller T, Madden H. A monoclonal "sandwich" chemiluminescent assay for thyroid stimulating hormone with paramagnetic particles as the solid phase. *Clin Chem* 1986;32:1165(A 572).

96. Sturges ML, Weeks I, Mpoko CN, Laing I, Woodhead JS. Chemiluminescent labeled-antibody assay for thyroxine in serum, with magnetic separation of the solid-phase. *Clin Chem* 1986;32:532–535.

97. Kohen F, Pazzagli M, Kim JB, Lindner HR, Boguslaski RC. An assay procedure for plasma progesterone based on antibody enhanced chemiluminescence. *FEBS Lett* 1979;104:201–205.

98. Kohen F, Pazzagli M, Kim JB, Lindner HR. An immunoassay for plasma cortisol based on chemiluminescence. *Steroids* 1980;36:421–438.

99. Kohen F, Kim JB, Lindner HR, Assay of gonadal steroids based on antibody-enhanced chemiluminescence, in McElroy WD, DeLuca MA (eds): *Bioluminescence and Chemiluminescence.* New York: Academic Press, 1981, pp 357–364.

100. Kohen F, Kim JB, Barnard G, Lindner HR. An assay for urinary estriol-16α-glucuronide based on antibody-enhanced chemiluminescence. *Steroids* 1980;36:405–419.

101. Campbell AK, Roberts PA, Patel A. Chemiluminescence energy transfer: A technique for homogeneous immunoassay, in Collins WP (ed): *Alternative Immunoassays.* New York: Wiley, 1985, pp 153–183.

102. Giles AF, Charles SA, De Vriendt JK, McIntyre A, Rimmer J, Sturley HN, Martin JK, Holian J. Amerlite assays for total T_4, T_3 and T_3 uptake. *Clin Chem* 1986;32:1160(A 544).

103. Arakaua H, Maed M, Tsuji A. Chemiluminescence enzyme immunoassay of cortisol using peroxidase as label. *Anal Biochem* 1979;97:248–254.

104. Spiller G, Tovey KC, Smith GFW, Mashiter K. Development of a highly sensitive assay for hCG based on enhanced luminescence. *Clin Chem* 1986;32:1164(A 567).

105. Douglas SG, Brockas AJ, Holian J, Mashiter K. Development of an assay for luteinizing hormone (LH) based on enhanced luminescence. *Clin Chem* 1986;32:1164(A 568).

106. Grundy MS, Brain M, Brockas AJ, Smith GFW, Holian J, Mashiter K. A supersensitive immunoassay for TSH using enhanced luminescence. *Clin Chem* 1986;32:1164(A 566).

107. Hughes J, Short F, James UHT. Synthesis of a novel bioluminescent conjugate of progesterone for immunoassay, in Kricka LJ, Stanley PE, Thorpe GHG, Whitehead TP (eds): *Analytical Applications of Bioluminescence and Chemiluminescence.* New York: Academic Press, 1984, pp 269–272.

108. Word WG, Fricke H, von Klitzing L, Strasburger CJ, Scriba PC. Solid phase antigen luminescent immunoassays for the determination of insulin, insulin antibodies and gentamicin levels in human serum. *J Clin Chem Clin Biochem* 1982;20:825–831.

109. Arakaua H, Maeda M, Tsuji A. Chemiluminescenece enzyme immunoassay of

17α-hydroxyprogesterone using glucose oxidase and bis(2,4,6-trichlorophenyl)-oxalate fluorescent dye system. *Chem Pharm Bull* 1982;30:3036–3039.

110. Cambiaso CL, Riccomi HA, Masson PL, Heremans JF. Automated nephelometric immunoassay. II. Its application to the determination of hapten. *J Immunol Methods* 1974;5:293–302.

111. Krieg AF. Wenk RE. Pregnancy tests and evaluation of placental function, in Henry JB (ed): *Clinical Diagnosis and Management*. Philadelphia: Saunders, 1984, pp 493–501.

112. Galvin JP, Looney CE, Leflar CC, Luddy MA, Litchfield WJ, Freytag JW, Miller WK. Particle enhanced photometric immunoassay systems, in Nakamura RM, Dito WR, Tucker ES (eds): *Clinical Laboratory Assays*. New York: Masson, 1983, pp 73–95.

113. Cambiaso CL, Leek AE, de Steenwinkel F, Billen J, Masson PL. Particle counting immnunoassay (PACIA). I. A general method for the determination of antibodies, antigens and haptens. *J Immunol Methods* 1977;18:33–44.

114. Mareschal J, Gilles J, Masson PL. Particle counting immunoassay of human choriogonadotropin beta subunit (β-hCG) in the Impact instrument. *Clin Chem* 1985;31:960(A 301).

115. Castracane CE, Cambiaso CL, Retegui LA, Gilbert I, Ketelslegers JM, Masson PL. Particle-counting immunoassay of human somatotropin. *Clin Chem* 1984;30:672–676.

116. Von Schulthess GK, Cohen RJ, Sakato N, Benedek GB. Laser light scattering spectroscopic immunoassay for hCG and hLH. *Immunochemistry* 1976;13:963–966.

117. Leuvering JAW, Thal PJHM, van der Waart M, Schuurs AHWM. Sol particle agglutination immunoassay for human chorionic gonadotropin. *Fresenius Z Anal Chem* 1980;301:132.

118. Leuvering JHW, Thal PJHM, van der Waart M, Schuurs AHWM. Sol particle immunoassay (SPIA). *J Immunoassay* 1980;1:77–91.

119. Cais M, Dani S, Eden Y, Gandolfi O, Horn M, Isaacs EE, Josephy Y, Saar Y, Slovin E, Snarsky L. Metalloimmunoassay. *Nature* 1977;270:534–535.

120. Haimovich J, Sela M. Antibody reactions with chemically modified bacteriophages. *Methods Immunol Immunochem* 1977;4:386–398.

121. Andrieu JM. Manas S, Dray F. Viroimmunoassays of steroids: Methods and principles, in Cameron EHD, Hillier SG, Griffiths K (eds): *Steroid Immunoassay—Proceedings of the Fifth Tenovus Workshop*. UK: Alpha Omega, 1975, pp 189–198.

122. Young M, Nichols AL. Bacteriophage immunoassay of hormones using β-galactosidase as a means of phage infectivity, in Langan J, Clapp JJ (eds): *Ligand Assay*. New York: Masson, 1981, pp 205–210.

123. Esser AF. Principles of electron spin resonance assays and immunologic applications, in Nakamura RM, Dito WR, Tucker ES (eds): *Immunoassays: Clinical Laboratory Techniques for the 1980s*. New York: Liss, 1980, pp 213–233.

124. Wei R, Almirez R. Spin immunoassay of progesterone. *Biochem Biophys Res Commun* 1975;62:510–516.

125. Sayo H, Hosokawa M. Spin immunoassay of urinary testosterone. *Yakugaker Zasshi* 1980;100:56–60.

126. Chan SW, Tan CT. Membrane immunoassay: Simplicity and specificity. *J Immunol Methods* 1978;21:185–195.

127. Boitieux JL, Lemay C, Desmet G, Thomas D. Use of solid phase biochemistry for potentiometric enzyme immunoassay of oestradiol-17β—Preliminary report. *Clin Chim Acta* 1981;113:175–182.

128. Gebauer CR, Rechmitz GA. Deaminating enzyme labels for potentiometric enzyme immunoassay. *Anal Biochem* 1982;124:338–348.

CHAPTER 8

COAGULATION

CURTIS LIU

*Memorial Medical Center of Long Beach
Long Beach, California*

INTRODUCTION

Quantitative coagulation assays are performed in the hematology section of most clinical laboratories. The development of synthetic substrates that allow assay of blood clotting and fibrinolytic enzymes on spectrophotometers has shifted this testing to the clinical chemistry section in many clinical laboratories (*1–4*). The use of commercially available synthetic substrates is routine in most clinical chemistry laboratories. This chapter gives the reader with a background in chemistry information to select and set up clinically useful assays and to be able to interpret and compare assay results with test results from the hematology section.

FUNDAMENTAL CONCEPTS OF HEMOSTASIS

Hemostasis is divided into two phases. The first or primary phase requires interaction between platelets and a blood vessel. The platelet membrane provides a scaffold for the second phase of coagulation. The second phase involves interactions of coagulation proteins that result in a cross-linked fibrin clot.

The second phase of the coagulation process is a linear sequence of proteolytic reactions. The nomenclature for the coagulation factors is listed in Table 1. The sequence of events which lead to conversion of fibrinogen to fibrin and the fibrin to cross-linked fibrin can be divided into intrinsic system reactions and extrinsic system reactions (see Figure 1). This series of reactions is initiated on platelet phospholipid membrane surfaces. At each step a biochemical reaction takes place in which an inactive zymogen or proenzyme is converted into an active enzyme. The plasma clotting factors may be divided into groups based on their general properties (Table 2) or their functional activity (Table 3).

197

Table 1. Nomenclature for Blood Coagulation Factors

Factor	Synonyms
I	Fibrinogen
II	Prothrombin
III	Tissue thromboplastin, tissue factor
IV	Calcium
V	Proaccelerin, labile factor, Ac globulin
VI	Not used
VII	Proconvertin, SPCA, stable factor, autoprothrombin I
VIII	Antihemophilic factor A (AHF), antihemophilic globulin (AHG)
IX	Christmas factor, plasma thromboplastin component (PTC) antihemophilic factor B
X	Stuart–Prower factor, autoprothrombin III
XI	Plasma thromboplastin antecedent (PTA), antihemophilic factor C
XII	Hageman factor
XIII	Fibrin-stabilizing factor, Laki–Lorand factor
Prekallikrein	Fletcher factor
HMWK	High molecular weight kininogen, Fitzgerald factor

The extrinsic system is a pathway where tissue factor or extract is necessary for conversion of prothrombin to thrombin. The intrinsic system is a pathway where conversion of prothrombin to thrombin takes place in the absence of tissue factor.

Both the extrinsic and intrinsic systems amplify or accelerate formation of a blood clot. Factor Va and factor VIIIa are cofactors which accelerate the step in their pathway 100-fold.

Blood clot formation is controlled and localized to an injury site by circulating antithrombins. The circulating antithrombins decelerate clotting. The circulating antithrombins are protease inhibitors. They are listed in Table 4.

Antithrombin III is the most important circulating antithrombin. The decreased plasma concentration of antithrombin III is proportional to an increased risk for deep venous thrombosis. Antithrombin is also known as heparin cofactor. Heparin interacts with antithrombin III in a 1:1 stoichiometric ratio. Antithrombin III is a slow, ineffective inhibitor of activated serine proteases. The antithrombin III–heparin complex is a fast, efficient inhibitor of serine proteases. The mechanism of the antithrombin III–heparin inactivation of serine proteases can be summarized in the following manner. Six of the 11 coagulation proteins are trypsin-like serine proteases. Activated

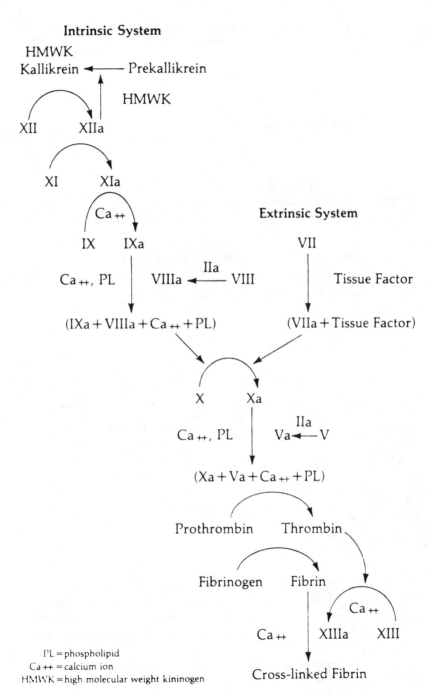

Figure 1. Sequence of events for the conversion of fibrinogen to fibrin. Reprinted with permission from ASCP Press, a division of the American Society of Clinical Pathologists.

Table 2. Division of Coagulation Factors Based on General Properties

Vitamin-K-Dependent Clotting Factors

Factor II (prothrombin)
Factor VII (proconvertin)
Factor IX (Christmas factor)
Factor X (Stuart factor, Stuart–Prower factor)

Contact Factors

Factor XII (Hageman factor)
Factor XI (plasma thromboplastin antecedent)
High molecular weight kininogen (Fitzgerald factor)
Prekallikrein (Fletcher factor)

Thrombin-Sensitive Clotting Factors

Factor V (proaccelerin, labile factor)
Factor VIII (antihemophilic factor)
Fibrinogen
Factor XIII (fibrin-stabilizing factor)

Table 3. General Functional Classification of Coagulation Factors

Serine Protease	Transamidase	Cofactor	Substrate
Factor XIIa	Factor XIIIa	Fitzgerald factor	Fibrinogen
Kallikrein		Factor VIII[a]	
Factor XIa		Factor V	
Factor IXa		Tissue factor	
Factor VIIa			
Factor Xa			
Thrombin			

[a]Recently found to have protease activity.

factors VII, IX, X, XI, and XII and prothrombin possess an active site serine. The activated serine proteases have a predilection for basic residues arginine or lysine adjacent to the peptide bond cleaved. Inactivated antithrombin III has an arginine site which is exposed and made available to serine proteases when the antithrombin III–heparin complex is formed. Heparin is localized at the endothelial surface; hence, the inactivation of activated clotting factors is membrane based *in vivo*.

Table 4. Major Circulating Antithrombins

Inhibitor	Proteases Inhibited	Potentiated by Heparin	Rate of Inhibition
α_1-Antitrypsin	Thrombin, XIa, kallikrein	No	Slow, may complete with α_2-macroglobulin
Antithrombin III	XIIa, XIa, IXa, Xa, VIIa, thrombin, kallikrein, plasmin	Yes	Slow
α_2-Macroglobulin	XIIa, XIa, thrombin, kallikrein, plasmin	No	Rapid
C' Inhibitor	XIIa, XIa, kallikrein, first component of complement	No	Slow
α_2-Antiplasmin	Plasmin	No	Slow
Protein C	Activated factors V and VIII	No	Slow

Protein C is a vitamin-K-dependent protein. It is the serine protease anticoagulant second in importance to antithrombin III. Protein C is activated by the thrombomodulin–thrombin complex localized to the endothelial membrane surface (Figure 2). Protein S is a cofactor for protein C and is also vitamin K dependent.

Fibrinolysis opposes the clotting process. It is a membrane-bound process mediated by tissue plasminogen activator and plasmin (Figure 3). In disease states associated with acute disseminated intravascular coagulation (DIC),

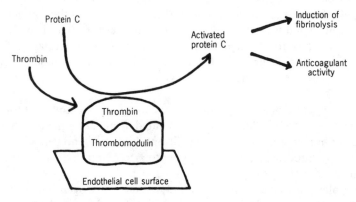

Figure 2. Activation of protein C by the thrombin–thrombomedullin complex. Reproduced from the Journal of Clinical Investigation, 1982, 70: 133 by copyright permission of the American Society for Clinical Investigation.

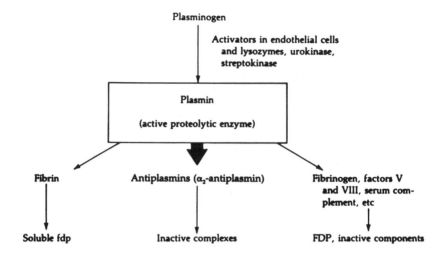

Figure 3. Role of plasmin in fibrinolysis. Reprinted with permission from ASCP Press, a division of the American Society of Clinical Pathologists.

there is widespread fibrin deposition throughout the vasculature with secondary, compensatory fibrinolysis. Elevation of fibrinogen–fibrin split products is characteristic of DIC and confirms the diagnosis.

Activation of fibrinolysis depends on conversion of the enzymatic zymogen plasminogen to the active enzyme plasmin. Intrinsic and extrinsic systems of plasminogen activation have been identified. Activation of the contact phase of the intrinsic pathway of coagulation also initiates the intrinsic pathway of fibrinolysis. Activated Hagemann factor (factor XIIa) generates kallikrein, which activates plasminogen. Kallikrein has a feedback function which generates factor XIIa. The extrinsic system involves tissue plasminogen activator.

Two therapeutic plasminogen activators are urokinase and streptokinase. Urokinase is a trypsin-like protease isolated from human urine and cell cultures of human embryonic kidney. Streptokinase is a nonenzyme protein produced by Lancefield C strains of streptococci. Streptokinase is antigenic and causes pyrogenic side effects.

Tissue plasminogen activator is a therapeutic plasminogen activator that is now commercially available. Experience is still being gained in its use for patients with myocardial infarction. It has a short half-life and must be delivered to the intravascular site of thrombosis.

Table 5. Fibrinogen–Fibrin Conversion

Step	Reaction[a]
Proteolysis	Fibrinogen–thrombin→FM + FP A and B
Polymerization	nFM $\rightleftarrows$ SFC
Clotting	mSFC $\rightleftarrows$ fibrin S
Cross-linking	Fibrin S–factor XIIIA, Ca^{2+} → fibrin I

[a] FM = fibrin monomer, FP = fibrinopeptides, SFC = soluble fibrin complexes, n and m = some large number, fibrin S = soluble (non-cross-linked) fibrin, and fibrin I = insoluble (cross-linked) fibrin.

Fibrinogen is a symmetrical dimer composed of six polypeptide chains— one pair of α chains, one pair of β chains, and one pair of γ chains—linked by covalent disulfide bonds. Fibrinogen is converted to fibrin when the thrombin cleaves fibrinopeptides A and B from the amino terminal ends of the α and β chains. The arising fibrin monomers polymerize by hydrogen bonding. The soluble fibrin polymer is stabilized by factor XIIIa, which introduces covalent bonds cross-linking γ chains to form γ-chain dimers and cross-linking γ chains to form γ-chain polymers (Table 5).

Plasmin digestion of fibrinogen is sequential. Fragments X and Y are early fibrin split products. Fragments D and E are late fibrin split products (Table 6). Plasmin digestion of non-cross-linked fibrin produces products similar to those produced by plasmin digestion of fibrinogen. Plasmin digestion of cross-linked fibrin produces γ-chain cross-linked D fragments referred to as D-dimers.

Table 6. Hydrolysis of Fibrinogen by Plasmin

Before (mol wt $\times 10^{-3}$)	After (mol wt $\times 10^{-3}$)
Fibrinogen (340)–plasmin→	Fragment X (240–280)[a]
Fragment X (240–280)–plasmin→	1 Fragment Y (130–160)[b] and 1 fragment D (80–100)[b]
Fragment Y (130–160)–plasmin→	1 Fragment D (80–100) and 1 fragment E (30–35)[b]

[a] Partly thrombin clottable.
[b] Not clottable by thrombin.

ADVANTAGES AND LIMITATIONS OF CHROMOGENIC ASSAYS

The advantages of chromogenic assay systems are several fold.

1. The assays can be automated.
2. The coefficient of variation is low under defined conditions and precise spectrophotometric analysis.
3. Automated chemical analyzers connected to calculators and printers permit the assay of a large number of samples.
4. The plasma requirements are small (10–30 μL).
5. The assays are independent of clotting-factor-deficient plasmas.

The limitations of chromogenic assay systems are more complex.

1. Synthetic substrates are preferentially split by a specific activated clotting factor and may be split by other activated clotting factors to some extent. Most assay systems are devised to prevent extraneous possible contributions to substrate splitting from disturbing the assay. Manipulations used to ensure a more or less specific reaction involve the addition of inhibitors to the assay system and the selection of the appropriate activation and reaction conditions. Deviation from the correct pH or ionic strength or absence of a necessary ion species can give inaccurate results.

2. The amidase or esterase activity for a given activated clotting factor toward a synthetic chromogenic substrate is not necessarily the same as the biological activity. The activity of a serine protease to its natural substrate is dependent on specific molecular sites that are involved in binding to a catalytic surface or substrate. More molecular determinants are necessary for biological function than for catalytic activity. To illustrate these points, we offer two examples.

Thrombin has an esterase and hence amidase activity which is not identical to the biological reaction of fibrinogen conversion to fibrin (5). The denatured thrombin molecule loses its clotting activity before it loses its esterase activity. This does not cause a problem when thrombin is freshly generated but may present a problem when a purified thrombin standard preparation has been denatured during processing.

Oral anticoagulation with warfarin compounds or vitamin K deficiency results in production of abnormal prothrombin that lacks γ-COOH-glutamic acid residues in its N-terminal end. These groups anchor prothrombin to a phospholipid surface. Physiological activation cannot take place without attachment to a phospholipid surface. Activation of the abnormal pro-thrombin induced by vitamin K absence or antagonists by *Echis carinates* venom or staphylocoagulase generates protease activity as readily from the abnormal prothrombin as the normal prothrombin (6).

3. There can be competition between artificial chromogenic substrates and normal substrates. Note that factor Xa catalyzes conversion of prothrombin to thrombin. Estimation of thrombin generation by the continuous measurement of color production from a chromogenic substrate specific for thrombin can be falsely decreased when binding of factor Xa is appreciable. When binding of factor Xa to the substrate occurs, prothrombin conversion will be slower in the presence of the substrate than in its absence.

GENERAL PRINCIPLES OF CHROMOGENIC SUBSTRATE ASSAYS

Chromogenic substrates (Table 7) are designed to mimic naturally occurring substrates. They are small peptides to which p-nitroaniline (pNA) is coupled to the C-terminal end. The sequence of the three to five amino acids preceding pNA is similar to the sequence of amino acids preceding the bond split in natural substrates (7,8). When an activated protease catalyzes the hydrolysis of the peptide–pNA bond, free pNA is released. The pNA differs in absorbance from the substrate at a wavelength of 405 nm. The substrate has an absorbance of less than 1% of the pNA absorbance at 405 nm.

The hydrolysis of the peptide–pNA bond must take place under conditions where the buffer system, pH substrate concentration and ionic strength have

Table 7. Chromogenic Substrates for the Assay of Enzymes

Substrate Code[a]	Chemical Structure[b]	Enzyme
S2222	Bz-Ile-Glu(γ-OR)-Gly-Arg-pNA[c]	Xa
S2337	Bz-Ile-Glu(γ-piperidyl)-Gly-Arg-pNA	Xa
S2302	H-D-Pro-Phe-Arg-pNA	Plasma–kallikrein
Chromozym PK	Bz-Pro-Phe-Arg-pNA	Plasma–kallikrein
S2238	H-D-Phe-Pip-Arg-pNA	Thrombin
S2160	Bz-Phe-Val-Arg-pNA	Thrombin
Chromozym TH	Tos-Gly-Pro-Arg-pNA	Thrombin
S2444	Pyroglutamyl-Gly-Arg-pNA	Urokinase
Chromozym UK	Bz-Val-Gly-Arg-pNA	Urokinase
S2251	H-D-Val-Leu-Lys-pNA	Plasmin
Chromozym PL	Tos-Bly-Pro-Lys-pNA	Plasmin
S2366	<Glu-Pro-Arg-pNA	Protein C

[a]The S series is produced by Kabi Diagnostica, Stockholm, and the Chromozym series by Pentapharm, Basel.
[b]Bz = benzoyl and Tos = tosyl.
[c]50% where R = H and 50% where R = CH_3.

been optimized so that the Michaelis–Menten law is followed (see Figure 1, Chapter 6) (9).

In a reaction system where E is the enzyme, S the substrate, and P the final product, the following reactions take place:

$$E + S \underset{k_4}{\overset{k_1}{\rightleftharpoons}} ES \underset{k_5}{\overset{k_2}{\rightleftharpoons}} EP \underset{k_6}{\overset{k_3}{\rightleftharpoons}} E + P$$

The assumptions in this system are that:

1. ES → EP takes place almost instantaneously, and
2. the reaction ES → E + P is considerably slower than E + S → ES.

When these assumptions are applied to the initial reaction system, the equation simplifies to:

$$E + S \underset{k_4}{\overset{k_1}{\rightleftharpoons}} ES \overset{k_2}{\longrightarrow} E + P$$

Since ES → E + P is the rate-limiting reaction, the reaction rate is proportional to the concentration of ES. The reaction curve of substrate concentration versus reaction velocity is hyperbolic. For initial reaction rates, first-order kinetics apply, and the initial velocity V_0 is proportional to substrate concentration. During the initial portion of reaction, a decrease in substrate concentration does not decrease the reaction rate. When these conditions are met, enzyme concentration E, can be estimated from the reaction velocity V. The following formulas apply when Michaelis–Menten principles hold (10):

$$V_{max} = k_3 \times E$$

$$V = \frac{k_3 \times E \times S}{K_m + S}$$

For a more complete discussion of enzyme kinetics, see Chapter 6.

CHROMOGENIC CLOTTING FACTOR ASSAYS

Tables 7 and 8 list commercially available analytes. Table 9 classifies the established chromogenic assay systems in terms of clinical utility.

Factor II assays can be used to monitor patients on oral anticoagulant therapy (11). The use of the chromogenic assay to replace the use of the prothrombin time for such patients needs further verification.

Table 8. Clinical Applications of Chromogenic Substrates

Substrate	Applications
S-2222	Factor Xa; factor X; heparin; factors VII and IX; Antithrom-
S-2337	bin III or antifactor Xa; platelet factor 4
S-2302	Kallikrein, prekallikrein, kallikrein inhibitor, urine kallikrein
Chromozym PK	Factor XII
S-2238	Monitoring of oral anticoagulants; vitamin-K-dependent
Chromozym Th	factors; heparin; quality control of procoagulants,
	prothrombin complex concentrates, and other plasma-
	based concentrates
S-2160	Thrombin; antithrombin III; prothrombin; platelet factor 3
S-2444	Urokinase; management of thrombolytic therapy
Chromozym UK	
S-2251	Plasmin; plasminogen; antiplasmin; plasminogen activators
Chromozym Th	urokinase inhibitor, antibrinase
S-2266	Glandular kallikrein
Chromozym Try	Trypsin; antitrypsin
S-2433	Endotoxin

Table 9. Clinical Usefulness of Chromogenic Assay Systems

Useful	Possibly Useful	Low Usefulness
Factor VIII		Kallikrein inhibitor
Factor IX		Prekallikrein
Factor X	Factor II	Factor VII
Protein C		Factor XII
Antithrombin III		
Heparin (anti-Xa)		
Plasminogen		
α_2-Antiplasmin		

Factor VII assay has no clinical applications because of the short half-life of factor VII and the difficulty of performing the assay. The factor VII assay could be used to monitor oral anticoagulant therapy.

The clinical value of factor XII, prekallikrein, and kallikrein inhibitor is low. These substances have been used in research to monitor critically ill patients in shock.

Factor VIII

Factor VIII assays can be useful in

1. diagnosis of hemophilia A,
2. detection of female heterozygotes for hemophilia A in family studies,
3. management of hospitalized hemophilia A patients,
4. standardization of factor VIII concentrate preparations,
5. cross-referencing of factor VIII concentrate preparations, and
6. quality control of factor VIII levels of cryoprecipitant for blood banks.

The chromogenic assay using S2222 substrate has a linear relationship between factor VIII concentration and reaction velocity. The reaction is an intrinsic pathway reaction. Factors IXa and X, phospholipid, and calcium are incubated with dilute test plasma. Factor VIII is rate limiting in the generation of factor Xa, which is quantitated by S2222 hydrolysis (12,13).

Test Principle

$$X \xrightarrow{\text{IXa} + \text{phospholipid} + \text{Ca}^{2+} + \text{VIII}} Xa$$

$$Xa + S2222 \rightarrow pNa$$

Factor IX

Factor IX assays can be used to:

1. diagnose and monitor hemophilia B patients,
2. monitor oral anticoagulant therapy,
3. standardize factor IX concentrate preparations,
4. cross-reference factor IX concentrate preparations, and
5. diagnose factor IX deficiency in patients with liver failure.

The assay using S2222 substrate is an intrinsic pathway assay similar to the factor VIII assay. Purified factor XIa, factor X, phospholipid, and calcium are incubated with dilute test plasma. Factor IX is rate limiting in the generation of factor Xa, which is quantitated by S2222 hydrolysis (14–16).

$$IX \xrightarrow{\text{XIa}} IXa$$

$$X \xrightarrow{\text{IXa} + \text{phospholipid} + \text{Ca}^{2+}} Xa$$

$$Xa + S2222 \rightarrow pNa$$

Factor X

Factor X assays can be useful in monitoring oral anticoagulant therapy. Assay using Russell's viper venom (RVV) as the activator and S2222 and S2337 as substrates have been developed (*14,15,17–23*).

Test Principle

$$X \xrightarrow{\text{RVV} + \text{Ca}^{2+}} Xa$$

$$Xa + \text{substrate} \rightarrow pNa$$

Protein C

Protein C assay is useful in

1. screening patients for protein C deficiency when there is history or evidence of thromboembolic disease at an early age, and
2. detection of acquired deficiencies that are present in oral anticoagulant treatment, liver disease, and disseminated intravascular coagulation.

The assay requires thrombin and thrombomodulin as activators S2266 is the substrate (*24–28*).

Test Principle

$$\text{protein C} \xrightarrow{\text{thrombin} - \text{thrombomodulin}} \text{activated protein C}$$

$$\text{activated protein C} + S2266 \rightarrow pNA$$

Antithrombin III (AT III)

Antithrombin III assay is useful in

1. treatment of patients who have a history of thromboembolic phenomenon at an early age, and
2. detection of acquired antithrombin III deficiency secondary to disseminated intravascular coagulation, proteinuria, or protein-losing gastroenteropathy.

The antithrombin III in test plasma combines with reagent heparin to inactivate a proportional amount of reagent thrombin, which has been added in excess. S2160, S2238, and Chromozyme TH can be used as substrates (*29–32*).

Test Principle

$$AT\ III + thrombin + heparin \rightarrow heparin - AT\ III - thrombin\ inactive$$
(excess)   (excess)   complex

$$residual\ thrombin + substrate \rightarrow pNA$$

Heparin

Quantitative assay of heparin levels can be useful in

1. monitoring of heparin therapy
2. monitoring mini-dose heparin therapy, where clot-based assays have minimal clinical value,
3. ensuring adequate protamine neutralization of heparin,
4. standardizing heparin preparations,
5. cross-referencing of heparin preparations, and
6. checking for contamination of specimens by heparin when an abnormal PTT is present with no evident reason.

The correlation of heparin values with clotting methods has produced evidence that the number of heparin international units per unit volume of plasma does not always correspond to therapeutic heparinization because of the varying therapeutic responses of patients to heparin therapy. Since the physiological actions of heparin are primarily modulated by antithrombin III and partially by platelet factor IV and fibronectin, patients with fluctuating concentrations of these proteins have varying therapeutic responses.

Reagent factor Xa in excess is inhibited by plasma heparin and reagent antithrombin III. Factor Xa activity is quantitated by hydrolysis of S2222. The appearance of pNA is linearly and inversely related to the heparin level (*33–36*).

Test Principle

$$Xa + AT\ III\ \xrightarrow{heparin}\ Xa + AT\ III - Xa\ inactive\ complex$$
(excess)

$$Xa + S2222 \rightarrow pNA$$

Plasminogen

Plasminogen assays can be used to monitor therapeutic thrombolysis. When plasminogen levels approach zero, administration of thrombolytic agents such as streptokinase, urokinase, or tissue plasminogen activator has low efficacy.

Reagent streptokinase added in excess forms an enzymatically active complex with plasminogen. The active complex hydrolyzes S2251 (*36–39*).

Test Principle

$$\text{plasminogen} + \text{streptokinase} \rightarrow \text{plasminogen–streptokinase}$$
$$\quad\text{(excess)} \qquad\qquad\qquad \text{(active complex)}$$

$$\text{plasminogen–streptokinase} + \text{S2251} \rightarrow \text{pNA}$$

α_2-Antiplasmin

α_2-Antiplasmin is the primary inhibitor of plasmin and is decreased during pathological and therapeutic fibrinolytic activity.

Excess reagent plasmin is incubated with test plasma. Plasmin activity after inactivation by α_2-antiplasmin has an inverse relationship with the concentration of α_2-antiplasmin. S2251 or chromozyme PL can be used as substrates (*40–43*).

Test principle

$$\text{plasmin} + \alpha_2\text{-antiplasmin} \rightarrow \text{plasmin} + (\alpha_2\text{-antiplasmin–plasmin})$$
$$\text{(excess)} \qquad\qquad\qquad\qquad\qquad \text{(inactive complex)}$$

$$\text{plasmin} + \text{S2251} \rightarrow \text{pNA}$$

INSTRUMENTATION

Assays using synthetic chromogenic substrates can be done manually on spectrophotometers or filter photometers with a band-width of 10 nm or less. A recorder is necessary for initial rate methods. End-point methods are simpler to perform and for this reason are the preferred method when manual techniques are used.

Table 10. Automated Instruments for Chromogenic Substrate Assays

Cobas Bio	FP 901 Sebia
Vitatron PA 800	1SMAT Isabiologie
Gemsaec	KEM.0.MAT Coultronics
Vitatron AKES	Gilford 203 S
LKB 2086 Mark II Kinetic Analyzer	
LKB 8600/2086	
Abbott VP	
Abbott ABA-100	
Gilford 3500	
Centrifichem	
Hitachi 705	

A number of automated instruments can be used for chromogenic substrate assays (Table 10), and the list is growing (*44,45*). Reagent packs for use on the du Pont aca are also available.

SUMMARY

Manufacturers have produced kits with proven, reliable chromogenic substrates and the appropriate bioreagents. Specific methods for use with manual procedures, microtiter plates, or automated analyzers are available. Kits are available for plasminogen, heparin, factor VIII, factor X, antithrombin III, antiplasmin, α_2-macroglobulin, α_1-antitrypsin, prekallikrein, kallikrein, protein C, and tissue plasminogen activator–tissue plasminogen activator inhibitor. The cost of the kits is reasonable. The number of assays obtained from a kit depends on the method used. A $120 kit for factor VIII assay can produce 60 to 240 test results. As kits become more widely available, they may replace coagulation assays.

Clinical studies are showing that chromogenic assays are suitable for clinical use. Improvements on the specificity of the synthetic chromogenic reagents by modifying the size, charge, and hydrophobicity of the low molecular weight substrates are under investigation. Increased specificity may be accomplished by (1) varying the amino acid sequence of present substrates, (2) altering cleavage sites, or (3) changing the structure of the chromophore. The second approach involves addition of an amino acid residue between the cleavage site and the chromophore. A peptide bond is cleaved and the amino acid–chromophore is then detected by an aminopeptidase reacting with the formed substrate. An example is:

$$\text{H-D-Phe-Pro-Arg-Leu-pNA} \xrightarrow{\text{thrombin}} \text{H-D-Phe-Pro-Arg} + \text{Leu-pNA}$$

$$\text{Leu-pNA} \xrightarrow{\text{aminopeptidase}} \text{Leu} + \text{pNA}$$

The third approach can involve the use of thioesterol (46), fluorogenic substrates (47), or fluorescent quench substrates (48). Also, 5-amino-2-nitrobenzoic acid (ANBA) is a parent chromophore from which derivative chromophores can be made by modification at the carboxyl group (49).

The current chromogenic assays are more precise and reproducible than conventional assays, and their coefficients of variation are as much as 10% below the conventional assays. They are less time-consuming to perform than most conventional assays. These advantages are responsible for their present use for clinical and diagnostic purposes.

REFERENCES

1. Triplett DA. Chromogenic substrates: A revolution in the diagnostic coagulation laboratory. *Clin Lab Ann* 1982;1:243–287.

2. Friberger P. Chromogenic substrates. *Scand J Clin Lab Invest* 1982; 42(suppl):162.

3. Lijnen HR, Collen D, Verstraete M (eds). Nijhoff, The Hague, 1980.

4. Fareed J, Messmore HL, Walenga JM, et al. Diagnostic efficacy of newer synthetic substrate methods for assessing coagulation variables: A critical overview. *Clin Chem* 1983;29:225–236.

5. Gaffney PJ, Lord K, Brasher M, et al. Problems in the assay of thrombin using synthetic peptides as substrates. *Thromb Res* 1977;10:549–556.

6. Stenflo J, Fernlund P, Egen W, et al. Vitamin K dependent modifications of glutamic acid residues in prothrombin. *Proc Natl Acad Sci* 1974;71:2730–2733.

7. Claeson G, Awell L, Karlsson G, et al. Design of chromogenic peptide substrates, in Scully MF, Kakkar VV (eds): *Chromogenic Peptide Substrates*. Edinburgh: Churchill & Livingstone, 1979, pp 20–31.

8. Blomback B. Theoretical considerations of substrate structures governing enzyme specificity, in Scully MF, Kakkar VV (eds): *Chromogenic Peptide Substrates*. Edinburgh: Churchill & Livingstone, 1979, pp 3–12.

9. Christensen U. Requirements for valid assays of clotting enzymes using chromogenic substrates. *Thromb Haemost* 1980;43:169–174.

10. Friberger P. Enzyme kinetics for serine proteases—Mathematical treatment. *Scand J Clin Lab Invest* 1982;42(appendix 3):82–83.

11. Baughman DJ, Lytwyn A. A novel chromogenic assay equivalent to the one-stage prothrombin time. *Thromb Haemost* 1979;42:291.

12. Segatchian MJ. The usefulness of chromogenic substrates in the diagnosis of haemophilia and control of blood products, in Scully MF, Kakkar VV (eds): *Chromogenic Peptide Substrates*. Edinburgh: Churchill & Livingstone, 1979, pp 102–118.

13. Rosen S, Andersson M, Blomback M, et al. Clinical application of a chromogenic substrate method for determination of factor VIII activity. *Thromb Haemost* 1985;54:818–823.

14. Aiach M, Schreiber N, Nussas C, et al. An automated amidolytic assay for testing factor X activity. *Thromb. Res* 1981;21:317–320.

15. Tans G, Janssen-Claessen T, van Dieijen G, et al. A spectrophotometric assay for factor IX in human plasma. *Thromb Haemost* 1982;48:127–132.

16. van Wijk EM, Kahle LH, ten Cate JW. A rapid manual chromogenic factor X assay. *Thromb Res* 1981;22:681–686.

17. Aurell L, Simonsson R, Airelly S, et al. Chromogenic peptide substrates for factor Xa. *Haemostasis* 1978;7:92–94.

18. Bergstrom K, Egberg N. Determination of vitamin K sensitive coagulation factors in plasma. Studies on three methods using synthetic chromogenic substrates. *Thromb Res* 1978;12:531–547.

19. van Wijk EM, Kahle LH, ten Cate JW. Mechanized amidolytic technique for determination of factor X and factor X antigen and its application to patients being treated with oral anticoagulants. *Clin Chem* 1980;26:885–890.

20. Erskine JG, Walker ID, Davidson JF. Maintenance control of oral anticoagulant therapy by a chromogenic substrate assay for factor X. *J Clin Pathol* 1980;33:445–448.

21. Latallo ZS, Thomson JM, Poller L. An evaluation of chromogenic substrates in the control of oral anticoagulant therapy. *Br J Haematol* 1981;47:307–318.

22. Italian CISMEL Study Group. Multicenter evaluation of a new chromogenic factor X assay in plasma of patients on oral anticoagulants. *Thromb Res* 1980;19:493–502.

23. Egberg N, Heedman PA. Simplified performance of amidolytic factor X assay. *Thromb Res* 1982;25:437–440.

24. Esmon NB, Owen WG, Esmon CT. Isolation of a membrane-bound cofactor for thrombin-catalysed activation of protein C. *J Biol Chem* 1982;257:859–864.

25. Thiel W, Preissner KT, Delvos U, et al. A simplified functional assay for protein C in plasma samples. *Blut* 1986;52:169–177.

26. Bertina RM, Brockmans AW, Krommenhoek-van Es C, et al. The use of a functional and immunologic assay for plasma protein C in the study of the heterogeneity of congenital protein C deficiency. *Thromb Haemost* 1984;51:1–5.

27. Sala N, Owen WG, Collen D. A functional assay of protein C in human plasma. *Blood* 1984;63:671–675.

28. Comp PC, Nixon RR, Esmon CT. Determination of functional levels of protein C,

an antithrombotic protein, using thrombin–thrombomodulin complex. *Blood* 1984;63:15–21.

29. Blomback M, Blomback B, Olsson P, et al. The assay of antithrombin using a synthetic chromogenic substrate for thrombin. *Thromb Res* 1974;5:621–632.

30. Odegard OR. Evaluation of an amidolytic heparin cofactor method. *Thromb Res* 1975;7:351–360.

31. Abildgaard U, Lie M, Odegard OR. Antithrombin (heparin cofactor) assay with new chromogenic substrates. *Thromb Res* 1977;11:549–553.

32. Kahle LH, Schipper HG, Jenkins CSP, et al. Antithrombin III. Evaluation of an automated antithrombin III method. *Thromb Res* 1978;2:1003–1014.

33. Teien AN, Lie M, Abildgaard V. Assay of heparin in plasma using a chromogenic substance for activated factor X. *Thromb Res* 1976;8:413–416.

34. Teien AN, Lie M. Evaluation of an amidolytic heparin assay method: Increased sensitivity by adding purified antithrombin III. *Thromb Res* 1977;10:399–410.

35. ten Cate H, Lamping R, Henry CHP, et al. Automated amidolytic method for determining heparin, a heparinoid and low M_r heparin fragment, based on their anti-Xa activity. *Clin Chem* 1984;30:860–864.

36. Friberger P. Chromogenic peptide substrates. Their use for the assay of factors in the fibrinolytic and plasma kallikrein–kinin system. *Scand J Lab Invest* 1982;42(suppl 162):49–54.

37. Soria J, Soria C, Samama MA. A plasminogen assay using a chromogenic synthetic substrate. Results from clinical work and studies of thrombolysis, in Davidson J, et al. (eds): *Progress in Chemical Fibrinolysis and Thrombolysis*, vol 4. Edinburgh: Churchill & Livingstone, 1978, pp 337–346.

38. Soria C, Soria J, Dunn F, et al. Comparison of the potentiating effect of fibrinogen, fibrinogen degradation products and fibrin degradation products on the amidolytic activity of the plasminogen–SK complex. Improvement of plasminogen determination in biological samples by decreasing the influence of fibrin degradation products. *Thromb Haemost* 1983;50:56.

39. Gram J, Jesperson J. A functional plasminogen assay utilizing the potentiating effect of fibrinogen to correct the overestimation of plasminogen in pathological plasma samples. *Thromb Haemost* 1985;53:255–259.

40. Edy J, Collen D, Verstraete M. Quantitation of plasma protease inhibitor antiplasmin with the chromogenic substrate S2251, in Davidson JF, et al. (eds): *Progress in Chemical Fibrinolysis and Thrombolysis*. New York: Raven, 1978, pp 315–322.

41. Teger-Nilsson AC, Friberger P, Gyzander E. Determination of a new rapid plasma inhibitor in human blood by means of a plasmin specific tripeptide substrate. *Scand J Clin Lab Invest* 1977;37:403–409.

42. Teger-Nilsson AC, Friberger P, Gyzander E. Antiplasmin determination by means of a chromogenic tripeptide substrate, in Davidson JF, et al. (eds): *Progress in Chemical Fibrinolysis and Thrombolysis*. New York: Raven, 1978, pp 305–314.

43. Friberger P. Chromogenic peptide substrates. Their use for the assay of factors in

the fibrinolytic and the plasma kallikrein–kinin systems. *Scand J Clin Lab Invest* 1982;42(suppl 162):41–48.

44. Bartl K, Becker U, Lill H. Application of several chromogenic substrate assays to automated instrumentation for coagulation analysis. *Sem Thromb Hemost* 1983;9:301–308.

45. Aiach M, Leon M, Michaud A, et al. Adaptation of synthetic peptide substrate-based assays on a discrete analyzer. *Sem Thromb Hemost* 1983;9:206–216.

46. Cho K, Tanaka T, Cook RC, et al. Active site mapping of bovine and human blood coagulation serine proteases using synthetic peptide 4-nitroanilide and thioester substrates. *Biochemistry* 1984;23:644–650.

47. Morita T, Kato H, Iwanaga S, et al. New fluorogenic substrates for α-thrombin, factor Xa, kallikrein, and urokinase. *J Biochem (Tokyo)* 1977;82:1495–1498.

48. Castillo MJ, Kurachi K, Nishino N, et al. Reactivity of bovine blood coagulation factor IXa$_B$, factor Xa$_B$, and factor XIa toward fluorogenic peptides containing the activation site sequences of bovine factor IX and factor X. *Biochemistry* 1983;22:1021–1029.

49. Kolde HJ, Eberle R, Heber H, et al. New chromogenic substrates for thrombin with increased specificity. *Thromb Haemost* 1986;56:155–159.

CHAPTER 9

THERAPEUTIC DRUG MONITORING

WILLIAM H. PORTER

University of Kentucky
Lexington, Kentucky

Therapeutic drug concentration monitoring is one of the fastest growing segments of the clinical laboratory. This growth has been spirited by advances in analytical methods and instrumentation, which have paved the way for broader and more routine application of the principles on which therapeutic drug monitoring is based.

RATIONALE

The rationale for the determination of the concentration in serum of therapeutically administered drugs rests on the existence of a relationship between this concentration and the magnitude and duration of drug binding at a specific receptor site in a target tissue. Thus, for certain drugs a correlation exists between the serum concentration range and the intensity of pharmacological response. When the drug concentration is within this range, therapeutic efficacy is maximized, while the incidence of dose-related side effects is minimal in most patients. Knowledge of the serum concentration is most useful when the drug requires individualized dosing for optimal therapeutic response and when clinical or other more routine parameters for measuring therapeutic success are not available. The necessity for monitoring the serum concentration of a particular drug is amplified when the therapeutic range for the drug is narrow, that is, when the difference between the concentration producing a desired therapeutic response and that resulting in toxicity is relatively small (Table 1).

PHARMACOKINETICS

Pharmacokinetics is the study of the rate processes of absorption, distribution, metabolism, and excretion of drugs. While a detailed discussion of the

Table 1. Drug Characteristics for Therapeutic Drug Monitoring

1. The drug should have an established therapeutic range.
2. The therapeutic range should be narrow.
3. No clearly observable therapeutic end point is evident.
4. The dose–response relationship is unpredictable.
5. Toxicity or lack of effectiveness may have severe consequences.
6. Accurate methods for determining the serum concentration must be readily available.

principles of pharmacokinetics is beyond the scope of this chapter, I highlight a few basic concepts central to the interpretation of serum drug concentrations. More complete discussions of pharmacokinetic principles may be found in an excellent review (*1*) or in a number of texts (*2–5*).

The serum concentration after drug administration reaches a maximum or peak value and then declines to a minimum or trough value just before the next dose (Figure 1). The time required for the serum concentration to decrease by 50% is defined as the drug's half-life. When the drug is administered at intervals approximately equal to its half-life, an equilibrium, or steady state will be reached after the fifth dosing interval (five half-lives). At steady state, the amount of drug entering the vascular compartment equals the amount eliminated during the dosing interval. Thus, both peak and

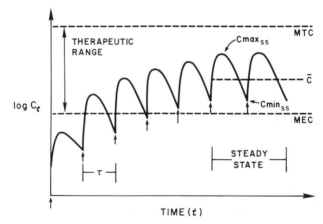

Figure 1. Illustration of drug accumulation during multiple-dosing showing achievement of steady state after approximately five half-lives. $Cmax_{ss}$ and $Cmin_{ss}$ = maximum (peak) and minimum (trough) steady-state concentrations, respectively; $\bar{c}$ = average steady-state concentration; τ = dosing interval; ↑ = dose; MTC = minimum toxic concentration; MEC = minimum effective concentration. (Moyer TP, et al, in Tietz NW (ed): *Clinical Chemistry*. Philadelphia: Saunders, 1986, p 1617, modified from Mayer SE et al in Gilman AG, Goodman LS, Gilman A, Eds.: *The Pharmacological Basis of Therapeutics*, 6th ed., Macmillan Publishing Co., NY, 1980, p. 24 with permission.)

trough concentrations are constant from one dosing interval to the next. It is clearly important for steady state to be achieved before interpreting serum drug concentrations.

The steady-state drug concentration achieved in serum after its administration and thus the corresponding pharmacological response will depend on a number of factors. The main determinants of the steady-state drug concentration are the drug dose, the dosing interval, the rate and extent of drug absorption (for drugs administered extravascularly), the distribution of the drug within the body, and the rate of drug elimination. Large individual variations in drug absorption, distribution, and elimination may result in sizable differences in final steady-state serum concentrations when equal drug doses are administered. These pharmacokinetic parameters may be influenced to varying degrees by such factors as sex, age, genetics, pregnancy, smoking, disease state, altered serum protein–drug binding, and concomitant drug therapy. Thus, not only may great individual variation in the major determinants of steady-state serum drug concentration occur, but these parameters may also be altered within an individual over the course of time.

DRUG–PROTEIN BINDING

Once in the vascular compartment, drugs will bind to plasma proteins to varying degrees depending on their individual physicochemical properties. In general, acid and neutral drugs are bound primarily to albumin, and basic drugs primarily to α_1-acid glycoprotein. It is generally accepted that only unbound (free) drug is available for extravascular distribution and for elimination. Moreover, only free drug is able to cross cellular membranes and interact with the drug receptor to elicit a pharmacological response. Thus, the extent of binding to plasma and tissue protein significantly influences a drug's volume of distribution, transport to the site of metabolism and elimination, and the magnitude of its pharmacological action. Disease states, concomitant drug therapy, and genetic and age-related factors can alter the extent of protein binding and thus affect the steady-state concentration of the pharmacologically active free drug.

It is general practice to routinely measure the total drug (free plus protein-bound) concentration in serum. For certain drugs, particularly those extensively bound to serum protein, a relatively small change in the protein-bound fraction may profoundly influence the interpretation of the measured total serum drug concentration. For instance, a decrease in the protein-bound fraction from 0.9 to 0.8 would initially result in a twofold increase in the concentration of free drug. The net effect of such an alteration would depend, among other factors, on the degree to which the drug's clearance from the circulation is influenced by the unbound (free) fraction. The pharmacokinetic concepts governing these changes are complex and clearly beyond the scope of this chapter. Suffice it to say that for drugs whose rate of clearance is *dependent* on the fraction unbound (e.g., phenytoin), the stated decrease in the protein-bound fraction would result in a new steady state wherein the concentration of free drug, and therefore the clinical response, would return to the original value, but the total drug concentration would be significantly reduced. In this instance, a change in drug dosage would not be warranted. For other drugs whose clearance is *independent* of the free fraction (e.g., lidocaine), a similar change in bound fraction would result in little change in the total drug concentration, but the free drug concentration and therefore the pharmacological response may be significantly increased. In this instance, a reduction in the drug dosage would be warranted.

It should be apparent that appropriate interpretation of the total serum drug concentration depends on a knowledge and understanding of the pharmacokinetic characteristics of the drug being monitored and on the clinical and physiological status of the patient. For certain drugs (phenytoin, valproic acid, disopyramide), measurement of the free rather than total drug concentration may significantly enhance optimization of therapeutic management for selected patients. Methods applicable for use in the clinical laboratory are now available for the determination of free drug concentration (see "Free Drug Measurements").

THERAPEUTIC RANGE

It is generally desirable to maintain the steady-state peak concentration below the minimal toxic (upper therapeutic) value and the corresponding trough value above the minimum effective concentration, thus assuring adequate but not toxic drug concentration throughout the dosing interval (Figure 1). Obviously, the measured drug concentration will depend on the time of blood sampling during the dosing interval. For many drugs, determination of the trough concentration provides useful information concerning therapeutic efficacy. Determination of peak serum drug concentrations may be useful for assessing possible toxic effects. For certain drugs, such as the aminoglycoside antibiotics, it is generally efficacious to measure drug concentrations at both peak and trough points. In this instance, the peak value should exceed the antibiotic's minimum inhibitory concentration for the susceptible organism, but drug accumulation that might lead to toxicity should be avoided. Thus, measurement of peak aminoglycoside concentrations may provide information on therapeutic efficacy, whereas the trough value may be useful to assess possible toxicity (accumulation). Table 2 lists the recommended therapeutic ranges for commonly monitored drugs.

In certain instances, it may be desirable to measure drug concentrations at several points during a dosing interval to provide data for the calculation of important pharmacokinetic parameters such as drug clearance, volume of distribution, and elimination half-life. This information may assist in determining appropriate individualized dosing regimens for selected patients.

Recommended therapeutic ranges are based on population mean responses, and thus individual variations in pharmacological response are to be expected. In general, interindividual variance in pharmacological response occurs to a lesser magnitude than do variations in drug absorption, distribution, and elimination. Nevertheless, some patients may experience effective therapeutic response at drug concentrations below the recommended therapeutic range, whereas other patients may require serum concentrations somewhat higher than the upper limit of the therapeutic range. Thus, it may be necessary to individualize the therapeutic range as well as the drug dosage schedule for a given patient. Only through a coordinated team effort involving laboratory measurement of serum drug concentration, an understanding and

Table 2. Therapeutic Range for Commonly Measured Drugs

Drug	Therapeutic Range (μg/mL)
Antiepileptic Drugs	
Carbamazepine	8–12
Ethosuximide	40–100
Phenobarbital	15–40
Phenytoin	10–20
Primidone	5–12
Valproic acid	50–100
Cardioactive Drugs	
Digoxin	0.8–2.0[a]
Disopyramide	2–5
Flecainide	0.2–1.0
Lidocaine	1.5–5.0
Quinidine	2–5
Procainamide	4–10
Procainamide and N-acetylprocainamide	10–30

Table 2. (Continued)

Drug	Therapeutic Range (μg/mL)
Antibiotics	
Amikacin	
Trough	1–8[b]
Peak	20–30
Gentamicin	
Trough	< 1–2
Peak	5–10
Tobramycin	
Trough	< 1–2
Peak	5–10
Vancomycin	
Trough	5–10
Peak	20–40
Analeptics, Bronchodilators	
Theophylline	10–20
Psychoactive Drugs	
Amitriptyline	120–250[a, c]
Desipramine	75–160[a]
Imipramine	150–250[a, d]
Nortriptyline	50–150[a]

[a] ng/mL.
[b] Less severe infection, 1–4 μg/mL; life-threatening infection, 4–8 μg/mL.
[c] Amitriptyline plus nortriptyline.
[d] Imipramine plus desipramine.

application of pharmacokinetic principles, and sound clinical acumen is drug therapy efficiently and effectively optimized.

THE ANALYTICAL CHALLENGE

Therapeutic drug concentration monitoring entails the accurate and precise measurement of a drug in a complex biological matrix. The analysis must be free not only from interference by matrix components, but also from endogenous compounds, coadministered therapeutic agents, and structurally similar drug metabolites. Moreover, the speed of analysis is an important consideration, since results should be available within a clinically relevant time frame. Finally, minimal sample volume requirements are desirable, and are paramount for pediatric patients.

Two main analytical approaches have been applied to meet this challenge: chromatography and immunoassays.

Chromatography

Both gas–liquid chromatography (GC) and high performance liquid chromatography (HPLC) are powerful analytical techniques, which have been used to establish the foundation of drug monitoring. The high resolving power and applicability for the rapid development of new assays for pharmacokinetic studies and for assessing the necessity for monitoring the serum concentration of a particular drug are major advantages of these techniques. Chromatographic methods also generally provide an analytical reference to which immunoassays are compared. Of the two, HPLC is the more versatile, since the liquid mobile phase composition may be varied to effect the separation of different drug classes using the same analytical column. Gas chromatography may require separate analytical columns for the analysis of diverse drug groups. Moreover, a derivatization step may be required before GC analysis.

Chromatographic techniques allow for the simultaneous measurement of several drugs; this is an advantage when it is desirable to measure a drug and its pharmacologically active metabolite (e.g., procainamide and N-acetylprocainamide) or when a patient is receiving multiple drug therapy (e.g., treatment with two or more anticonvulsant drugs). An example of the determination of several anticonvulsant drugs by HPLC is presented in Figure 2.

Disadvantages of chromatography include the complexity of instrumentation, which requires a highly skilled and trained analyst, the relatively large sample volume requirements, the necessity in most instances for an extraction step prior to analysis, and the relatively slow sample throughput.

Recent advances in column technology (e.g., capillary GC and microbore HPLC columns) have not only enhanced sensitivity, thereby reducing sample volume requirements, but have also increased considerably the speed of chromatographic analysis (6,7). Moreover, microprocessor-controlled instruments have greatly simplified chromatographic analyses. A commercial HPLC system (Waters QA-1 Analyzer, Water Associates, Milford, MA) designed for ease of operation has been marketed for the drug monitoring field.

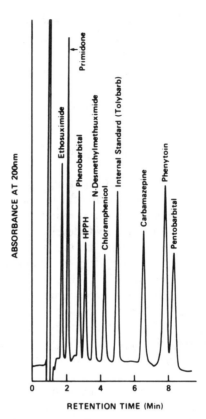

Figure 2. Chromatographic separation of a standard mixture of 10 drugs. (Ou CN, Rognerud CL. *Clin Chem* 1984;30:1668 with permission. Copyright American Association for Clinical Chemistry, Inc.)

Another analytical challenge is imposed by the chiral nature of some therapeutic drugs. Although they may be administered as racemic mixtures, only one of the enantiomers may have significant pharmacological and/or toxicological activity. Moreover, the enantiomers may have markedly different rates of metabolism and pharmacokinetic characteristics. Clearly it would be appropriate to measure only the concentration of the active antipode rather than the total racemate. However, since the enantiomers of a chiral compound have identical physical properties, they cannot be resolved by conventional chromatographic methods. In one analytical approach to address this issue, the racemate is first reacted with a chiral derivatizing agent to form a pair of diastereomers which, because of their differing physical properties, may subsequently be separated by conventional chromatography.

An example of this technique is the separation of the enantiomers of propranolol as their N-trifluoroacetyl-(S)-prolyl amide diastereomers by conventional HPLC (8). Another approach uses a chiral stationary phase—for example, in the resolution of the same propranolol enantiomers, as the racemic oxazolidone derivatives, with an HPLC column in which (R)-N-(3,5-dinitrobenzoyl)phenylglycine has been incorporated as a chiral discriminator (9). A highly promising chiral stationary phase consisting of immobilized α_1-acid glycoprotein appears to have broad application for the resolution of racemic drugs and does not require prior derivatization of the enantiomers (10,11). Undoubtedly, techniques such as these will have increasing influence and application in the therapeutic drug monitoring arena.

Immunoassays

The development of immunoassays for drug quantitation has had a major impact in the field of therapeutic drug monitoring. The high specificity of interaction between an antibody and its hapten, in this case a drug, circumvents the need to physically separate the compound of interest from other components of the biological matrix to effect quantitation. A variety of techniques have been employed to assess binding of the drug to its specific antibody. In general, these techniques are rapid and relatively simple to perform, and they may be automated. Their development, however, is neither rapid nor simple, and thus they frequently follow chromatographic techniques as second-generation methods. Most drugs are not immunogenic. To develop antibodies against them, therefore, chemical coupling as a hapten to a carrier protein, usually bovine serum albumin, is necessary. Using modern techniques of molecular biology, monoclonal antibodies with narrow, defined specificity can be produced from a single clone of specifically prepared antibody-forming hybridoma cells in seemingly inexhaustible supply (12). Monoclonal antibodies have recently been employed in selected drug immunoassays (discussed below). Immunoassay development is generally beyond the capability of most, if not all, laboratories engaged in therapeutic drug monitoring; therefore they must rely on the commercial availability of immunoassay reagent kits.

Radioimmunoassay

Radioimmunoassay (RIA) combines the specificity of antibody–hapten binding with the exquisite sensitivity for measurement of an added radiolabeled tracer hapten. The radiolabeled tracer drug competes with drug present in the sample for antibody binding sites. After separation of radiolabeled drug bound to antibody from that free in solution, the radioactivity present in either fraction may be measured and the unknown drug concentration computed from the response curve obtained with known standards.

A primary advantage of RIA methods is their sensitivity, for which detection limits in the picogram range are common. This order of sensitivity is normally not required for most therapeutic drugs (see Table 2). Disadvantages include the requirement for the handling and disposal of radioactive materials, the short reagent storage life, and because of the separation step involved, the lack of suitable automated procedures. (See Chapter 7 for a more complete discussion of RIA.)

The major application of RIA in the drug monitoring field is for the measurement of digoxin (and digitoxin). The dominance, until recently, of RIA methods for digoxin was fostered by the lack of suitable chromatographic techniques and by digoxin's relatively low therapeutic concentration. Both RIA and the newer nonisotopic immunoassay methods for measuring digoxin all suffer to varying degrees from interference by protein, especially albumin, present in the sample, and more importantly, from cross-reactivity with digoxin-like immunoreactive factors (DLIF) present in cord serum from newborns, in the serum from pregnant women, or from patients who have liver disease or are in renal failure (13,14). It has recently been reported that interference by DLIF is dramatically reduced by ultrafiltration of serum at 4°C prior to digoxin immunoassay (15).

Enzyme-Multiplied Immunoassay Technique (EMIT)

The EMIT (Syva, Palo Alto, CA) method was the forerunner of homogeneous nonisotopic immunoassays and until recently the dominant analytical method in use for therapeutic drug monitoring. In this technique, the indicator drug is covalently linked to (i.e., labeled with) the enzyme glucose-6-phosphate dehydrogenase. When the enzyme-labeled drug binds to a drug-specific antibody, the activity of the enzyme is inhibited. Drug present in the patient's serum will compete with the enzyme-labeled drug for the available antibody binding sites. Consequently, the greater the concentration of drug present in the sample, the greater the enzyme activity, which may be conveniently monitored by measuring the increase with time in the absorbance by NADH at 340 nm (Figure 3). The binding of each mole of drug makes available an equivalent amount of unbound, active enzyme-labeled drug, which can then catalyze the reaction of many moles of substrate. Thus, these assays are referred to as "enzyme multiplied." Moreover, separation of bound and unbound enzyme-labeled drug is not required and therefore the assays are termed "homogeneous."

EMIT drug assays in general are rapid, may be easily automated using instrumentation which does not require a highly specialized operator, require

$$D + D\text{–}E + Ab \rightleftharpoons Ab \cdot D + Ab \cdot D\text{–}E$$

$$\text{glucose-6-P} + NAD^+ \xrightarrow[\quad D-E \quad]{Ab \cdot D-E} \begin{array}{l} NR \\ \text{gluconolactone} + NADH + H^+ \\ \quad\text{(absorbs at 340 nm)} \end{array}$$

Figure 3. Enzyme-multiplied immunoassay technique (EMIT). Nonstandard abbreviations: D, drug; D–E, drug covalently linked to glucose-6-phosphate dehydrogenase (E); Ab, drug-specific antibody.

a small sample volume, and generally correlate well with chromatographic methods (16). In addition to these attributes, the wide range of available drug assays (Table 3) has led to their ready acceptance in the clinical laboratory. Disadvantages include the need to calibrate instrumentation relatively

Table 3. Selected Immunoassay Systems and Reagents Used in Therapeutic Drug Monitoring

Commonly Monitored Drugs	Systems[a]					
	Syva EMIT	Abbott TDx FPIA	Ames TDA/ Optimate SLFIA	Dade Stratus	du Pont aca EMIT[b]	Beckman ICS NINIA
Carbamazepine	×	×	×	×	×	×
Ethosuximide	×	×	×		×	
Phenobarbital	×	× M	×	×	×	×
Phenytoin	× M	×	×	×	× M	×
Primidone	×	×	×	×	×	×
Valproic acid	× M	×	×		×	
Digoxin	×	×		×	ACMIA	
Lidocaine	×	×		×	×	
Quinidine	× M	×	×	×	×	×
Procainamide	×	×	×	×	×	
N-Acetylprocain-amide	×	×	×	×	×	
Amikacin	×	×	×		×	
Gentamicin	×	×	× M	×	×	×
Tobramycin	×	×	×	×	×	×
Vancomycin		×				
Theophylline	×	× M	× M	×	PETINIA; M	× M
Methotrexate	×	×				

[a] M = Monoclonal antibody.
[b] Unless otherwise indicated, assays on the du Pont aca are based on Syva EMIT reagents.

frequently because of the instability of the enzyme/substrate reagents, spectral interference from high concentrations of lipids or hemoglobin, and, in common with all immunoassays, the necessity of a separate assay for each drug (e.g., procainamide and N-acetylprocainamide). Antibody cross-reactivity with coadministered drugs or drug metabolites is always a potential occurrence with any immunoassay. Prior EMIT assays for phenytoin, which used a polyclonal antibody, were particularly prone to interference by the phenytoin metabolite 5-(p-hydroxyphenyl)-5-phenylhydantoin (HPPH), present in especially high concentrations in the serum from patients with end-stage renal disease (17). Newer EMIT reagent formulations for phenytoin quantitation, which use a more specific monoclonal antibody, demonstrate significantly less interference from HPPH (18,19). The EMIT theophylline assay may also be subject to interference by substances, perhaps the theophylline metabolite 1,3-dimethyluric acid, present in increased concentration in the sera of patients with renal disease (20).

Fluorescence Polarization Immunoassay (FPIA)

Fluorescence occurs when a molecule is excited by a beam of light and its high energy electron emits radiant energy of a longer wavelength as the electron returns to the ground state. The time interval between the light absorption and emission is the fluorescence lifetime. If the incident light is plane-polarized, absorption and emission will occur only when the molecule's absorption dipoles are parallel to the plane of vibration of the exciting light. Moreover, the plane of vibration of the emitted light will remain parallel to the emission dipoles (21).

The fluorescence lifetimes of many low molecular weight molecules in aqueous solution are long relative to their rates of Brownian rotation. Thus, small molecules will become randomly oriented during the interval between excitation and emission and thus will emit randomly oriented (depolarized) light when excited by a polarized incident beam. Because their rotational rates are slower, large molecules undergo only a few degrees of rotation during the same time interval, and the emitted light therefore remains largely polarized in the same plane with the incident polarized light (21).

In fluorescence polarization immunoassay (22), the drug of interest is labeled with a fluorescent tracer such as fluorescein. This indicator fluorescein-labeled drug competes with drug present in patient sera for antibody binding sites. Since the antibody is a large molecule, labeled drug which is bound to the antibody will emit largely polarized light when excited with a polarized incident beam. The unbound fluorescein-labeled drug is small and therefore emits light which is depolarized. As the serum concentration of drug increases, the ratio of unbound indicator drug to antibody-bound indicator drug increases, and thus the degree of fluorescence polarization diminishes.

Adaptation of this analytical concept for use in the clinical laboratory was hampered by the lack of convenient instrumentation to measure the change in fluorescence polarization. This situation changed dramatically with the introduction of the highly automated Abbott TDx (Abbott Laboratories, Chicago), an instrument for performing fluorescence polarization immuno-assays (23,24). The TDx uses a polarizer–liquid crystal combination to rotate the plane of polarization of incident light between the vertical and horizontal axes. Incident light from the fixed horizontal polarizer will be rotated by 90° when it traverses the liquid crystal. When a voltage is applied to the liquid crystal, no rotation occurs and the incident light that impinges the sample remains horizontally polarized. Only emitted light which passes through a fixed vertical polarizer is detected, and these intensity measurements are taken at the same frequency as the voltage changes in the liquid crystal.

The degree of polarization P of the fluorescent sample is determined from the equation

$$P = \frac{I_{vv} - I_{hv}}{I_{vv} + I_{hv}}$$

where I_{vv} is the intensity of emitted light measured in the fixed vertical plane after excitation of the sample with vertically polarized light, and I_{hv} is the vertical emission intensity after excitation with horizontal light. Thus, I_{vv} represents the antibody-bound, fluorescein-labeled drug that retains the polarization of the incident beam and I_{hv} represents the unbound labeled drug which will randomly orient (depolarize) the incident light. When drug concentration in the sample is low, a large fraction of the labeled-drug will be bound by antibody; I_{vv} will be large relative to I_{hv} and P will approach 1. When the drug concentration is high, the fraction of unbound labeled drug will be high; I_{vv} and I_{hv} will be of similar magnitude, and P will approach 0.

Reagent kits for use with the Abbott TDx are available for many therapeutic drugs including digoxin (Table 3). The instrument is highly automated and simple to operate. The assays are rapid and precise, sample volume requirements are reasonably low (50 μL), and results generally compare favorably with chromatographic techniques (25). Moreover, reagent stability is very good, and thus calibration curves remain usable for several weeks.

Falsely elevated values for theophylline were observed when sera from patients with renal disease were assayed using FPIA reagents containing polyclonal antitheophylline antibody (26–28). Newer theophylline kits, which contain a more specific mouse monoclonal antibody, were reported to demonstrate significantly improved results for uremic patients (*29,30*). Nevertheless, high theophylline values in uremic patients have been reported even with this monoclonal antitheophylline antibody (*20*). Likewise, monoclonal antibodies are now used for the determination of phenobarbital to reduce but not completely eliminate cross-reactivity with its major metabolite, *p*-hydroxyphenobarbital. This metabolite, and perhaps others, may accumulate to significant concentrations in patients with chronic renal failure and lead to falsely high phenobarbital values when assayed with less specific polyclonal antibody reagents (*31*).

The Abbott TDx digoxin assay is a popular non-RIA digoxin immunoassay in wide use. Because of the high sensitivity requirements for this assay, it is necessary to precede the immunoassay by achieving a reduction in the background fluorescence produced by the serum protein matrix via a protein precipitation step. This precipitation step does result in a protein concentration-dependent loss of digoxin (*32*). To minimize this protein effect, Abbott altered the precipitating reagent; however, the modification apparently has resulted in increased interference by DLIF (*33*).

Substrate-Labeled Fluorescence Immunoassay (SLFIA)

The concept that fluorescence quenching may occur upon chemical derivatization of a natural fluorophore forms the basis for immunoassays using fluorogenic enzyme substrates as developed by Ames Laboratories (Elkhart, IN). In this approach, the drug of interest is conjugated with β-galactosyl-umbelliferone (G-U) to form a substrate-labeled drug complex (G-U-D; Figure 4). This conjugate has weak fluorescence until acted on by the enzyme β-galactosidase. Upon hydrolysis of the galactose moiety by β-galactosidase, the resulting umbelliferone-labeled drug (U-D) exhibits strong fluorescence.

$$G\text{-}U\text{-}D \xrightarrow{\ \beta\text{-galctosidase}\ } \underset{\textbf{fluorescent}}{U\text{-}D} + G$$

The utility of such a fluorogenic substrate-labeled drug in a homogeneous immunoassay rests on the protection from enzymatic hydrolysis afforded when the substrate-labeled drug binds to anti-drug antibody:

$$Ab \cdot G\text{-}U\text{-}D \xrightarrow{\ \beta\text{-galactosidase}\ } no\ reaction$$

Thus, drug present in the sample and substrate-labeled drug compete for a limiting number of antibody binding sites. Upon addition of β-galactosidase,

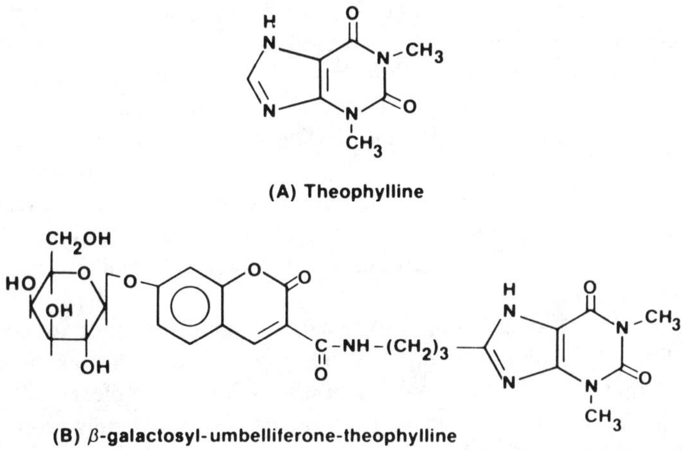

(A) Theophylline

(B) β-galactosyl-umbelliferone-theophylline

Figure 4. Chemical structure of (A) theophylline and (B) β-galactosyl-unbelliferone-theophylline (G-U-theophylline): 8-[3-(7-β-galactosylcoumarin-3-carboxyamido)propyl] theophylline. (Li, TM, et al. *Clin Chem* 1981;27:22 with permission. Copyright American Association for Clinical Chemistry, Inc.)

only unbound fluorogenic substrate-labeled drug is hydrolyzed to the fluor-escent product. As the concentration of drug present in the sample increases, more unbound substrate-labeled drug becomes available for enzymatic hydrolysis, resulting in a proportionate increase in measured fluorescence:

$$\left.\begin{array}{c} G\text{-}U\text{-}D + Ab + D \\ \downarrow \quad \uparrow \\ G\text{-}U\text{-}D \cdot Ab + D \cdot Ab \end{array}\right\} \xrightarrow{\beta\text{-galactosidase}} U\text{-}D + G$$

Reagent kits (Ames Laboratories) for the measurement of several therapeutic drugs, some of which employ monoclonal antibodies, are available for use on an automated SLFIA system (Ames TDA/Optimate) as well as any other suitable fluorometer (34–36), including a centrifugal analyzer with fluorescence capability (37). These reagent kits have a shelf life of up to 18 months, and the calibration curves generally remain stable for at least 2 weeks. Results using SLFIA reagents are generally comparable to other reference methods (35,36,38).

Nephelometric Inhibition Immunoassay (NINIA)

Antigen–antibody soluble complexes, before they separate out of solution as immunoprecipitates, are large enough to scatter incident light. Thus, the formation of these complexes may be determined using sensitive nephelo-metric techniques to measure the scattered incident light.

In rate–nephelometric inhibition immunoassays (*39–41*), multiple drug (hapten) molecules are covalently linked to a developer antigen (e.g., equine apoferritin or albumin). Reaction of this developer antigen with drug-specific antibody results in the formation of soluble light-scattering complexes (Figure 5). The rate of this complex formation is accelerated, hence assay sensitivity improved, by including a nonionic hydrophilic polymer such as polyethylene glycol, which increases the probability of protein–protein interaction by excluding water (*42*).

The presence of a small amount of drug in the sample or standard competes for the limited number of antibody binding sites and results in a large reduction in the rate of formation of the soluble complexes. Thus, the maximum rate of change in light-scattering intensity is inversely proportional to the drug concentration in the sample.

Rate–nephelometric inhibition assays for use in therapeutic monitoring of drugs have been developed for both the semiautomated and automated immunochemistry systems "ICS" (Beckman Instruments, Fullerton, CA) (*41*). These instruments measure the maximum rate of the light-scattering intensity

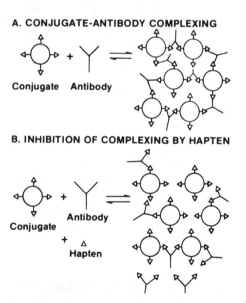

Figure 5. Principle of inhibition immunoassay. (Polito AJ. *Therapeutic Drug Monitoring Continuing Education*, October 1981. Reprinted with permission. Copyright American Association for Clinical Chemistry, Inc.)

and automatically compute the equivalent drug concentration in the sample. The rate assays require no sample or reagent blanking to correct for background light scattering. Since, however, the signal-to-noise ratio, hence the sensitivity of the assay, is affected by nonspecific light scatter, serum samples are generally diluted before assay. These inhibition immunoassays are rapid (30–50 seconds reaction time), they generally correlate well with other immunoassays and chromatographic methods, and the reagents are very stable (43–45).

Other manufacturers have recently developed reagent kits based on similar concepts of inhibition of antibody agglutination, but they have employed more traditional turbidimetric rather than nephelometric measurements of antibody agglutination. Included among these are a turbidimetric rate inhibition assay (46) developed by Coulter Diagnostics (Hialeah, FL), assays based on the inhibition of the rate of agglutination of antibody-coated latex particles by Ficoll-bound drug (Technicon Corporation, Tarrytown, NY) (47), and drug assays based on sequential latex agglutination inhibition (Instrumentation Laboratory, Lexington, MA) (48).

Radial Partition Immunoassay

In radial partition immunoassay, a solid phase procedure developed by American Dade (Miami, FL), anti-drug antibody is immobilized in the center portion of a glass fiber paper tab (49). Serum is premixed with an enzyme-labeled drug (drug conjugated with E. coli alkaline phosphatase) and then applied to the center portion of the glass fiber tab. Portions of drug present in the sample and enzyme-labeled drug compete for a limited number of drug binding sites on the antibody molecules. Addition of a substrate wash solution (4-methylumbelliferyl phosphate) removes excess unbound enzyme-labeled drug from the center of the tab via radial elution and at the same time initiates the enzymatic reaction. The rate of appearance of the fluorescent 4-methylumbelliferone product, generated by the action of alkaline phosphatase on the nonfluorescent 4-methylumbelliferyl phosphate substrate, is measured in the center portion of the filter paper tab by front surface fluorescence (Figure 6). The rate of increase in fluorescence intensity is inversely proportional to the drug concentration in the sample.

With the appropriate sample handler accessory, the entire procedure is automated using a microprocessor controlled front surface fluorometer (Stratus) and requires approximately 7 minutes for the entire reaction sequence. Additional samples are analyzed at a rate of about one per minute. The stored calibration curves may generally be used for 2 weeks or more before recalibration is required.

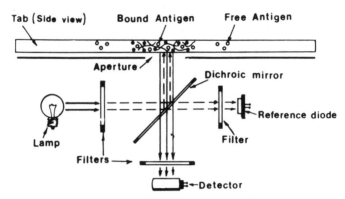

Figure 6. Schematic diagram of front-surface fluorometer. (Geigel JL, et al. *Clin Chem* 1982;28:1895 with permission. Copyright American Association for Clinical Chemistry, Inc.)

To achieve the required sensitivity for the measurement of digoxin and digitoxin, these two assays are based on a sequential saturation methodology. In the case of digoxin (*49*), undiluted serum is placed on the antibody tab and digoxin is allowed to bind to the immobilized anti-digoxin antibody. The remaining unbound antibody sites are then reacted with an excess of the enzyme–digoxin conjugate. The remaining steps in the assay are identical to those described previously for other drugs. The Stratus digoxin assay was reported to compare reasonably well with RIA procedures (*50,51*), but both falsely increased (*52*) and decreased (*53*) values have been observed. The performance of other drug assays on the Stratus, in comparison to HPLC and RIA, was reported to be good (*54*).

Particle-Enhanced Turbidimetric Inhibition Immunoassay (PETINIA)

The PETINIA methodology developed by du Pont (*55*) employs microscopic latex particles to which drug molecules are covalently bound via a synthetic spacer polymer (Figure 7). Binding of these particles by anti-drug antibody results in aggregation and the formation of complexes that can be detected by light-scattering turbidimetric measurements. Drug present in the sample competes for the limited number of antibody binding sites, thus reducing the degree of particle aggregation (Figure 8). The rate of particle agglutination is measured and is inversely proportional to the concentration of drug present in the sample.

A PETINIA assay for theophylline is available for use on the du Pont aca (*56*) and is also formulated separately for use on other suitable instrumentation (*57*). Since no enzyme activity measurements are involved, these

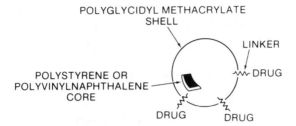

POLYGLYCIDYL METHACRYLATE
SHELL

LINKER

DRUG

POLYSTYRENE OR
POLYVINYLNAPHTHALENE
CORE

DRUG DRUG

Figure 7. Diagram of a particle reagent: high refractive index cores of either polystyrene or polyvinylnaphthalene surrounded by a thin shell of polyglycidyl methacrylate to which drug-linked conjugates are attached. (Litchfield WJ, et al. *Clin Chem* 1984;30:1491 with permission. Copyright American Association for Clinical Chemistry, Inc.)

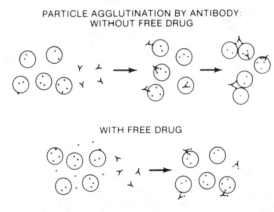

PARTICLE AGGLUTINATION BY ANTIBODY:
WITHOUT FREE DRUG

WITH FREE DRUG

Figure 8. Schematic representation of the PETINIA principle. Specific antibody (Y) aggregates latex particles coated with drug. Free drug (*) from the patient's sample inhibits both the rate and extent of aggregation. (Litchfield WJ, et al. *Clin Chem* 1984;30:1491 with permission. Copyright American Association for Clinical Chemistry, Inc.)

reagents have excellent stability and the assays demonstrate good precision. The theophylline assay employs a monoclonal antibody with negligible cross-reactivity toward caffeine and most other xanthines. Nevertheless, a small degree (13%) of cross-reactivity is observed with 1,3-dimethyluric acid, a theophylline metabolite that may be detected in serum from patients with renal disease (56). Moreover, interference by other unidentified factors present in the serum of uremic patients has been noted with this and other immunoassays for theophylline (20).

Although most drug assays available on the du Pont aca use the EMIT methodolgy (see Table 3), du Pont markets reagent kits based on the

PETINIA method for use on other discrete analyzers. In addition to theophylline, PETINIA kits are currently available for the assay of gentamicin (58), tobramycin (59), phenobarbital (60), and phenytoin (61).

Affinity-Column-Mediated Immunometric Assay (ACMIA)

Because of the design restraints imposed by the du Pont aca analyzer (5-mL reaction volume), du Pont developed an especially sensitive immunometric assay for the measurement of digoxin (62,63). For the assay, an antibody–enzyme conjugate was prepared by the covalent attachment of the F(ab')$_2$ fragment of anti-digoxin antibody with β-galactosidase. The F(ab')$_2$ fragment was selected because it minimizes nonspecific (Fc-region-dependent) binding due to rheumatoid factor and also demonstrates efficient separation of digoxin-bound and free fractions in subsequent steps of the procedure. An excess of this antibody–enzyme conjugate is first incubated with serum to allow all the digoxin present to bind to the antibody. Excess unbound antibody–enzyme conjugate is then removed by passing the mixture through an affinity column composed of the digoxin analogue, oubain, covalently attached by a protein spacer to Sephadex G-10. Unbound antibody–enzyme conjugate remains on the column, whereas digoxin-bound antibody–enzyme conjugate elutes from the column. Hydrolysis of o-nitrophenyl-β-D-galactopyranoside, mediated by the eluted enzyme conjugate, is measured spectrophotometrically and the rate of formation of o-nitrophenol is directly proportional to the concentration of digoxin in the sample (Figure 9). This assay is approximately 1000-fold more sensitive than the previously described PETINIA method but it does require fivefold greater sample volume. Reagent kits for digoxin measurement based on the ACMIA principle have been marketed by du Pont for use on suitable automated instruments (64). The high degree of sensitivity afforded by this saturation immunometric assay exceeds the requirements for most therapeutically monitored drugs. This property, and the necessity of the separation step, will limit the general application of the ACMIA method in the therapeutic drug monitoring field.

Apoenzyme-Reactivated Immunoassay System (ARIS)

For the competitive immunoassay called ARIS, developed by the Ames Division, Miles Laboratories, Inc. (Elkhart, IN), a drug conjugate is formed by the covalent attachment of the drug with the enzyme prosthetic group flavin adenine dinucleotide (FAD) (Figure 10). This drug conjugate competes with drug in the sample for a limited number of anti-drug antibody binding sites. When drug–FAD is bound to the antibody, reactivation of the apoenzyme, apoglucose oxidase, is prevented. Increasing concentrations of drug in

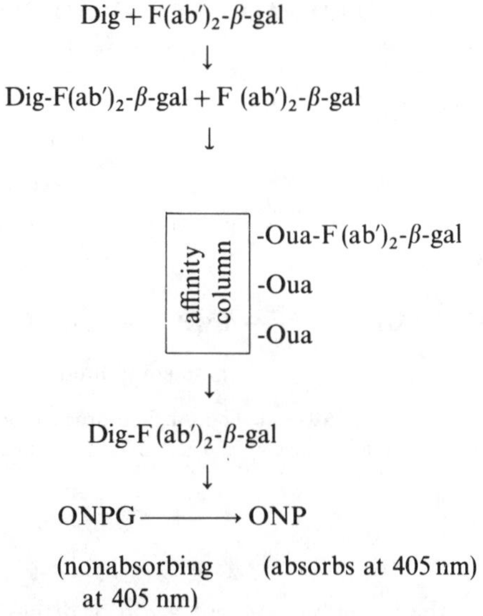

Dig + F(ab')$_2$-β-gal

↓

Dig-F(ab')$_2$-β-gal + F (ab')$_2$-β-gal

↓

-Oua-F (ab')$_2$-β-gal

-Oua

-Oua

↓

Dig-F (ab')$_2$-β-gal

↓

ONPG ⟶ ONP

(nonabsorbing   (absorbs at 405 nm)
at 405 nm)

Figure 9. Principle of affinity-column-mediated immunometric assay (ACMIA). Dig, digoxin; F(ab')$_2$-β-gal, β-galactosidase covalently coupled to the F (ab')$_2$ fragment of anti-digoxin antibody; Oua, ouabain covalently bound to Sephadex G-10; ONPG, o-nitrophenyl-β-D-galactopyranoside; ONP, o-nitrophenol.

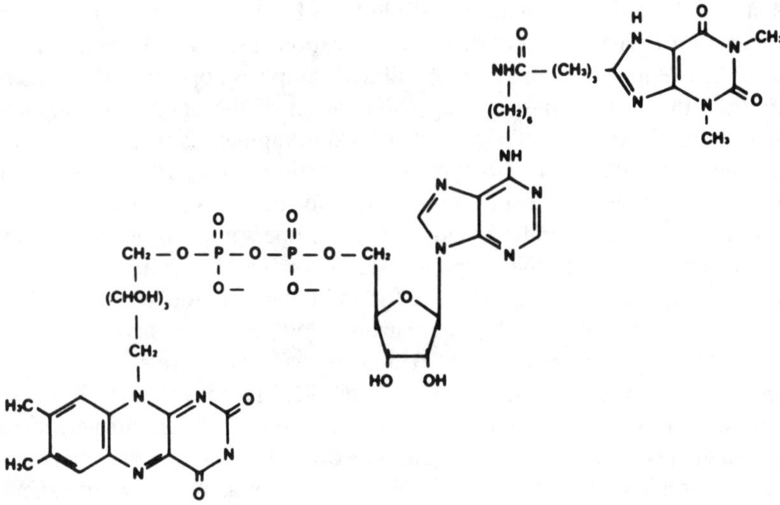

Figure 10. The FAD label used with the theophylline ARIS. (Greenquist AC. *Therapeutic Drug Monitoring Continuing Education* June 1984. Reprinted with permission. Copyright American Association for Clinical Chemistry, Inc.)

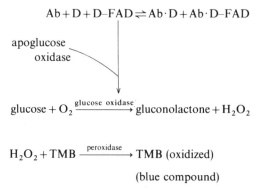

$$Ab + D + D\text{-}FAD \rightleftharpoons Ab \cdot D + Ab \cdot D\text{-}FAD$$

apoglucose
oxidase

$$glucose + O_2 \xrightarrow{\text{glucose oxidase}} gluconolactone + H_2O_2$$

$$H_2O_2 + TMB \xrightarrow{\text{peroxidase}} TMB \text{ (oxidized)}$$

(blue compound)

Figure 11. Reaction sequence for the ARIS method. Ab, anti-drug antibody; D, drug; D-FAD, drug conjugated with flavin adenine dinucleotide; TMB, 3,3',5,5'-tetramethylbenzidine.

the sample increases the available concentration of drug–FAD, which reactivates the apoenzyme. The activated glucose oxidase converts glucose to gluconolactone and hydrogen peroxide. In the presence of peroxidase, the H_2O_2 oxidizes 3,3',5,5'-tetramethylbenzidine to a blue product (Figure 11). Since reactivated apoglucose oxidase catalyzes the oxidation of many substrate molecules, substantial amplification of the response is achieved.

Reagents based on the ARIS principle have been incorporated into a dry strip form for measurement of drug concentrations using the Ames Seralyzer desktop reflectance photometer (65). Diluted sample is applied to the reagent strip and, after a lag phase during reactivation of the apoglucose oxidase (generally 60–70 seconds), the rate of color development is measured over a 20-second interval. This rate is directly proportional to the drug concentration in the sample. This drug immunostrip format is especially applicable when rapid testing, generally by non laboratory personnel, is desirable, such as the emergency room, the outpatient clinic, or the physician's office.

The performance of reagent strips for the determination of theophylline (66,67), phenytoin (68), and phenobarbital (69) compare favorably with HPLC. Although the phenytoin strip demonstrates relatively low cross-reactivity with the phenytoin metabolite 5-(p-hydroxyphenyl)-5-phenyl-hydantoin, this metabolite may accumulate in the sera of patients with renal impairment (17) and thus may potentially produce erroneous phenytoin values. A monoclonal antibody with minimal cross-reactivity toward caffeine is used in the reagent strip for theophylline measurement. Nevertheless, interference with the theophylline assay by a substance, perhaps 1,3-dimethyl-uric acid, present in the sera of patients with renal impairment has been

observed (*26, 70*), and interference by 8-chlorotheophylline (present in dimen-
hydrinate) may also occur (*66*).

Enzyme Immunochromatography

Enzyme immunochromatography is a novel noninstrumental test strip
immunoassay (*71*) consisting of (1) a dry paper strip to which has been added
immobilized drug-specific antibody, (2) an enzyme reagent consisting of
glucose oxidase plus a drug–horseradish peroxidase conjugate, and (3) a
color-developer solution containing substrate for both enzymes.

The patient sample is mixed with the enzyme solution, and then the end of
the antibody strip is immersed into this solution to allow the liquid
components to migrate the length of the strip by capillary action (Figure 12).
During this migration, drug present in the sample and the drug–peroxidase
conjugate are bound by the immobilized antibody. Since drug and
drug–peroxidase compete for antibody binding sites, the height of migration
of the drug–enzyme conjugate is dependent on the concentration of drug in

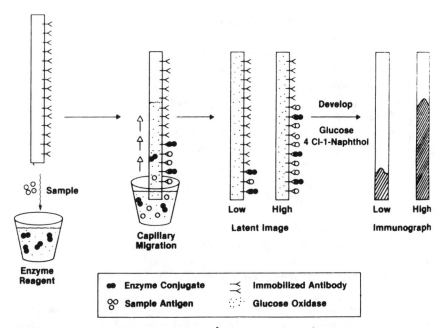

Figure 12. Schematic representation of the enzyme immunochromatographic test strip assay.
(Zuk RF, et al. *Clin Chem* 1985;31:1144 with permission. Copyright American Association for
Clinical Chemistry, Inc.)

the sample. Glucose oxidase, on the other hand, is distributed homogeneously throughout the strip.

The antibody-bound drug–peroxidase conjugate is visualized in a second step in which the test strip is immersed in the developer solution containing glucose and a chromogenic substrate for horseradish peroxidase. The *in situ* generation of hydrogen peroxide by the glucose-oxidase-catalyzed oxidation of glucose obviates the need for relatively unstable peroxide-containing developer reagents. This enzyme-generated hydrogen peroxide then mediates the peroxidase-catalyzed oxidation of 4-chloro-1-naphthol to form an insoluble blue-gray product.

$$\text{glucose} + O_2 \xrightarrow{\text{glucose oxidase}} \text{gluconolactone} + H_2O_2$$

$$H_2O_2 + 4\text{-Cl-1-naphthol} \xrightarrow{\text{Ab} \cdot \text{drug-peroxidase}} \text{blue-gray product}$$

In this way, the position of the antibody-bound drug–peroxidase conjugate is localized, and the height of the color front is proportional to the drug concentration in the sample. Immunospecific quantitation is thus dependent only on the location of the enzyme-label rather than on immunomodulation of its activity. Therefore, matrix interference and variations due to temperature, timing, and enzyme instability are minimized. Quantitative results may be obtained in 15 minutes without instrumentation and whole blood samples may be analyzed. Enzyme immunochromatogrphy is thus especially well suited for on-site drug monitoring in nonlaboratory settings such as the physician's office, the emergency room, or the outpatient clinic.

Enzyme immunochromatography test strips (AccuLevel) were developed and are marketed by Syntex Medical Diagnostics Division of Syna (Palo Alto, CA).

Catalytic Activity Recovery Immunoassay

Two conceptually similar homogeneous immunoassays that have recently been described depend on immunomodulation of the recovery of β-galactosidase catalytic activity resulting from the spontaneous assembly of genetically engineered inactive complementary β-galactosidase polypeptides (72,73).

In the more completely described technique (72), recombinant DNA technology is used to produce an *E. coli* β-galactosidase protein which contains small amino acid sequence deletions. As such, these so-called enzyme acceptors (EA) are enzymatically inactive. When combined with small polypeptides (called enzyme donors, ED), which contain some of the sequence omitted in the enzyme acceptors, aggregation into active tetrameric β-galactosidase spontaneously occurs.

For the immunoassay, the drug to be measured is covalently attached to the ED polypeptide in a manner that does not inhibit its combination with EA. In the presence of anti-drug antibody, the drug–ED conjugate is bound by antibody, thereby preventing assembly of active enzyme. Drug and drug–ED conjugate compete for available antibody binding sites, and thus formation of active enzyme is directly proportional to drug concentration in the sample. The amount of active enzyme formed may be monitored by measuring the rate of hydrolysis of a suitable β-galactosidase substrate such as o-nitrophenyl-β-D-galactopyranoside. The initial application of this technique to the immunoassay of digoxin produced results comparable to those obtained by RIA (72).

Time-Resolved Fluoroimmunoassay (TR-FIA)

Europium-β-diketone chelates have fluorescent characteristics which make them attractive immunoassay labels. Included among these are their high quantum yield, the large differential between excitation (330–350 nm) and emission (613 nm) wavelengths (Stokes shift), and their exceptionally long fluorescence decay time (0.1–1 ms), which is more than 10^4 times longer than the average background fluorescence decay of biological specimens. The selective detection of this long-decay fluorescence markedly reduces interference from background light scattering and fluorescence, factors which limit the sensitivity of conventional fluoroimmunoassays (74). Thus, the time-resolved fluorometric measurement of europium chelates has a theoretical sensitivity similar to that of radioisotopic methods (75).

A recently described time-resolved fluoroimmunoassay for digoxin (76) uses anti-digoxin antibody labeled with a europium chelate. A solid phase antigen is prepared by immobilization of digoxin-conjugated albumin to the surface of polystyrene microtitration strip wells. The Eu-labeled antibody is competitively distributed between this solid phase and the sample digoxin. After an appropriate incubation period (30 minutes), the strips are washed to remove soluble Eu-labeled antibody, a fluorescence enhancement solution is added to release the Eu-chelate from the surface-bound antibody, and fluorescence is then measured in a time-resolved fluorometer. The digoxin assay performance characteristics were comparable to an RIA procedure.

FREE DRUG MEASUREMENTS

The monitoring of free rather than total serum drug concentration is beneficial when the total drug concentration inappropriately reflects the pharmacologically active free drug concentration. Thus, for drugs with high degrees of protein binding (bound fraction ≥ 0.7), alterations in drug protein binding may significantly influence the free drug concentration (see "Drug–Protein Binding").

Factors which may influence the degree of drug binding include pathophysiological changes in the concentration of binding proteins (albumin and α_1-acid glycoprotein), concentration-dependent alterations in the free fraction due to binding saturation by the drug (valproic acid, disopyramide), competitive displacement from binding site by endogenous substances (free fatty acids, bilirubin) or other drugs (salicylate), or alteration in the binding affinity, such as occurs in chronic renal failure (77,78).

The two most widely used techniques to measure free drug concentrations involve the physical separation of the free and protein-bound drug by either equilibrium dialysis or ultrafiltration.

Equilibrium Dialysis

In equilibrium dialysis (78,79), serum is allowed to equilibrate with an isotonic buffer solution across a semipermeable membrane of suitable pore size to allow the passage of low molecular weight drug molecules but the retention of larger protein molecules. At equilibrium, the concentration of free drug on each side of the membrane is equivalent. Measurement of drug concentration in the dialysate and the retentate (fraction containing the retained protein) provides a measure of the free fraction:

$$\text{free fraction} = \frac{[\text{free drug}]}{[\text{total drug}]}$$

where retentate [total drug] = [free drug] + [protein-bound drug].

While the free and total drug concentrations are altered from the original values by the dialysis process, the free fraction remains constant for most drugs. To calculate the original free drug concentration, the free fraction must be multiplied by the original total drug concentration. Therefore, three separate analytical determinations are required to derive the desired free drug concentration.

The time required to reach equilibrium may vary from 1 to 24 hours, depending on the binding characteristics of the drug and on the dialysis system and thus must be established in each case. Moreover, various factors such as pH and temperature may influence drug binding and thus must be adequately controlled. For drugs that demonstrate saturable binding characteristics (valproic acid, disopyramide), equilibrium dialysis will underestimate the original free drug concentration because of the dilution effect of the dialysis process. Thus, the free fraction for these drugs will not be constant but will change as the total drug concentration in the retentate is reduced. This dilution effect may be minimized by use of dialysate buffer volumes equal to or less than the retentate volume.

Ultrafiltration

In ultrafiltration (78,79), the serum sample is placed above a semipermeable membrane and a centrifugal force is applied to cause the movement of water and low molecular weight molecules into a filtrate collection device. Measurement of drug concentration in the filtrate directly provides the free drug concentration. Although the protein concentration changes during the ultrafiltration process, both unbound protein and protein-bound drug are similarly affected. Thus, if the binding constant (K) does not change during filtration, the filtered free drug concentration is also constant:

$$\text{free drug} + \text{unbound protein} \rightleftharpoons \text{protein bound drug}$$

$$[\text{free drug}] = \frac{[\text{protein-bound drug}]}{K\,[\text{unbound protein}]}$$

As with equilibrium dialysis, temperature is a critical variable in the binding of many drugs but is not as easy to control with ultrafiltration. Ultrafiltration devices suitable for free drug determinations are commercially available from Amicon and Syva. With these devices, an ultrafiltrate of sufficient volume for subsequent drug analysis may typically be generated after about 10 minutes of centrifugation. This advantage, combined with the requirement of only a single drug concentration determination, makes ultrafiltration better suited for use in the clinical laboratory than equilibrium dialysis. Ultrafiltration has been demonstrated to provide free drug concentrations equivalent to those determined by equilibrium dialysis for phenytoin (80), valproic acid (81), and carbamazepine (81).

CONCLUSIONS

The field of therapeutic drug monitoring continues to grow at an amazing pace. We have witnessed in just a few short years the development of an astonishing array of highly innovative methods in immunoassay technology. There is no reason to suspect that advances in diverse disciplines such as molecular biology, immunology, engineering, computer science, and analytical and clinical chemistry will not continue to be applied in the drug monitoring arena. New, highly sensitive detection systems such as chemiluminescence will undoubtedly be exploited, and there will be greater use of monoclonal antibody technology. Versatile, high efficiency chromatographic systems will continue to be used for the initial study of the pharmacokinetics of new therapeutic agents and for the establishement of the need for drug monitoring. Highly sensitive and specific immunoassays will provide for rapid drug analyses in hospital, clinic, and reference laboratory settings. The advent of dry reagents and quantitative drug immunoassays without instrumentation ("dipsticks") will provide the means for drug monitoring in the physician's office and perhaps even in the patient's home.

REFERENCES

1. Levy RH, Bauer LA. Basic pharmacokinetics. *Ther Drug Monit* 1986;8:47–58.
2. Rowland M, Tozer TN. *Clinical Pharmacokinetics: Concepts and Applications.* Philadelphia: Lea & Febiger, 1980.
3. Benet LZ, Massoud N, Gambertoglio JC (eds). *Pharmacokinetic Basis for Drug Treatment.* New York: Raven, 1984.
4. Winter ME, Katcher BS, Kada-Kimble MA. *Basic Clinical Pharmacokinetics.* San Francisco: Applied Therapeutics, 1980, pp 5–67.
5. Taylor WJ, Diers Caviness MH (eds). *A Textbook for the Clinical Application of Therapeutic Drug Monitoring.* Irving, TX: Abbott Laboratories, 1986.
6. Wong SHY. Microbore HPLC in drug monitoring and toxicology: An overview. *Lab Manage* 1985;Oct:59–64.
7. Ehresman DJ, Price SM, Lakatua DJ. Screening biological samples for underivatized drugs using a splitless injection technique on fused silica capillary column gas chromatography. *J Anal Toxicol* 1985;9:55–62.
8. Silber B, Riegelman S. Stereospecific assay for (−)- and (+)-propranolol in human serum and dog plasma. *J Pharmacol Exp Ther* 1980;215:643–648.
9. Wainer IW, Doyle TD. The direct enantiomeric determination of (−)- and (+)-propranolol in human serum by high-performance liquid chromatography on a chiral stationary phase. *J Chromatogr* 1984;306:405–411.
10. Hermansson J, Eriksson M. Direct liquid chromatographic resolution of acidic drugs using a chiral α_1-acid glycoprotein column (Enantiopac). *J Liquid Chromatogr* 1986;9:621–639.
11. Schill G, Wainer IW, Barkan SA. Chiral separation of cationic drugs on an α_1-acid glycoprotein bonded stationary phase. *J Liquid Chromatogr* 1986;9:641–666.
12. Polin RA, Wasserman RL. Monoclonal antibodies: Progress and promise. *Lab Manage* 1983;Oct:33–44.

13. Valdes R. Endogenous digoxin-like immunoreactive factors: Impact on digoxin measurements and potential physiological implications. *Clin Chem* 1985; 31:1525–1532.

14. Soldin SJ. Digoxin—Issues and controversies. *Clin Chem* 1986;32:5–12.

15. Graves SW, Sharma K, Chandler AB. Methods for eliminating interferences in digoxin immunoassays caused by digoxin-like factors. *Clin Chem* 1986; 32:1506–1509.

16. Dito WR. Immunoassays employing enzymes for therapeutic drug monitoring, in Baer DM, Dito WR (eds): *Interpretations in Therapeutic Drug Monitoring.* Chicago: American Society of Clinical Pathologists, 1981:235–252.

17. Sawchuk RJ, Matzke GR. Contribution of 5-(4-hydroxyphenyl)-5-phenyl-hydantoin to the discrepancy between phenytoin analysis by EMIT and high-pressure liquid chromatography. *Ther Drug Monit* 1984;6:97–103.

18. Raisys VA, Opheim KE, Thorson CS, Ainardi V. Determination of serum phenytoin in uremic and non-uremic patients using EMIT monoclonal assay. *Clin Chem* 1985;31:931 (abstract).

19. Lewis SC. Monoclonal antibody immunoassay for phenytoin: An evaluation of performance in cases with uremia. *Clin Chem* 1985;31:931 (abstract).

20. Breiner R, McComb R, Lewis S. Positive interference with immunoassay of theophylline in serum of uremics. *Clin Chem* 1985;31:1575–1576 (letter).

21. Weber G. Rotational Brownian motion and polarization of the fluorescence of solutions. *Adv Protein Chem* 1953;8:415–459.

22. Dandlinker WB, Kelly RJ, Dandlinker J, Farquhar J, Levin J. Fluorescence polarization immunoassay. Theory and experimental method. *Immunochemistry* 1973;10:219–227.

23. Popelka S, Miller DM, Holen JT, Kelso DM. Fluorescence polarization immuno-assay. II. Analyzer for rapid, precise measurement of fluorescence polarization with use of disposable cuvettes. *Clin Chem* 1981;27:1198–1201.

24. Jolley ME, Stroupe SD, Schwenzer KC, et al. Fluorescence polarization immuno-assay. III. An automated system for therapeutic drug determination. *Clin Chem* 1981;27:1575–1579.

25. Jolley ME. Fluorescence polarization immunoassay for the determination of therapeutic drug levels in human plasma. *J Anal Toxicol* 1981;5:236–240.

26. Opheim KE, Ainardi V, Raisys V. Increase in apparent theophylline concentration in the serum of two uremic patients as measured by some immunoassay methods (caused by 1,3-dimethyluric acid?). *Clin Chem* 1983;29:1698–1699 (letter).

27. Nelson KM, Matthews SE, Bowers LD. Theophylline concentrations may be falsely high in serum of uremic patients. *Clin Chem* 1983;29:2125–2126 (letter).

28. Patel JA, Clayton LT, LeBel CP, McClatchey KD. Abnormal theophylline levels in plasma by fluorescence polarization immunoassay in patients with renal disease. *Ther Drug Monit* 1984;6:458–460.

29. Ross CA, Kraft CJ, Lee MH, Haughey DB. Evaluation of a mouse monoclonal antibody for the determination of serum theophylline by fluorescence polarization immunoassay. *Ther Drug Monit* 1985;7:355–357.

30. Compton R, Lichti D, Ladenson JH. Influence of uremia on four assays for theophylline: Improved results with a monoclonal antibody in the TDx procedure. *Clin Chem* 1985;31:152–154 (letter).

31. Bridges RB, Jennison TA. Spurious phenobarbital levels by fluorescence polarization immunoassay using TDx analyzer in patients with renal disease. *Ther Drug Monit* 1984;6:368–370.

32. Porter WH, Haver VM, Bush BA. Effect of protein concentration on the determination of digoxin in serum by fluorescence polarization immunoassay. *Clin Chem* 1984;30:1826–1829.

33. Gault MH, Vasdev S, Longerich L. Higher values for digitalis-like factors with TDx digoxin II. *Clin Chem* 1986;32:2000–2001 (letter).

34. Li TM, Benovic JL, Buckler RT, Burd JF. Homogeneous substrate-labeled fluorescent immunoassay for theophylline in serum. *Clin Chem* 1981;27:22–26.

35. Johnson PK, Messenger LJ. Homogeneous substrate-labeled fluorescent immunoassay for disopyramide in human serum: Semi- and fully automated procedures. *Clin Chem* 1985;32:378–381.

36. Klotz U. Performance of a new automated substrate-labeled fluorescence immunoassay system evaluated by comparative therapeutic monitoring of five drugs. *Ther Drug Monit* 1984;6:355–359.

37. Tosoni S, Signorini C, Albertini A. Drug monitoring by fluoroimmunoassay, with use of a centrifugal analyzer. *Clin Chem* 1983;29:991–992.

38. Sheehan M, Caron G. Evaluation of substrate-labeled fluorescent immunoassays for 9 drugs on automated fluorometer. *Clin Chem* 1983;29:1236 (abstract).

39. Nishikawa T, Kubo H, Saito M. Competitive nephelometric immunoassay method for antiepileptic drugs in patient blood. *J Immunol Methods* 1979; 29:85–89.

40. Nishikawa T, Kubo H, Saito M. Competitive nephelometric immunoassay of theophylline in plasma. *Clin Chim Acta* 1979;91:59–65.

41. Finley PR, Dye JA, Williams RJ, Lichti DA. Rate–nephelometric inhibition immunoassay of phenytoin and phenobarbital. *Clin Chem* 1981;27:405–409.

42. Hellsing K. The effects of different polymers for enhancement of the antigen–antibody reaction as measured with nephelometry, in Peters H (ed): *Protides and Biological Fluids*, vol 21. Oxford: Pergamon, 1974, pp 579–583.

43. Farber SJ, Goldgorin M, Repique EV. Performance of a rate–nephelometric inhibition immunoassay for primidone. *Clin Chem* 1982;28:1665 (abstract).

44. Jones T, Joseph R, Polito C, et al. Clinical evaluation of a monoclonal-based nephelometric immunoassay for theophylline. *Clin Chem* 1983;29:1156 (abstract).

45. Davenport L, Lepoff RB, Jones T, et al. Clinical evaluation of a rate–nephelometric inhibition immunoassay for carbamazepine. *Clin Chem* 1983;29:1274 (abstract).

46. Lucas F, Bedevia J, McRae B, Shenkin M. Turbidimetric rate inhibition assay for theophylline using a monoclonal antibody. *Clin Chem* 1986;32:1082 (abstract).

47. Reichberg S, Levey S, Miller R, et al. Gentamicin: Performance of the Technicon

latex particle immunoassay on Technicon RA systems. *Clin Chem* 1986;32:1113 (abstract).

48. Eranio S, Chan TH, Soybel J, et al. A rapid automated method for determination of phenobarbital on the IL Multistat and Monarch systems. *Clin Chem* 1986;32:1080 (abstract).

49. Giegel JL, Brotherton MM, Cronin P, et al. Radial partition immunoassay. *Clin Chem* 1982;28:1894–1898.

50. Evans S, Brotherton M, Cronin P, et al. Radial partition immunoassay: Monitoring digoxin levels in serum and plasma. *Clin Chem* 1983;29:1209 (abstract).

51. Cilissen J, Hooymans PM, Merkus FWHM. Modified fluorescence polarization immunoassay compared with radial partition immunoassay and a radioimmunoassay for digoxin. *Clin Chem* 1986;32:2100.

52. Clark DR, Inloes RL, Kalman SM, Sussman HH. Abbott TDx, Dade Stratus, and du Pont aca automated digoxin immunoassays compared with a reference radioimmunoassay method. *Clin Chem* 1986;32:381–385.

53. Verstraeta AG, Wieme RJ. An enzymatic factor may interfere with the digoxin assay on the Stratus analyzer. *Ther Drug Monit* 1986;8:244 (letter).

54. Henkel E. Evaluation of the Stratus radial partition immunoassay analyzer—Comparison with HPLC and RIA. *Clin Chem* 1985;31:922 (abstract).

55. Litchfield WJ, Craig AR, Frey WA, et al. Novel shell/core particles for automated turbidimetric immunoassays. *Clin Chem* 1984;30:1489–1493.

56. Opheim KE, Glick MR, Ou C-N, et al. Particle-enhanced turbidimetric inhibition immunoassay for theophylline evaluated with the du Pont aca. *Clin Chem* 1984;30:1870–1874.

57. Gotelli G, Mitchell M. Particle-enhanced turbidimetric inhibition immunoassay for theophylline with a centrifugal analyzer. *Clin Chem* 1985;31:1085–1086 (letter).

58. Ou CN, Armbruster MA, Rogneurd CL, et al. Clinical evaluation of du Pont gentamicin PETINIA reagent on Cobas-Bio centrifugal analyzer. *Clin Chem* 1986;32:1083 (abstract).

59. Armbruster MA, Ou CN, Lewis LM, et al. Evaluation of the du Pont PETINIA tobramycin assay on the Cobas-Bio. *Clin Chem* 1986;32:1078 (abstract).

60. Poto EM, Rugg AE. Measurement of serum phenobarbital levels on open reagent analyzers using du Pont phenobarbital PETINIA reagents. *Clin Chem* 1986;32:1083 (abstract).

61. Kassai MM. Measurement of serum phenytoin levels on open reagent analyzers using du Pont phenytoin PETINIA reagents. *Clin Chem* 1986;32:1081 (abstract).

62. Leflar CC, Freytag JW, Powell LM, et al. An automated, affinity-column-mediated, enzyme-linked immunometric assay for digoxin on the du Pont aca discrete clinical analyzer. *Clin Chem* 1984;30:1809–1811.

63. Demers LM, Wenk RE, Abbott LB, Pippenger CE. An evaluation of the digoxin method for the du Pont aca. *Clin Chem* 1985;31:930 (abstract).

64. Masulli IS, Poto EM. Measurement of serum digoxin levels on open reagent analyzers using du Pont ACMIA reagents. *Clin Chem* 1985;31:929 (abstract).

65. Tyhach RJ, Rupchock PA, Pendergrass JH, et al. Adaption of prosthetic group-label homogeneous immunoassay to reagent strip format. *Clin Chem* 1981;27:1499–1504.

66. Rupchock P, Sommer R, Greequist A, Tyhach R, Walter B, Zipp A. Dry-reagent strips used for determination of theophylline in serum. *Clin Chem* 1981;31:737–740.

67. Lindberg R, Ivaska K, Irjala K, Vanto T. Determination of theophylline in serum with the Seralyzer ARIS reagent strip test evaluated. *Clin Chem* 1985;31:613–614.

68. Sommer R, Nelson C, Greenquist A. Dry-reagent strips for measuring phenytoin in serum. *Clin Chem* 1986;32:1770–1774.

69. Burnett D, Goudie JH, Tabossi-Reynolds C. Seralyzer reagent-strip system evaluated for measurement of phenobarbital in serum. *Clin Chem* 1987;33:191.

70. Jenny RW, Jackson KY, Thompson SG. Two types of error found with the Seralyzer ARIS assay of theophylline. *Clin Chem* 1986;32:2122–2123 (letter).

71. Zuk RF, Ginsberg VK, Houts T, et al. Enzyme immunochromatography— A quantitative immunoassay requiring no instrumentation. *Clin Chem* 1985;31:1144–1150.

72. Henderson DR, Friedman SB, Harris JD, Manning WB, Zoccoli MA. CEDIA, a new homogeneous immunoassay system. *Clin Chem* 1986;32:1637–1641.

73. Kiser EJ, Davis JC, Orf JW, Puckett LD, Coleman PM. A homogeneous enzyme immunoassay based on enzyme recombination. *Clin Chem* 1986;32:1068 (abstract).

74. Hemmila I, Dakuku S, Mukkala V-M, Siitari H, Lovgren T. Europium as a label in time-resolved immunofluorometric assay. *Anal Biochem* 1984;137:335–343.

75. Soini E, Kojola H. Time-resolved fluorometer for lanthanide chelates—A new generation of nonisotopic immunoassays. *Clin Chem* 1983;29:65–68.

76. Helisingius P, Hemmila I, Lovgren T. Solid-phase immunoassay of digoxin by measuring time-resolved fluorescence. *Clin Chem* 1986;32:1767–1769.

77. Wandell M, Wilcox-Thole WL. Protein binding and free drug concentrations, in Mungall DR (ed): *Applied Clinical Pharmacokinetics*. New York: Raven, 1983, pp 17–48.

78. Kwong TC. Free drug measurements: Methodology and clinical significance. *Clin Chim Acta* 1985;151:193–216.

79. Friel P. Methods for free drug level analysis. Therapeutic Drug Monitoring Continuing Education and Quality Control Program. Washington DC: American Association for Clinical Chemistry, June pp. 1–5, 1983.

80. Koike Y, Magnusson A, Steiner E, Rane A, Sjoqvist F. Ultrafiltration compared with equilibrium dialysis in the determination of unbound phenytoin in plasma. *Ther Drug Monit* 1985;7:461–465.

81. Levy RH, Friel PN, Johno I, et al. Filtration for free drug level monitoring: Carbamazepine and valproic acid. *The Drug Monit* 1984;6:67–76.

CHAPTER 10

THE CLINICAL LABORATORY EVALUATION OF VITAMIN NUTRITIONAL STATUS

CHARLES P. TURLEY

University of Arkansas for Medical Sciences
Little Rock, Arkansas

INTRODUCTION

A variety of techniques can be used to evaluate the nutritional status of individuals. Clinical assessment, anthropometric measurements, and nutritional intake studies are but some of the approaches. This chapter is devoted to the role that the clinical laboratory can play in evaluating nutritional status.

Vitaminologists constantly seek new and better methods for evaluating vitamin status. Not only do they measure the vitamin concentrations in body fluids and tissues, they also look to tests that measure biochemical function. The advent of parenteral nutritional therapy has caused a resurgence in vitamin nutritional analysis, as has the practice of megadose consumption of vitamins. Whereas laboratorians were once almost exclusively called on to look for vitamin deficiencies, they are now sometimes asked to test for vitamin toxicity.

What follows is an overview of some of the analytical approaches commonly used in clinical laboratories, with some limited discussion of newer analytical techniques that may see more use in the future. Not all vitamins are covered in this chapter. Some vitamins are not included because their deficiency states (or toxicities) are not often encountered in clinical practice, at least in developed countries. I have tried to focus on techniques that use instrumentation, such as spectrophotometry, fluorometry, radioisotope counting, and high pressure liquid chromatography (HPLC). From this potpourri of instrumentation, the clinical laboratorian should be able to develop just about any vitamin assay. For more comprehensive reviews of vitamin analysis, the reader is referred to two excellent resources (*1,2*).

VITAMIN B₁

Background

Thiamine, or vitamin B_1, is a pyrimidyl-substituted thiazole compound whose biologically active cofactor forms are phosphate esters. Thiamine deficiency causes beriberi, and it was in pursuing this disease that thiamine was discovered. Clinically, beriberi appears as a constellation of symptoms including poor appetite, fatigue, and peripheral neuritis (dry beriberi), and sometimes edema and cardiac failure (wet beriberi). Beriberi is now generally limited to developing countries, particularly in Southeast Asia, where there is consumption of thiaminase, a microbial substance that hydrolyzes thiamine in the intestinal tract. Beriberi has also reappeared in developed countries in adolescents. Wernicke's encephalopathy or Wernicke–Korsakoff's psychosis is seen in thiamine-deficient alcoholics. In adults, thiamine toxicity causes fatty liver, sweating, tachycardia, and perhaps hypotension (3).

Thiamine appears as free thiamine or as phosphorylated cofactor forms. Thiamine pyrophosphate (TPP) is the predominant tissue form and is the biologically active cofactor that participates in decarboxylation and ketol formation reactions. Thiamine triphosphate (TTP) appears to be the cofactor form that participates in sodium ion conduction. Inhibition of TTP synthesis by a factor that can be measured in urine has been linked to Leigh's encephalopathy (4). The major circulating form of the vitamin is non-phosphorylated thiamine.

Biochemical Evaluation

A variety of analytical techniques have been used to measure thiamine in body fluids. A microbiological procedure using Lactobacillus viridescens has proven efficacious but is susceptible to the same limitations as all microbiological approaches, namely difficulty in standardizing results between laboratories, interference from antibiotics, and requirement of specialized skills (5). A chemical method based on the oxidation of thiamine to the thiochrome derivative by alkaline ferricyanide has been a popular approach (6). Thiochrome is then extracted into an organic solvent and measured fluorometrically.

Thiamine can also be measured by HPLC. In one HPLC approach thiamine was measured in 0.1 mL of blood (7). Thiamine phosphate esters were converted to free thiamine with Aspergillus oryzae carboxyl proteinase (Takadiastase) and an aliquot applied to a column (Shodex OH-Pak, M-414) and eluted with 0.2 mol/L NaH_2PO_4. Thiamine was converted on-line to thiochrome and detected fluorometrically. The reaction was linear from 10.0 ng/dL to 50.0 μg/dL and recovery was $97.0 \pm 2.1\%$. The blood thiamine concentration in 20 human controls was 4.62 ± 0.23 μg/dL (mean $\pm$ SD). Correlation with the conventional thiochrome method was: Y (conventional) $= 0.98$ X (HPLC) $+ 0.07$ ($r = 0.94$). Conventional thiochrome methods require 3 mL of blood, while this HPLC approach requires only 0.1 mL of blood, thus rendering the technique useful for pediatric applications.

In another HPLC approach the thiochrome derivative was formed before injection (8). In this procedure 2 mL of serum or whole blood was added to 3 mL of trichloroacetic acid and the thiamine phosphate esters were hydrolyzed by a 2-hour incubation in clara-diastase. Urine was directly subjected to the thiochrome reaction. The thiochrome derivative was separated on a Nucleosil-NH_2 column using an isocratic elution with 25% potassium phosphate buffer in acetonitrile at a flow rate of 1.8 mL/min. The thiochrome derivative was detected fluorometrically with excitation at 370 nm and emission at 425 nm. Thiamine concentrations in volunteers were: urine $= 0.31 \pm 0.21$ mg/day; whole blood $= 3.52 \pm 0.74$ μg/dL; serum $= 0.33 \pm 0.07$ μg/dL (mean $\pm$ SD).

There is a good correlation between the urinary excretion of thiamine and dietary intake. Excretion of greater than 100 μg in 24 hours or 66 μg/g creatinine is considered adequate in adults. Adults who excrete less than 27 μg of thiamine per gram of creatinine are considered to be at high risk for deficiency. Children excrete more thiamine per gram of creatinine than do adults, and the excretion is developmentally dependent, as shown in Table 1.

Measurement of erythrocyte thiamine concentrations may someday prove to be a valuable approach. One group showed that erythrocyte TPP concentrations decreased in thiamine-deficient rats before changes in a functional test of thiamine deficiency, the erythrocyte transketolase activity (9).

One of the more popular means of assessing thiamine nutritional status is by a functional test using the erythrocyte transketolase activity and *in vitro* stimulation with TPP (10). Transketolase catalyzes the following two reactions of the hexose monophosphate shunt:

1. xylulose-5-P + ribose-5-P $\rightleftharpoons$ sedoheptulose-7-P + glyceraldehyde-3-P
2. xylulose-5-P + erythrose-4-P $\rightleftharpoons$ fructose-6-P + glyceraldehyde-3-P

Transketolase activity can be assessed by colorimetric procedures that measure the formation of sedoheptulose or fructose or by procedures that measure the disappearance of ribose (11). Measurement of sedoheptulose formation has been used in a micromethod requiring only 0.05 mL of whole blood (12). Alternatively, transketolase (TK) activity can be measured kinetically (13) by monitoring NADH oxidation as follows:

$$\text{ribose-5-PO}_4 + \text{xylulose-5-PO}_4 \overset{\text{TK}}{\rightleftharpoons} \text{sedoheptulose-7-PO}_4$$
$$+ \text{D-glyceraldehyde-3-PO}_4 \qquad (1)$$

$$\text{D-glyceraldehyde-3-PO}_4 \overset{\text{TIM}}{\rightleftharpoons} \text{dihydroxyacetone-PO}_4 \qquad (2)$$

$$\text{dihydroxyacetone-PO}_4 + \text{NADH} \overset{\text{GDH}}{\rightleftharpoons} sn\text{-glycerol-3-PO}_4 + \text{NAD}^+$$

$$(3)$$

Variants of transketolase have been found in erythrocytes, but the effects of these on assessing thiamine nutritional status remain to be evaluated (*14*). Xylulose-5-phosphate, one of the reaction components, is supplied endogenously through the conversion of ribose-5-phosphate by D-ribose-5-phosphate ketol-isomerase and D-ribulose-5-phosphate 3-epimerase present in the erythrocyte hemolysate.

Table 1. Guidelines for the Interpretation of Thiamine Nutritional Status

	Urinary Excretion (μg/g creatinine)		
Subjects	Deficient (high risk)	Low (medium risk)	Acceptable (low risk)
1–3 years	< 120	120–175	≥ 176
4–6 years	< 85	85–120	≥ 121
7–9 years	< 70	70–180	≥ 181
10–12 years	< 60	60–180	≥ 181
13–15 years	< 50	50–150	≥ 151
Adults	< 27	27–65	≥ 66
Pregnant			
2nd trimester	< 23	23–54	≥ 55
3rd trimester	< 21	21–49	≥ 50
Other Interpretive Guidelines			
Adults			
μg/24 hours	< 40	40–99	≥ 100
μg/6 hours	< 10	10–24	≥ 25
ETK Activity Coefficient[a]			
Acceptable	1.00–1.15		
Low	1.16–1.20		
Deficient	≥ 1.20		

Source: Reprinted with permission from Sauberlich HE, Skala JH, Dowdy RP. *Laboratory Tests for the Assessment of Nutritional Status*, 1974, pp 24–25. Copyright CRC Press, Inc, Boca Raton, FL.

[a]ICNND classification.

Transketolase activity can also be measured by incubating erythrocyte hemolysates with [1-^{14}C]ribose-5-phosphate and measuring the incorporation of label into sedoheptulose-7-phosphate (15).

Leukocyte transketolase activity has been measured in rats with success (16). Measurement of enzyme activity in human leukocytes may become more popular as techniques for isolating leukocytes improve.

Many laboratories prefer to measure erythrocyte transketolase activity and its in vitro stimulation with TPP (17). This is called the TPP effect or the erythrocyte transketolase activity coefficient (ETK AC). The ETK AC is a good indicator of experimentally induced thiamine deficiency. Laboratories should not rely completely on the ETK AC however, since prolonged thiamine deficiency lowers apo-ETK and it is possible that TPP added in vitro would not bind ETK. This situation would yield an ETK AC within the normal range despite the low apo-ETK activity. While depletion of other vitamins may lower ETK activity, the ETK AC is unaffected. Cancer patients have a low ETK activity but elevated ETK AC, suggesting an in vivo defect in conversion of thiamine to TPP. Diabetics appear to have low levels of apo-ETK, a situation that leads to low ETK activity but a normal TPP effect. The TPP effect disappears within about 2 hours after parenteral administration of the vitamin. Reference values for the ETK AC are shown in Table 1. ETK activity is a poor indicator of response to thiamine therapy, since it takes some time for the activity to return to normal.

Transketolase is not the only enzyme that is thiamine dependent. Pyruvate decarboxylase activity has been measured in rats by monitoring the formation of $^{14}CO_2$ from [1-^{14}C]pyruvic acid in isolated leukocytes (18). Although pyruvate decarboxylase activity decreased in the thiamine-deficient rats, it did so 2 weeks after a change in ETK; thus this approach may not elicit strong support in clinical laboratory settings.

VITAMIN B$_2$

Background

Riboflavin, also called vitamin B$_2$, is a yellow fluorescent pigment having the structure 7,8-dimethyl-10-(1'-D-ribityl) isoalloxazine. Many derivatives of this compound are found in nature, including the cofactor active forms riboflavin-5'-phosphate (flavin mononucleotide: FMN) and flavin adenine dinucleotide (FAD). While FAD is the predominant tissue form, nonphosphorylated riboflavin is the primary excretory product.

Ariboflavinosis is not unique to developing countries. Depending on the method used and on the population studied, riboflavin deficiency has a prevalence of from 5 to 47% (19). Since riboflavin deficiency is often accompanied by inadequate intake of other nutrients as well, pure, uncomplicated riboflavin deficiency is rare. Clinical findings of deficiency are usually noticed only after body stores have been depleted. Symptoms include but are not limited to angular stomatitis, glossitis, blepharospasm, and conjunctival congestion. Itching and paresthesias have been linked to excess riboflavin.

Biochemical Evaluation

The microbiological assays are not discussed in detail here. Organisms used with success include *Lactobacillus casei*, *Leuconostoc mesenteroides* (20), and the protozoan *Tetrahymena pyriformis* (21). Flavin compounds can also be measured fluorometrically (22). A luminometric assay specific for FAD has been described and is based on formation of holo-D-amino-acid oxidase from apo-D-amino-acid oxidase and FAD (23). Urinary riboflavin has also been measured by fluorometric titration with an aporiboflavin binding protein isolated from chicken eggs (24).

HPLC methods are now being used in many laboratories. In most of these procedures the flavins in urine or serum are separated on reversed-phase C_{18} columns and the eluted vitamins detected fluorometrically. In one procedure, riboflavin was measured by directly injecting urine onto a 3.9 mm × 30 cm μBondapak C_{18} column, eluted with methanol–water (34:66, v/v) and detected fluorometrically with excitation at 450 nm and emission at 530 nm (25). At a flow rate of 1.0 mL/min, riboflavin eluted at approximately 7 minutes. In another procedure the internal standard isoriboflavin was added to urine (0.5 mL) or serum (2.0 mL) and the proteins precipitated with trichloroacetic acid (TCA) (26). Precipitation with TCA not only removes proteins which might damage the HPLC column, but also enhances the recovery of riboflavin, since the vitamin is more stable at a low pH. The serum TCA supernate was purified over a C_{18} Sep-pak column, and the flavins were separated on a 0.32 × 15 cm ROSIL C_{18} column and detected fluorometrically. Urine was injected directly. HPLC methods using other internal standards such as nicotinamide (27), 2,2'-diphenic acid (28), and p-hydroxybenzoic acid (29) have been described.

Measurement of riboflavin excretion in urine has been used extensively. The urine specimen can be collected randomly, in which case the results should be expressed as micrograms of riboflavin per gram of creatinine. Alternatively, the specimen can be collected over a period of time such as 6 or 24 hours. Age-adjusted reference values are provided in Table 2. Negative nitrogen balance, stress, and antibiotic administration increase excretion of riboflavin.

Table 2. Guidelines for the Interpretation of Erythrocyte Levels and Urinary Excretion of Riboflavin

Subjects	Urinary Excretion (μg/g creatinine)		
	Deficient (high risk)	Low (medium risk)	Acceptable (low risk)
1–3 years	< 150	150–499	> 500
4–6 years	< 100	100–299	> 300
7–9 years	< 85	85–269	> 270
10–15 years	< 70	70–199	> 200
Adults	< 27	27–79	> 80
Pregnant			
2nd trimester	< 39	30–119	> 120
3rd trimester	< 30	30–89	> 90
Other Interpretive Guidelines			
Adults			
μg/24 hours	< 40	40–119	> 120
μg/6 hours	< 10	10–29	> 30

Source: Reprinted with permission from Sauberlich HE, Skala JH, Dowdy RP. *Laboratory Tests for the Assessment of Nutritional Status*, 1974, p 31, Copyright CRC Press, Inc, Boca Raton, FL.

Flavin nutritional status can also be assessed by measuring riboflavin, FMN, and FAD in blood, serum, and erythrocytes. Blood riboflavin concentrations reflect recent dietary intake. The guidelines of the Interdepartmental Committee on Nutrition for National Defense (ICNND), expressed as micrograms of riboflavin per deciliter of cells, are: deficient < 10 μg riboflavin, low 10–14.9 μg riboflavin, and normal > 15 μg riboflavin (*17*). In one study subjects were found to have more than 15 μg riboflavin even though clinical symptoms of deficiency were present and a functional test, the erythrocyte glutathione reductase activity coefficient (discussed below), was abnormal (*30*).

One of the more popular functional tests for assessing riboflavin nutritional status involves measuring glutathione reductase activity. Glutathione reductase catalyzes the reduction of oxidized glutathione (GSSG) as shown:

$$NADPH + H^+ + GSSG \xrightarrow{FAD} NADP^+ + 2GSH$$

Kinetic methods involve monitoring the rate of NADPH oxidation, while colorimetric procedures measure the amount of reduced glutathione formed (*31*). One group reviewed the kinetic methods and tendered suggestions for optimizing the assay (13). They showed that the concentration of glutathione used in some procedures is low and suggested a final optimal concentration of 2.0 mmol/L. When the reaction is started with glutathione, a one-hour preincubation of hemolysate with FAD is necessary. When started with NADPH, preincubation is reduced to 30 minutes or less. Glutathione reductase has also been measured successfully in leukocytes and has been shown to be an acceptable predictor of riboflavin status in rats (32). Improved techniques for isolating lymphocytes may make this a more popular procedure in the future.

Although enzyme activity may be measured directly, a more common approach is to measure enzyme activity in the presence or absence of *in vitro* FAD to arrive at the erythrocyte glutathione reductase activity coefficient (EGR AC):

$$EGR\ AC = \frac{\text{activity with added FAD}}{\text{activity without added FAD}}$$

In healthy subjects the EGR AC is close to 1.0 (17). Values lower than 1.20 indicate a low risk of developing riboflavin deficiency. Individuals with EGR AC between 1.20 and 1.40 are considered to be at marginal risk and should be monitored closely. Values greater than 1.40 indicate a high risk for developing clinical symptoms of riboflavin deficiency. The validity of the test in individuals with glucose-6-phosphate dehydrogenase (G6PD) deficiency has been questioned because erythrocyte glutathione reductase has an increased avidity for FAD in this disease. G6PD deficiency should therefore be ruled out in susceptible individuals who have an elevated EGR AC (17).

VITAMIN B$_6$

Background

The B$_6$ vitamins are comprised of six predominant physiological forms: pyridoxine, pyridoxamine, pyridoxal, and their respective 5'-phosphate esters. Pyridoxine is found mainly in plants, whereas pyridoxal and pyridoxamine are found in animal tissues. All three nonphosphorylated vitamin forms are metabolically converted to their phosphate ester forms in the mucosal cell and in other peripheral tissues. The synthesis of one of these phosphorylated forms, pyridoxal phosphate (PLP), depends on a flavin-dependent enzyme, pyridoxine (pyridoxamine)-5'-phosphate oxidase, hence the relationship between riboflavin and vitamin B$_6$ metabolism. Pyridoxal is metabolized to 4-pyridoxic acid (4PA) in the liver. The 4PA metabolite is found in urine. PLP participates in numerous reactions involving the metabolism of amino acids, glycogen, and lipids.

Isolated B$_6$ deficiency is rare and is more commonly found in association with deficits of other B-complex vitamins. Even when diets deficient in vitamin B$_6$ are administered, they rarely produce clinical signs of deficiency unless pyridoxine antagonists such as penicillamine and the tuberculostatic drug isoniazid are also administered. Symptoms include seborrheic dermatitis, cheilosis, anemia, and CNS changes. Deficiency of the vitamin during pregnancy secondary to increased fetal demand has been linked to suboptimal birth outcomes. Vitamin B$_6$ excess appears to increase the metabolism of several neurotransmitters and has caused permanent paralysis.

Biochemical Evaluation

Vitamin B$_6$ nutritional status can be assessed by a variety of techniques such as quantitation of plasma B$_6$ concentrations, measurement of urinary excretion of intact vitamin or the 4PA metabolite, assessment of erythrocyte aminotransferase activity, and metabolic response to load tests.

Direct quantitation of the vitamin can be conducted with the yeast microbiological assay using *Saccharomyces carlsbergensis*, also known as *S. uvarum*. *Streptococcus faecium* has been used to measure pyridoxal and pyridoxamine concentrations, and *Lactobacillus casei* has been used to quantitate pyridoxal (*33*).

Chemical methods for measuring the vitamin forms and 4PA have historically been of limited practical use. Most of these have been fluorometric assays with a variety of chromatographic steps to enhance specificity. HPLC methods have improved the analysis. In one HPLC procedure, PLP was extracted from blood, eluted, and reacted on-line with semicarbazide to form the fluorescent semicarbazone derivative (*34*), and 4PA has also been measured by HPLC (*35*). Trichloroacetic acid supernates of urine were injected directly onto the HPLC column (C$_{18}$ μBondapak) and 4PA was eluted with 0.033 M phosphate buffer/5% methanol (pH 2.2). The vitamin was detected fluorometrically with excitation at 355 nm and emission at 436 nm. The chromatographic run time was approximately 6 minutes.

Various enzymatic methods for PLP have also been described but are rarely used in clinical laboratories since they are laborious and technique dependent. More than 50 enzymes require PLP for activation but only a few of these have been used to measure the vitamin. Tyrosine apodecarboxylase and apoaspartate aminotransferase are two of the more popular enzymatic procedures. The radiotyrosine apodecarboxylase assay, based on the conversion of [^{3}H]tyrosine to [^{3}H]tyramine appears to be a reliable indicator of B$_6$ status (*36*).

Table 3. Guidelines for the Interpretation of Urinary Excretion of Vitamin B$_6$

Age Group (years)	Urinary Excretion (μg/g creatinine)	
	Unacceptable Level	Acceptable Level
1–3	<90	≥90
4–6	<75	≥75
7–9	<50	≥50
10–12	<40	≥40
13–15	<30	≥30
Adults	<20	≥20

Source: Reprinted with permission from Sauberlich HE, Skala JH, Dowdy RP. *Laboratory Tests for the Assessment of Nutritional Status*, p 41. Copyright CRC Press, Inc, Boca Raton, FL.

Urinary pyridoxine excretion correlates with dietary intake. Between 20 and 50% of dietary pyridoxine is excreted as 4PA in the adult. In children up to 6% of excreted B$_6$ is the 4PA metabolite (*37*). Reference ranges for total vitamin B$_6$ excretion using the yeast assay are age dependent, as shown in Table 3 (*38*). Normal adults have 0.46–7.84 μg 4PA per milliliter of urine as measured by HPLC (*35*).

The concentration of pyridoxine is higher in plasma than in red cells, the reverse of the distribution seen with the other B-complex vitamins. Adult plasma concentrations of the vitamin are 59 ± 13 ng/ml (mean $\pm$ SD) by the microbiological assay (*39*) and 5–23 ng/mL by the tyrosine apodecarboxylase procedure (*36*). Breast-fed premature infants have plasma PLP concentrations of 1.75 ± 0.70 ng/mL, and formula-fed infants have levels of 25.8 ± 4.13 ng/mL (mean $\pm$ SD) at 17 days after birth (*40*). Adult whole blood PLP by HPLC is 12.4 to 29.6 ng/mL.

Load tests have proven useful in assessing B$_6$ nutritional status. Substances which have been used include tryptophan, methionine, alanine, and kynurenine sulfate. In the tryptophan load test, an oral dose of 2–5 g of tryptophan (100 mg per kilogram of body weight in children) is administered, and the excretion of xanthurenic acid, kynurenine, and other metabolites is measured in a 24-hour urine sample. In adults the net increase in excretion of xanthurenic acid should be less than 25 mg/day. Net increases greater than 50 mg/day are considered to be marginal or inadequate (*41*).

Measurement of erythrocyte alanine aminotransferase (EALT) and aspart-ate aminotransferase (EAST) activities and activity coefficients upon *in vitro* addition of PLP are commonly used to evaluate B_6 status. Enzyme activities can be measured colorimetrically or by coupled enzymatic techniques (*41*). EALT activity is roughly one-tenth that of EAST. The procedure has been optimized for reaction components and conditions (*13*). EAST measurement has been adapted to centrifugal analysis and continuous-flow systems (*42*).

Reliable guidelines for interpreting EAST activity coefficients are not available. According to one group, individuals with an activity coefficient of less than 1.5–2.0 are deficient, but other laboratories have used higher discriminating points (*43*). Reference values appear to be method dependent, with some indication that kinetic approaches yield higher activity coefficients than colorimetric approaches (*43*). Numerous drugs and diseases are known to affect serum transaminase activity, but their effects on erythrocyte activities have not been explored in detail.

ASCORBIC ACID

Background

Vitamin C, or ascorbic acid, is a water-soluble vitamin that is also a strong reducing compound. It is reversibly oxidized to dehydroascorbic acid, which is also biologically active. Dehydroascorbic acid can be converted to the inactive diketogulonic acid metabolite (Figure 1). The vitamin functions in hydroxylating the proline and lysine residues of collagen and thereby maintains connective tissue. Ascorbic acid also participates in the dopamine β-hydroxylase reaction in the conversion of tyrosine to catecholamines. Deficiency of vitamin C leads to the well-known disease scurvy, characterized by swollen gums, rough and dry skin, and osteoporosis. The popular interest in cosuming large amounts of ascorbic acid has led to some concern about the toxicity of this vitamin. Except for the few individuals who develop kidney stones and hemolysis, there appears to be little toxic effect.

Biochemical Evaluation

Chemical assessment is usually approached by the measurement of ascorbic acid (and sometimes dehydroascorbic acid) in serum and circulating cells. The chemical methods rely primarily on two approaches: (1) the reducing proper-

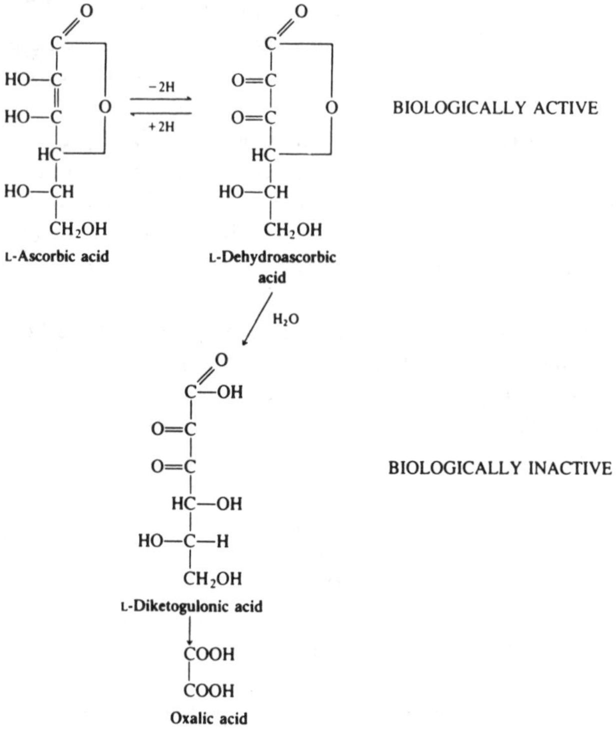

Figure 1. Structure of ascorbic acid and metabolites. [Reprinted by permission from Brewster MA, in Pesce AJ, Kaplan LA (eds): *Clinical Chemistry: Theory, Analysis, and Correlation.* St. Louis: CV Mosby, 1984, p 667.]

ties of the 1,2-enediol group of vitamin C that lead to absorbance changes in indicator dyes, and (2) the formation of hydrazones or fluorophores.

The 2,6-dichloroindophenol method uses the reducing properties of ascorbic acid to convert the dye from the oxidized form to the colorless leuko form, with the change in color monitored at 520 nm (*44*). Dehydroascorbic acid does not reduce the 2,6-dichloroindophenol dye and is thus not measured in this procedure. The reaction must be conducted at a pH of less than 4.0 to prevent interference from endogenous sulfhydryl compounds and phenols. Since cysteine and thiosulfate are not completely inhibited at the lower pH, urinary ascorbic acid concentrations tend to be falsely elevated by about 15% unless chloromercuribenzoic acid is added to the reaction mixture. Although not usually a problem when measuring the vitamin in serum, these interferences should be considered when assessing ascorbate excretion.

Both ascorbic acid and dehydroascorbic acid are measured in the 2,4-dinitrophenylhydrazine approach (45). In this method ascorbic acid is oxidized by copper to dehydroascorbic acid and diketogulonic acid. Upon addition of the dye, the 2,4-dinitrophenylosazone derivative is formed. Thiourea is included in the assay to reduce interference from fructose and glucuronic acid.

In the α,α'-dipyridyl approach, ascorbic acid reduces ferric iron to ferrous iron, which in turn reacts with the dye to form an orange-red color absorbing at 525 nm (46). Dehydroascorbic acid is not measured in this procedure. The reaction is conducted at a low pH established by the addition of orthophosphoric acid, the purpose of which is to reduce interference from glutathione, tocopherol, acetaminophen, and creatinine.

Ascorbic acid can also be measured fluorometrically (47). In this approach ascorbic acid is oxidized to dehydroascorbic acid and reacted with o-phenylenediamine to form a fluorescent quinoxaline derivative. Fluorescence intensity is measured with excitation at 348 nm and emission at 423 nm. Fluorescence from interfering compounds is measured in a "blank" specimen produced by adding boric acid to the reaction mixture to inhibit quinoxaline formation. The fluorometric approach can be used to measure ascorbic and dehydroascorbic acids in both serum and urine.

HPLC with electrochemical detection has been used to measure vitamin C in body fluids and tissues (48). Ascorbic acid is separated on reversed-phase C_{18} columns with an acetate buffer as a mobile phase. The ion-pair reagent n-octylamine can be added to the mobile phase to improve ascorbic acid retention. HPLC has been used successfully to measure vitamin C in leukocytes (49).

Interpretation of serum vitamin C concentrations is hampered by the observation that serum levels are not indicative of tissue stores (50). Individuals with serum concentrations below 2.0 mg/L are considered at high risk for developing scurvy. Levels between 2.0 and 2.9 mg/L are considered a medium risk, while concentrations above 3.0 mg/L are adequate. When tissues are saturated with vitamin C, serum concentrations of 10–15 mg/L are often seen. Clinical symptoms of scurvy have been noted in some individuals with serum ascorbic acid concentrations above 2.0 mg/L, but tissue stores of the vitamin tend to be depleted.

Some investigators have advocated the use of leukocyte ascorbic acid concentrations, since cellular levels may more closely approximate tissue stores of the vitamin. Leukocyte ascorbic acid concentrations measured by HPLC in healthy volunteers are 26.4–44.0 mg/L in polymorphonuclear leukocytes and 52.8–105.6 mg/L in mononuclear lymphocytes (49).

Urine ascorbic acid concentrations tend to reflect recent dietary intake and are of little diagnostic use except to confirm depressed serum concentrations.

VITAMIN B$_{12}$

Background

Vitamin B$_{12}$ is an organometallic compound consisting of a corrin ring, a ribonucleotide, and various substituents attached to a central cobalt atom. In mammalian systems there are three major coenzymes of vitamin B$_{12}$. They are hydroxy (OH-Cbl), methyl (Me-Cbl), and adenosyl (Ado-Cbl) cobalamins. A fourth cobalamin, cyanocobalamin (CN-Cbl), is sometimes found in humans but is not properly a coenzyme. Tissues and sera also contain a variety of biologically inactive cobalamin analogues.

The cobalamin coenzymes participate in a host of intracellular metabolic reactions. Cobalamin is taken up by the cell as the OH-Cbl form and is distributed to the mitochondria for enzymatic conversion to Ado-Cbl or to the cytoplasm for conversion to Me-Cbl. Ado-Cbl participates as a coenzyme in the methylmalonyl CoA mutase reaction that takes L-methylmalonyl CoA to succinyl CoA (51). Leucine 2,3-aminomutase, an enzyme that converts leucine to β-leucine, also has a requirement for Ado-Cbl (52). Me-Cbl participates in the homocysteine–methionine methyltransferase reaction, and it is at this point that cobalamin interrelates with folate metabolism (53).

Cobalamin deficiency is usually encountered as a result of inadequate intestinal absorption. Since there is a significant enterohepatic reabsorption of the vitamin, it may take up to 12 years for clinical symptoms to appear in strict vegetarians. Clinical symptoms of deficiency include megaloblastic anemia and various neurological abnormalities.

Biochemical Evaluation

A variety of analytical approaches have been used to measure total vitamin B$_{12}$ and coenzymes. These include microbial assays, competitive binding radioassays, radioimmunoassays, chromatography–bioautography, and HPLC.

The microbial assays are based on the observation that certain organisms require cobalamin as a growth factor. Two organisms have been used with success: *Lactobacillus leichmanni* and *Euglena gracilis* (54). Elevated levels of folates inhibit microbial growth, as do antibiotics. These assays are rarely used in routine clinical laboratories because they are laborious and technique dependent.

The competitive binding radioassays are based on the principle that cobalamin competes with [^{57}Co]CN-Cbl for binding to specific proteins such as porcine intrinsic factor. A variety of competitive binding methods have been developed; they differ in the choice of binding protein, in the method of removing or blocking R-protein, and in techniques for separating bound from free radiolabeled cobalamin (55). Binding proteins other than porcine intrinsic factor include intrinsic factor prepared from human sources, transcobalamins, and salivary proteins. The transcobalamins are a class of cobalamin binding proteins that transport cobalamin in the circulation and participate in the cellular uptake of the vitamin. When it was discovered that serum cobalamin concentrations measured by competitive binding radioassay were higher than levels determined by microbial assays, there was a concerted effort to develop assays free from interference by cobalamin analogues (56). At that time many of the commercial competitive binding kits contained a contaminating cobalamin binding protein called R-protein (because of its rapid electrophoretic mobility). The R-protein bound to not only biologically active cobalamin but to the inactive cobalamin analogues as well. Two approaches for eliminating this interference have been developed: preparation of R-protein-free intrinsic factor and saturation of R-protein with cobalamin analogues. In a large method comparison study, one group showed that competitive binding radioassays using R-protein containing binders (and without analogue saturation) correlated well with microbial assays and suggested that spurious differences between the microbial and competitive binding assays are more likely to be due to improper reference ranges for the two types of assay (57). Nevertheless, many of the commerical B$_{12}$ kits still use techniques to correct for cobalamin analogue interference. A variety of techniques have been used to separate bound from free cobalamin. These include adsorption on albumin-coated and uncoated charcoal, precipitation, and covalent attachment of the binding protein onto solid phase supports (55).

Serum total cobalamin concentrations are method dependent and laboratories are strongly urged to develop their own reference ranges. Source of binding protein, standard preparation, and bound from free separation are all factors which can affect the reference range for that particular assay. The following ranges are rough guidelines only. With the microbial assays, values less than 150 pg/mL are usually considered to be deficient and those above 200 pg/mL acceptable (58). Using the competitive binding radioassay that measures "true" cobalamin (not the inactive analogues), values in normals are 220–940 pg/mL. Deficient individuals generally have levels below 170 pg/mL (59).

A radioimmunoassay for CN-Cbl has been developed that reacts with the biologically active cobalamin coenzymes as well (60). The radioimmunoassay yields lower total serum vitamin B$_{12}$ concentrations than does the competitive binding radioassay.

The cobalamin coenzymes have been measured by thin-layer chromatography–bioautography (TLCB) and HPLC. In the TLCB approach the coenzymes are separated by two-dimensional TLC and the plate overlayed with a B_{12}-dependent organism and a tetrazolium dye (61). Areas of growth corresponding to cobalamin coenzyme migration are scanned photometrically to quantify the cobalamin present. Since areas of growth are dependent on the microorganism, the inactive cobalamin analogues are not identified. A gradient reversed-phase HPLC approach with detection of the eluted cobalamins by competitive binding radioassay has been used to measure the coenzymes in tissues (62). In this procedure the cobalamin coenzymes are extracted from tissues and purified by C_{18} minicolumn chromatography. The purified extracts are injected onto a C_{18} column and the coenzymes separated by isocratic elution for 2 minutes with 77% phosphate buffer/23% methanol, followed by a linear gradient to 70% methanol by 10 minutes. Fractions collected postcolumn are purified again by C_{18} minicolumn chromatography, reconstituted in cobalamin-free serum, and subjected to competitive protein binding analysis. HPLC analysis has not been used to measure the coenzymes in serum. Using TLCB, one group showed that Me-Cbl accounts for about 60–80% of total cobalamin in plasma, while children have up to 90% Me-Cbl (63). In pernicious anemia the Me-Cbl falls to less than 10% of total and Ado-Cbl is the predominant circulating coenzyme. The reduction in Me-Cbl is seen before the decrease in total cobalamin concentrations. CN-Cbl increases from about 2% to 40% of total cobalamin in pernicious anemia, but the reason for this change is not known.

Methylmalonic acid excretion is elevated in vitamin B_{12} deficiency. Excretion is normally less than 12 mg/day in individuals sufficient in cobalamin (64). Methylmalonic acid can be measured colorimetrically (65) or by gas–liquid chromatography (66).

FOLATE

Background

The folate compounds are a group of substances structurally related to pteroylglutamic acid (PGA) that function metabolically in the transfer of one-carbon units. The naturally occurring forms, found primarily in green and leafy vegetables, exist mostly as folate polyglutamates. The folate polyglutamates are hydrolyzed to monoglutamates in the intestinal mucosa. The liver converts some of these monoglutamates to polyglutamates for storage. The major circulating form is N^5-methyltetrahydrofolate (MeTHF) monoglutamate. After cellular uptake, MeTHF is converted to THF in a cobalamin-dependent reaction that establishes the interrelationship between vitamins B_{12} and folate. In the absence of B_{12}, folate is "trapped" in the MeTHF form, making it unavailable for the one-carbon transfer reactions.

The major clinical manifestation of folate deficiency is megaloblastosis. Other clinical findings that respond to folate therapy include cervical pathology and decreased resistance of the gums to local irritants. Affective disorders have also been linked to folate deficiency (67).

Biochemical Evaluation

The organisms *Lactobacillus casei* or *Streptococcus faecalis* are generally used in the microbiological assays (68). The *S. faecalis* assay does not respond to MeTHF, the predominant circulating form of folate. *L. casei* responds to all forms of folate mono- and diglutamates but not to polyglutamates. Since folate polyglutamates are abundant in erythrocytes, pretreatment to release the monoglutamates is required when the *L. casei* procedure is used. Antibiotic or antifolate administration may hamper test interpretation, as will bacterial contamination of the test organism. The microbiological procedures have been automated (69).

The competitive binding assays have become a popular clinical laboratory tool for assessing folate status, particularly since many of these have been developed for the simultaneous quantitation of vitamins B_{12} and folate (70). The binder used in the folate assays is usually β-lactoglobulin isolated from milk. Endogenous folates in the sample compete with ^{125}I-labeled folate for binding to this protein. Vitamin B_{12}, on the other hand, competes with [57]Co-labeled cobalamin for binding to a B_{12} binding protein. Folate is released from endogenous binding proteins by boiling or by increasing the pH and denaturing the proteins. Dithiothreitol is added to reduce the folates.

HPLC has been used successfully to measure folates in food and pharmaceutical preparations. MeTHF has been measured in serum and CSF using a two-column HPLC with electrochemical detection (71). Other folate forms could not be detected with this assay. Folate monoglutamates have also been quantitated by combined reversed-phase HPLC–microbiological assay (72). Although several forms of folate can be separated and quantitated with this assay, it is limited by the problems inherent in the total folate microbiological assays.

Measurement of serum folate is a popular method of evaluating folate nutritional status. Serum folate concentration becomes low after about 3 weeks of deprivation, even though tissue stores may be adequate. Serum folate concentrations also fluctuate according to recent dietary intake. Adult fasting serum folate concentrations are 1.8–9.0 $\mu g/L$, while erythrocyte folate is 150–450 $\mu g/L$ (73).

Erythrocyte folate concentrations are considered to be a superior indicator of depleted tissue stores (67). Depressed concentrations are observed 17 weeks after beginning a folate-deficient diet and approximately 6 weeks after onset of neutrophil hypersegmentation. Erythrocyte folate can also be reduced in vitamin B_{12} deficiency, since folate storage occurs after the B_{12}-dependent methyltransferase reaction. It is for this reason that serum folate assays are of more utility in differentiating the two vitamin deficiency states.

Urinary excretion of formiminoglutamic acid (FiGlu) and urocanate, both degradation products of histidine metabolism, has been used in some studies to assess folate status (67). Elevated FiGlu excretion is observed after 13 weeks of folate deprivation. After an oral load of histidine (2–15 g), urinary FiGlu excretion is normally less than 30 mg in 8 hours, while folate-deficient subjects excrete 5–10 times that amount. Since FiGlu excretion is also elevated in vitamin B_{12} deprivation, this test is not specific for folate deficiency.

RETINOL

Background

Vitamin A, or retinol, is a fat-soluble vitamin having a structure that consists of an unsaturated polyene chain and a trimethylcyclohexanyl group. Dietary vitamin A is supplied from free retinol, retinyl esters, and β-carotene. Deficiency is commonly seen in undernourished individuals and in patients with fat malabsorption. Clinically, hypovitaminosis A is first recognized by a decrease in night vision that progresses to irreversible blindness. Dermatological changes such as dry, scaly skin and papule formation are also observed. Vitamin A toxicity, on the other hand, is sometimes seen in individuals consuming megadose quantities of the vitamin as a dietary regimen and in some patients consuming excess vitamin A as a treatment for acne. Clinical symptoms of toxicity include anorexia, hepatosplenomegaly, personality disturbances, and bone pain (74).

Biochemical Evaluation

Vitamin A status is usually assessed by measuring the concentration of retinol in serum, although quantitation of retinol binding protein, its transport protein, has some clinical utility. The most commonly used methods for measuring serum retinol include spectrophotometry, fluorometry, and HPLC.

One of the more popular approaches for many years has been the Carr–Price method and its modifications, in which free retinol and esters react with antimony trichloride (75), trifluoroacetic acid (76), or trichloroacetic acid (77) to form a blue complex absorbing at 620 nm. In these procedures retinol is extracted into hexane, with or without prior saponification of the retinyl esters. β-Carotene is also extracted and reacts with the color reagent, causing falsely elevated results. Correction for β-carotene interference is usually obtained by differential absorbance measurements. There is also an interferent that has been found in sera frozen for longer than 6 weeks (78). The trifluoroacetic acid reaction is suitable for pediatric applications, since only 0.05 mL serum is required (76).

An additional chromogenic assay for retinol uses 1,3-dichloro-2-propanol (DCP), which forms a blue color absorbing at 550 nm (79). Pure DCP must be used for the color to be stable. Purification is conducted by aluminum oxide chromatography and vacuum distillation. β-Carotene interference is accounted for by measuring its absorption at 450 nm.

In the fluorometric approaches, serum proteins are precipitated with ethanol and the vitamin extracted into an organic solvent such as hexane (80). The fluorescent intensity of the extract is measured with excitation at 340 nm and emission at 485 nm. β-Carotene does not interfere with the fluorometric assays, but phytofluene does. Phytofluene is a pigment found in vegetables such as tomatoes, and can cause spurious elevations ($\leqslant$ twofold) in vitamin A levels. Fluorescence measurement at two different wavelengths (81) and silicic acid column binding (82) are two approaches used for correcting phytofluene interference. Since there is no correlation between serum phytofluene and retinol concentrations, correction by one of these approaches is mandatory. Fluorometric approaches have been designed to provide simultaneous quantitation of vitamin E (80).

A variety of HPLC approaches have been developed for measuring retinol, retinyl esters, and retinol analogues. Some of these also allow simultaneous measurement of vitamin E. Quantitation of the retinyl esters is useful in cases of vitamin A toxicity. The retinol analogues such as tretinoin, isotretinoin, and etretinate are administered in various dermatological disorders, and measurement is helpful in gauging toxicity and in studying pharmacokinetics (74). Conditions for some of the chromatographic procedures are outlined in Table 4. In the American Association for Clinical Chemistry Proposed Selected Method, 0.1 mL of serum or plasma is deproteinized with ethanol containing the internal standards retinyl acetate and tocopheryl acetate (85). The vitamins are extracted into hexane, evaporated, and reconstituted in ether–methanol for injection onto a C_{18} reversed-phase column. The vitamins are eluted with 95% methanol and monitored at 292 nm (Figure 2). Recovery of the vitamin by the Proposed Selected Method is excellent, but the analyst is

Table 4. HPLC Vitamin A Methods

Detection	Column	Solvent	Specimen Volume	Extraction	Retinoids Detected	Ref.
Ultraviolet 324 or 360 nm	Partisil, 10 μm, C_{18} (ODS-2, Whatman)	Acetic acid–water–acetonitrile 0.5:20.0:79.5)	1 mL serum	0.025 mL of retinyl acetate in butanol–acetonitrile (1:1); 0.4 mL of butanol–acetonitrile (1:1); 0.3 mL of K_2HPO_4 (1.2 kg/L)	Isotretinoin, tretinoin, retinol, retinal, etretinate, retinyl acetate	83
Ultraviolet 365 nm	Partisil, 10 μm, silica (Whatman)	Methylene chloride–glacial acetic acid (99.5:0.5)	1 mL whole blood or urine	2.5 mL of 1 M (pH 6) phosphate buffer; 6 mL of diethyl ether; evaporate; 0.1 mL of solvent	Tretinoin, isotretinoin; etretinate can be detected with a change in extraction procedure	84
Ultraviolet 280 or 292 nm	C_{18} 10 μm (μBondapak) (Waters)	Methanol–water (95:5)	0.1 mL serum	0.1 mL of ethanol containing retinyl acetate–tocopheryl acetate; 1 mL of hexane	Retinol, retinyl acetate	85
Ultraviolet 292 nm	C_{18} 10 μm (μBondapak) (Waters)	Methanol–water (96:4)	0.1 mL serum	0.1 mL of ethanol containing retinyl acetate; 0.2 mL of hexane	Retinol, retinyl acetate	86
Ultraviolet 292 nm	C_{18} 10 μm (μBondapak) (Waters)	Methanol–water (93:7)	0.1 mL serum	0.05 mL of ethanol containing retinyl acetate; 0.05 mL of 0.125% butylated hydroxytoluene (BHT); 0.2 mL of heptane containing 0.025% BHT	Retinol, retinyl acetate	87

Detection	Column	Sample	Mobile phase	Procedure	Analytes	
Ultraviolet 350 nm	Partisil, 10 μm, C$_{18}$ (ODS-2, Whatman)	0.5 mL of plasma	Acetonitrile–1% ammonium acetate (65:35)	0.05 mL of buffer (0.028 M sodium ascorbate, 0.014 M trisodium EDTA); 0.25 μg of trimethyl-methoxyphenyl analogue of tretinoin; lyophilized and reconstituted twice with 1 mL of methanol containing 50 μg BHT/mL	Tretinoin, isotretinoin	88
Ultraviolet 350 nm	Lichrosorb, 10 μm, C$_{18}$ (Altex)	1 mL of plasma	Acetonitrile–water (with 1% ammonium acetate	1 mL of methanol (containing 0.5 μg of retinyl acetate); 1 mL of 0.2 M acetate buffer (pH 3.0); 2 mL of hexane–methylene chloride–isopropanol (80:19:1); evaporate; dissolve in 0.1 mL of acetonitrile)	Tretinoin, isotretinoin, retinyl acetate, retinol	89
Ultraviolet 330 nm	C$_{18}$ (with 18% bonded organic material), 10 μm (RSL, Belgium)	0.2 mL serum	Methanol	0.6 mL of H$_2$O; 2 mL of methanol containing retinyl propionate; 1 mL of chloroform; 1 mL of H$_2$O; 1 mL of chloroform; evaporate chloroform phase, dissolve residue in 0.1 mL of methanol–chloroform (4:1); sonicate 10 minutes and inject 0.05 mL	Retinol, retinyl palmitate, retinyl stearate, retinyl propionate, retinyl laurate, retinyl myristate, retinyl linoleate, retinyl oleate	90

Source: Taken in part, by permission, from Turley CP, Brewster MA, Vitamin A, in Pesce AJ, Kaplan LA (eds): *Methods in Clinical Chemistry.* St. Louis: CV Mosby, 1987; p 553.

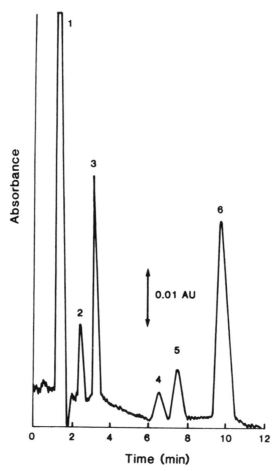

Figure 2. Chromatogram of the AACC Proposed Selected Method for vitamins A and E (*85*). 1, solvent front; 2, retinol; 3, retinyl acetate; 4, $\beta + \gamma$-tocopherol; 5, α-tocopherol; 6, tocopheryl acetate. [Reprinted by permission from Turley CP, Brewster MA, Vitamin E, in Pesce AJ, Kaplan LA (eds): *Methods in Clinical Chemistry*. St. Louis: CV Mosby, 1987, p 588.]

cautioned to conduct recovery studies, especially since other methods have yielded poor recoveries in the absence of antioxidants (*86*).

Using fluorometry with silicic acid phytofluene correction, the plasma retinol concentration is 0.25–0.43 mg/L in children and 0.32–0.90 mg/L in adults (*91*). Serum retinol concentrations in adult males is 0.45–0.80 mg/L and in adult females is 0.34–0.75 mg/L, as measured by HPLC (*92*). Deficiency of retinol binding protein sometimes causes depressed circulating vitamin A levels despite adequate hepatic stores of the vitamin. Retinol binding protein deficiency is seen in malnourished individuals, in patients with liver disease, and in patients with zinc deficiency. In these cases, treatment of the hypoproteinemia or hypozincemia restores the circulating plasma retinol concentrations to normal (93).

TOCOPHEROL

Background

Tocopherol, also called vitamin E, is a lipid-soluble vitamin that is found in nature as several isomers that are distinguishable by methyl substituents as shown in Figure 3. The isomers α- (AT), β- (BT), γ- (GT) and δ- (DT) tocopherol have different degrees of biological activity, with AT being the most active. There appear to be two roles for vitamin E in physiological systems. The major role is as an antioxidant, with the vitamin preventing peroxidation of unsaturated fatty acids (94). Tocopherol may also have a regulatory role, since it has been found to bind to a cytoplasmic protein that carries it to the cell nucleus, where it may enhance protein synthesis (95).

Deficiency is seen in individuals with fat malabsorption and in newborn infants. Premature newborns are often treated with vitamin E to prevent hemolytic anemia. The vitamin has also been used in treating retrolental fibroplasia and bronchopulmonary dysplasia.

Biochemical Evaluation

Functional tests of vitamin E deficiency include the measurement of erythrocyte hemolysis and erythrocyte or serum malondialdehyde. The erythrocyte hemolysis test is based on the observation that red cells from tocopherol-deficient individuals have an increased sensitivity to oxidant-induced stress (96). In these procedures, washed erythrocytes are incubated in a hemolyzing reagent such as 2% hydrogen peroxide or dialuric acid. The quantity of hemoglobin realeased is indexed to the amount of hemoglobin released from cells incubated in distilled water. Glucose is sometimes added to correct for non-tocopherol-dependent hemolysis, such as might be encountered in selenium deficiency (97). Although there is an inverse correlation between serum tocopherol concentrations and peroxide hemolysis, overlap in hemolysis values between deficient and nondeficient subjects imposes limitations on the interpretation of this test.

Malondialdehyde is an end product of polyunsaturated fatty acid metabolism and is increased in conditions of oxidative stress. Malondialdehyde

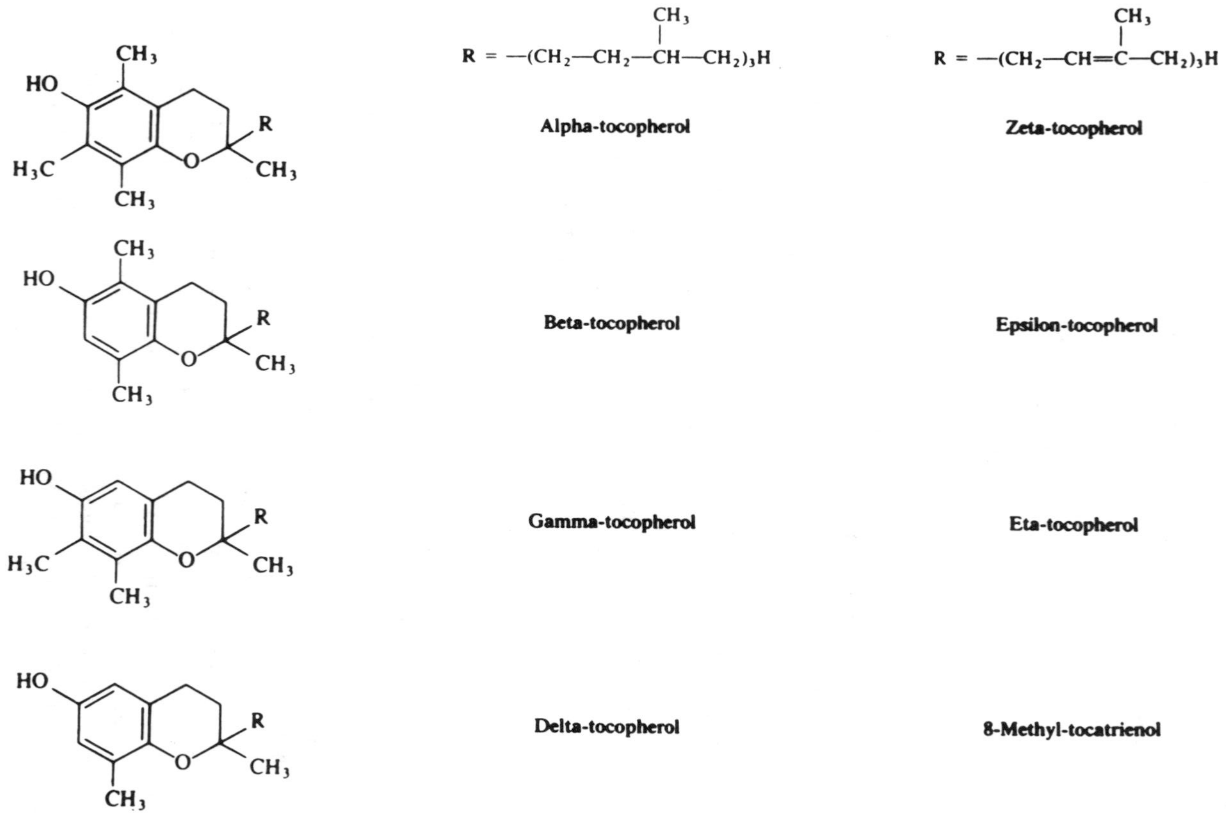

$R = -(CH_2-CH_2-CH-CH_2)_3H$
                    |
                   CH_3

Alpha-tocopherol

Beta-tocopherol

Gamma-tocopherol

Delta-tocopherol

$R = -(CH_2-CH=C-CH_2)_3H$
                    |
                   CH_3

Zeta-tocopherol

Epsilon-tocopherol

Eta-tocopherol

8-Methyl-tocatrienol

Figure 3. Structures of the tocopherol isomers. [Reprinted by permission from Brewster MA, in Pesce AJ, Kaplan LA (eds): *Clinical Chemistry: Theory, Analysis, and Correlation.* St Louis: CV Mosby, 1984, p. 663.]

can be measured fluorometrically, spectrophotometrically, and by HPLC. Fluorometric procedures yield higher reference values (3.27 ± 0.89 µmol/L) than spectrophotometric (0.61 ± 0.11 µmol/L) and HPLC (0.60 ± 0.113 µmol/L) (mean $\pm$ SD) approaches (98).

Vitamin E can also be measured directly in serum or in cells. Approaches include colorimetric techniques based on the Emmerie–Engel reaction, fluorometric techniques, and HPLC. All approaches have been used to measure total vitamin E or the individual tocopherol isomers.

In the Emmerie–Engel reaction tocopherols reduce ferric iron to ferrous iron which is then reacted with α,α'-dipyridyl to give a red-orange color with maximum absorbance at 510 nm. The colorimetric approaches are subject to interference from carotene and retinol and must include measures to correct for this, such as chromatography to remove the interferents (99) or blank correction to account for them (100). The AT isomer has been measured colorimetrically following its separation from the other tocopherol isomers by silica gel G–thin-layer chromatography. Carotene and retinol do not interfere in this chromatographic approach because they have distinct retention characteristics. BT and GT can also be removed from the thin-layer plate and quantitated, but results obtained from summing all three zones are about 10% lower than total vitamin E concentration as measured by direct colorimetry (99).

The enhanced sensitivity of the fluorometric approaches has been particularly useful in pediatric settings, where vitamin E deficiency is common. In the Hansen and Warwick procedure, vitamin E is extracted into hexane from 0.1 mL of serum and tocopherol fluorescence is measured with excitation at 295 nm and emission at 340 nm (101). Carotene and retinol do not interfere in the fluorometric approaches. The method has been adapted for the simultaneous determination of vitamins A and E in 0.2 mL of serum.

The HPLC approaches can also be used to measure vitamins A and E simultaneously (Table 5). Normal phase methods use hexane as the mobile phase, and the order of elution is AT-acetate > AT > BT > GT > DT. Reversed-phase systems commonly have a methanol–water mobile phase, and the order of elution is DT > BT = GT > AT > AT–acetate. BT and GT are not resolved in reversed-phase systems, but this usually poses no analytical constraints because BT is a small component of the total serum tocopherol content. Extraction conditions vary, but one popular approach is to first precipitate serum proteins with methanol and extract the lipid-soluble substances with hexane or heptane. Some investigators have recommended including an antioxidant such as butylated hydroxytoluene in the extraction mixture to improve analytical recovery, while others have achieved good recoveries without the use of antioxidants. In one study of rat and human plasma in the absence of antioxidants, the recovery of AT was 34% and 84%

Table 5. HPLC Vitamin E Methods

Detection	Column	Solvent	Specimen Volume	Extraction	Simultaneous Analysis of Vitamin A	Tocopherol Isomers Resolved	Ref.
Fluorescence ex: 295 nm em: 340 nm	Silica (Partisil PXS10)	Hexane (0.3% methanol)	0.05 mL	0.2 mL of 10% ascorbic acid; 2 mL of H_2O, 1 mL of ethanol; 2 mL of hexane	No	AT, BT, GT, DT	104
Fluorescence ex: 295 nm em: 370 nm	Silica (μPorasil, 10 μm)	Hexane–diiso-propyl ether (92:8)	0.5 mL	0.5 mL of ethanol containing DL-tocol; 1 mL of hexane	No	AT, BT, GT, DT	105
Ultraviolet, 280 or 292 nm	C_{18}, 10 μm (μBondapak)	Methanol–water (95:5)	0.1 mL	0.1 mL of ethanol containing retinyl acetate–tocopheryl acetate; 0.1 mL of hexane	Yes	AT, B+GT, DT	85
Ultraviolet, 292 nm	C_{18} (μBondapak)	Methanol–water (96:4)	0.1 mL	0.05 mL of ethanol containing retinyl acetate; 0.2 mL of hexane	Yes	AT, B+GT, DT	107
Ultraviolet, 292 nm	C_{18} (μBondapak)	Methanol–water (93:7)	0.1 mL	0.05 mL of ethanol containing retinyl acetate; 0.05 mL of 0.125% butylated hydroxytoluene (BHT); 0.2 mL of heptane containing 0.025% BHT	Yes	AT, GT,	102
Fluorescence ex: 205 nm em: 340 nm	C_{18}, 10 μm (μBondapak)	Methanol–water (95:5)	0.1 mL	2 mL of 2% pyrogallol in ethanol; incubate at 70 C for 2 minutes; 0.3 mL of saturates KOH; incubate 70 C for 30 minutes; 1 mL of water; 4 mL of hexane	No	AT, B+GT, DT	103

Source: Taken in part, with permission, from Turley CP, Brewster MA. Vitamin E, in Pesce AJ, Kaplan LA (eds): *Methods in Clinical Chemistry.* St. Louis: CV Mosby, 1987, p 583.

respectively (*102*). Others showed that saponification is necessary to achieve respectable recoveries (*103*).

These observations dictate that one should carefully evaluate the performance of vitamin E methods during assay development and adaptation to particular analytical problems. The eluted vitamins are detected spectrophotometrically or fluorometrically. AT has a maximum absorbance at 292 nm. Sensitivity with ultraviolet detection is around 0.5 mg/L (*85*). Fluorometric detection can be conducted with excitation at 295 nm and emission at 340 nm with sensitivity approaching 9 ng/L (*104*). A 20-fold enhancement in sensitivity can be achieved by setting excitation at 205 nm (*103*). HPLC methods also vary in the choice of internal standards used. Some use DL-tocol, a tocopherol isomer having no methyl substituents at positions 5, 7, or 8 (*105*). Another internal standard used is AT–acetate (*85*). Although suitable for population surveys and when it is certain that AT–acetate has not been administered therapeutically, this internal standard should not be used where there is reason to suspect its presence in the circulation. Because of its enhanced storage stability, AT–acetate is frequently used in parenteral vitamin formulations and can be found in the serum of patients receiving this form of therapy (*106*). In lieu of using AT–acetate, tocopherol can instead be indexed to the retinyl acetate internal standard (*107*).

In the Proposed Selected Method advanced by the American Association for Clinical Chemistry, AT–acetate is the internal standard and the vitamins are extracted without the use of antioxidants or saponification (*85*). The internal standard in ethanol is added to 0.1 mL of serum, and the lipid-soluble materials are removed by extraction into hexane. The hexane layer is removed and evaporated, and the vitamins are reconstituted in ether–methanol and injected. Chromatography run time is about 8 minutes, but this could be shortened by using retinyl acetate as the vitamin E internal standard (Figure 2).

The reference range for serum total tocopherol in adults is 5–20 mg/L. Since tocopherol circulates in the plasma associated with lipid, some investigators have recommended indexing vitamin E as a ratio of milligrams of total tocopherol per grams of total lipid. Adequate ratios are defined as 0.8 in adults (*108*) and 0.6 in children (*109*). Newborn infants often have a total tocopherol concentration below the normal 5 mg/L, but appear to be sufficient in the vitamin, with a tocopherol-to-lipid ratio greater than 0.6. Rapid physiological changes in the premature infant make the tocopherol-to-lipid ratio uninterpretable (*110*).

Total tocopherol concentrations may not always be an appropriate measure of functional vitamin E deficiency. Individuals on diets containing substantial amounts of BT and GT have abnormal erythrocyte hemolysis despite total tocopherol concentrations within reference limits (*111*).

Particularly susceptible to this are patients receiving lipid emulsions parenterally. Although vitamin E methods using chromatography to separate the isomers will alert the analyst to this situation, interpretation is difficult because the relationship of non-AT isomers to "adequacy" has not been defined. In this situation one might wish to use a functional test of antioxidant status such as erythrocyte hemolysis or serum malondialdehyde quantitation.

Reference values for the AT isomer are not as well defined. Using thin-layer chromatography to separate and the Emmerie–Engel reaction to quantitate the AT isomer, one group found 9.16 ± 3.05 mg/L (*99*), while another (*112*) found 5.07 ± 1.95 mg/L (mean ± SD). A recent study showed that the 90th percentile range for AT in adults is 5.9–12.9 mg/L as determined by HPLC with an AT–acetate internal standard (*92*). In normal adult serum AT accounts for 82.6–93.3%, BT for 0–2.3%, and GT for 6.7–15.7% of total tocopherols.

REFERENCES

1. Bamji MS. Laboratory tests for the assessment of vitamin nutritional status, in Briggs MH (ed): *Vitamins in Human Biology and Medicine.* Boca Raton, FL: CRC Press, 1981, pp 1–27.

2. Sauberlich HE. Newer laboratory methods for assessing nutriture of selected B-complex vitamins. *Annu Rev Nutr* 1984;4:377–407.

3. Barness LA. Adverse effects of overdosage of vitamins or minerals. *Pediatr Rev* 1986;8:20–24.

4. Pincus JH, Cooper JR, Pirus K, Turner V. Specificity of the urine inhibitor test for Leigh's disease. *Neurology* 1974;24:885–889.

5. Pearson WN. Thiamin, in Gyorgy P, Pearson WN (eds): *The Vitamins*, vol 3. New York: Academic Press, 1967, p 53.

6. Pelletier O, Madere R. New automated method for measuring thiamin (vitamin B_1) in urine. *Clin Chem* 1972;18:937.

7. Kimura M, Fujita T, Itokawa Y. Liquid-chromatographic determination of total thiamin content of blood. *Clin Chem* 1982;28:29–31.

8. Botticher B, Botticher D. Simple rapid determination of thiamin by a HPLC method in foods, body fluids, urine and faeces. *Int J Vit Nutr Res* 1986;56:155–159.

9. Warnock LG, Prudhomme CR, Wagner C. The determination of thiamin pyrophosphate in blood and other tissues, and its correlation erythrocyte transketolase activity. *J Nutr* 1979;108:421–427.

10. Warnock LG. Transketolase activity of blood hemolysate, a useful index for diagnosing thiamin deficiency. *Clin Chem* 1975;21:432–436.

11. Warnock LG. A new approach to erythrocyte transketolase measurement. *J Nutr* 1970;100:1057–1062.

12. Basu TK, Patel DR, Williams DC. A simplified microassay of transketolase in human blood. *Int J Vit Nutr Res* 1974;44:319–326.

13. Bayoumi RA, Rosalki SB. Evaluation of methods of coenzyme activation of erythrocyte enzymes for detection of deficiency of vitamins B_1, B_2 and B_6. *Clin Chem* 1976;22:327–335.

14. Kaczmarek MD, Nixon PF. Variants of transketolase from human erythrocytes. *Clin Chim Acta* 1983;130:349–356.

15. Reijnierse GL, Van Der Horst AR, De Kloet K, Voorhorst CD. A radiochemical method for the determination of transketolase activity in erythrocyte hemolysates. *Clin Chim Acta* 1978;90:259–268.

16. Cheng, CH, Koch M, Shank, RE. Leukocyte transketolase activity as an indicator of thiamin nutriture in rats. *J Nutr* 1976;106:1678–1685.

17. Sauberlich HE, Skala JH, Dowdy RP. Thiamin (vitamin B_1), in *Laboratory Tests for the Assessment of Nutritional Status.* Boca Raton, FL: CRC Press, 1974, pp 22–30.

18. Hathcock JN. Thiamin deficiency effects on rat leukocyte pyruvate decarboxylation rates. *Am J Clin Nutr* 1978;31:250–252.

19. Komindr S, Nicholalds GE. Clinical significance of riboflavin deficiency, in Brewster MA, Naito HK (eds): *Nutritional Elements and Clinical Chemistry.* New York: Plenum, 1980, pp 15–68.

20. Kornberg HA, Langdon RS, Cheldelin VH. Microbiological assay for riboflavin. *Anal Chem* 1948;20:81–83.

21. Baker H, Frank P, Feingold S, et al. A riboflavin assay suitable for clinical use and nutritional surveys. *Am J Clin Nutr* 1966;19:17–26.

22. Slater EC, Morrell DB. The fluorometric determination of riboflavin in urine. *Biochem J* 1946;40:652–657.

23. Decker K, Hinkkanen A. Luminometric determination of flavin adenine dinucleotide. *Methods Enzymol* 1986;122:185–192.

24. Tillotson JA, Bashor MM. Fluorometric titration of urinary riboflavin with an apoflavoprotein. *Methods Enzymol* 1986;122:234–237.

25. Gatautis VJ, Naito HK. Liquid–chromatographic determination of urinary riboflavin. *Clin Chem* 1981;27:1672–1675.

26. Lambert WE, Cammaert PM, De Leenheer AP. Liquid–chromatographic measurement of riboflavin in serum and urine with isoriboflavin as an internal standard. *Clin Chem* 1985;31:1371–1373.

27. Pietta P, Calatroni A, Rava H. Hydrolysis of riboflavin nucleotides in plasma monitored by high performance liquid chromatography. *J Chromatogr Biomed Appl* 1982;229:445–449.

28. Wittmer D, Haney WG. Analysis of riboflavin in commercial multivitamin preparations by high-speed liquid chromatography. *J Pharm Sci* 1974;63:588–590.

29. Walker MC, Carpenter BE, Cooper EL. Simultaneous determination of niacin-amide, pyridoxine, riboflavin and thiamine in multivitamin products by high-pressure liquid chromatography. *J Pharm Sci* 1981;70:99–101.

30. Bamji MS, Sharma KVR, Radhaiah G. Relationship between biochemical and clinical indices of B-vitamin deficiency. A study in rural school boys. *Br J Nutr* 1979;41:431–441.

31. Garry PJ, Owen GM. An automated flavin adenine dinucleotide dependent glutathione reductase assay for assessing riboflavin nutriture. *Am J Clin Nutr* 1976;28:663–674.

32. Muller EM, Bates CJ. The effect of riboflavin deficiency on white cell glutathione reductase in rats. *Int J Vitam Nutr Res* 1977;47:46–51.

33. Miller LT, Edwards M. Microbiological assay of vitamin B_6 in blood and urine, in Leklem JE, Reynolds RD (eds): *Methods in Vitamin B_6 Nutrition*. New York: Plenum, pp 45–55.

34. Schrijver J, Speek A, Schreurs WHP. Semiautomated fluorometric determination of pyridoxal-5'-phosphate in whole blood by high performance liquid chromato-graphy (HPLC). *Int J Vitamin Nutr Res* 1981;51:216–222.

35. Gregory JF, Kirk JR. Determination of urinary 4-pyridoxic acid using high performance liquid chromatography. *Am J Clin Nutr* 1979;32:879–883.

36. Shin YS, Rasshofer R, Friedrich B, Enders W. Pyridoxal-5'-phosphate determi-nation by a sensitive micromethod in human blood, urine and tissues; its relation to cystathioninuria in neuroblastoma and biliary atresia. *Clin Chim Acta* 1983;127:77–85.

37. Ritchey SJ, Feeley RM. The excretion patterns of vitamin B_6 and B_{12} in preadolescent girls. *J Nutr* 1966;89:411.

38. Sauberlich HE, Skala JH, Dowdy RP. Vitamin B_6, *Laboratory Tests for the Assessment of Nutritional Status*. Boca Raton, FL: CRC Press, 1974, pp 37–49.

39. Reynolds RD. Nationwide assay of vitamin B_6 in human plasma by different methods. *Fed Proc* 1983;42:665..

40. McCoy EE, Drebit R, Strynadka K, Schiff D. Assessment of vitamin B_6 status in infants and children: Serial pyridoxal phosphate levels in premature infants, in Leklen JE, Reynolds RS (eds): *Methods in Vitamin B_6 Nutrition*. New York: Plenum, 1981, pp 253–267.

41. Sauberlich HE. Vitamin B_6 status assessment: Past and present, in Leklen JE, Reynolds RS (eds): *Methods in Vitamin B_6 Nutrition*. New York: Plenum, 1981, pp 203–239.

42. Skala JH, Waring PP, Lyons MF, et al. Methodology for determination of blood aminotransferases, in Leklen JE, Reynolds RS (eds): *Methods in Vitamin B_6 Nutrition*. New York: Plenum, 1981, pp 171–202.

43. Bamji, MS. Laboratory tests for the assessment of vitamin nutritional status, in Briggs MH (ed): *Vitamins in Human Biology and Medicine*. Boca Raton, FL: CRC Press, 1981, pp 1–28.

44. Farmer CJ, Abt AF. Determination of reduced ascorbic acid in small amounts of blood. *Proc Soc Exp Biol Med* 1936;34:146–150.

45. Lloyd B, Sinclair HM, Webster GR. The estimation of ascorbic acid for clinical purposes by the hydrazine method. *Biochem J, Proc Biochem Soc* 1945;39:xvii–xviii (abstract).

46. Zannoni V, Lynch M, Goldstein S, Sato P. A rapid micromethod for the determination of ascorbic acid in plasma and tissues. *Biochem Med* 1974;11:41–48.

47. Deutsch MJ, Weeks CE. Microfluorometric assay for vitamin C. *J Assoc Off Anal Chem* 1965;48:1248–1256.

48. Rose RC, Nahrwold DL. Quantitative analysis of ascorbic acid and dehydro-ascorbic acid by high performance liquid chromatography. *Anal Biochem* 1981;114:140–145.

49. Lee W, Hamernyik P, Hutchinson M, et al. Ascorbic acid in lymphocytes: Cell preparation and liquid-chromatographic assay. *Clin Chem* 1982;28:2165–2169.

50. Sauberlich HE, Skala JH, Dowdy RP. Vitamin C (ascorbic acid), in *Laboratory Tests for the Assessment of Nutritional Status*. Boca Raton, FL: CRC Press, 1974, pp 13–22.

51. Wood HG, Kellermeyer RW, Stjernholm R, Allen SHG. Metabolism of methyl-malonyl CoA mutase and the role of biotin and B_{12} coenzymes. *Ann NY Acad Sci* 1964;112:661–679.

52. Poston JM. Cobalamin-dependent formation of leucine and β-leucine by rat and human tissues. *J. Biol Chem* 1980;255:10067–10072.

53. Poston JM, Stadtman TC. Cobamides as cofactors, in Babior BM (ed): *Cobalamin Biochemistry and Pathophysiology*. New York: Wiley, 1975, pp 111–140.

54. Grasbeck R, Salonen EM. Vitamin B_{12}. *Prog Food Nutr Sci* 1976;2:193–231.

55. Lee DSC, Griffiths BW. Human serum vitamin B_{12} assay methods. *Clin Biochem* 1985;18:261–266.

56. Kolhouse JF, Kondo H, Allen NC, et al. Cobalamin analogues are present in human plasma and can mask cobalamin deficiency because current radioisotope dilution assays are not specific for true cobalamin. *N. Engl J Med* 1978;299:785–792.

57. Herbert V, Colman N, Palat D, et al. Is there a "gold standard" for human serum vitamin B_{12} assay? *J Lab Clin Med* 1984;104:829–841.

58. Sauberlich HE, Skala JH, Dowdy RP. Vitamin B_{12} (cobalamin, corrinoids), in *Laboratory Tests for the Assessment of Nutritional Status*, Boca Raton, FL: CRC Press, 1974, pp 60–70.

59. Tietz NW. *Clinical Guide to Laboratory Tests*. Philadelphia: Saunders, 1983, pp 506–507.

60. Rothenberg SP, Marcoullis GP, Schwarz S, Lader E. Measurement of cyano-cobalamin in serum by a specific radioimmunoassay. *J Lab Clin Med* 1984;176:1463–1464.

61. Linnell JC, Mackenzie HM, Wilson J, Matthews DM. Patterns of plasma cobalamins in control subjects and in cases of vitamin B_{12} deficiency. *J Clin Pathol* 1969;22:545–550.

62. Turley CP, Brewster MA, Taylor H. Combined liquid chromatographic–competitive binding radioassay for measurement of cobalamin coenzymes. *Clin Chem* 1986;32:1194–1195.

63. Linnell JC, Matthews DM. Recent advances in cobalamin metabolism: Abnormalities in coenzyme distribution in tumour development and in inherited metabolic disease, in *Vitamin B_{12}*. New York: Walter de Gruyter, 1979, pp 1101–1111.

64. Barness LA. Vitamin B_{12} deficiency with emphasis on methylmalonic acid as a diagnostic aid. *Am J Clin Nutr* 1967;20:573–577.

65. Giorgio AJ, Plaut GWE. A method for the colorimetric determination of urinary methylmalonic acid in pernicious anemia. *J Lab Clin Med* 1965;66:667.

66. Giorgio AJ, Malloy E, Black T. A clinical laboratory GLC method for urine methylmalonic acid. *Anal Lett* 1972;5:13–19.

67. Colman N. Laboratory assessment of folate status, in Labbe RF (ed): *Clinics in Laboratory Medicine*. Saunders: Philadelphia, 1981, pp 775–796.

68. Scott JM, Ghanta V, Herbert V. Trouble-free microbiological serum and red cell folate assays. *Am J Med Technol* 1974;40:125–134.

69. Tennant GB. Continuous flow automation of the *Lactobacillus casei* serum folate assay. *J Clin Pathol* 1977;30:1168–1174.

70. Jacob E, Colman N, Herbert V. Evaluation of simultaneous radioassay for two vitamins: Folate and vitamin B_{12}. *Am. J Clin Nutr* 1977;30:6165.

71. Lankelma J, Van Der Kleijn E, Jansen MJ. Determination of 5-methyltetrahydrofolic acid in plasma and spinal fluid by high-performance liquid chromatography, using on-column concentration and electrochemical detection. *J Chromatogr* 1980;182:35–54.

72. McMartin KE, Virayotha V, Tephly TR. High-pressure liquid chromatography separation and determination of rat liver folates. *Arch Biochem Biophys* 1981;209:127–136.

73. Fairbanks VF, Klee GG. Biochemical aspects of hematology, in Tietz NW (ed): *Textbook of Clinical Chemistry*. Philadelphia: Saunders, 1986, pp 1495–1588.

74. Turley CP, Turley KO. The retinoids in dermatology. AACC TDM-TOX Laboratory Improvement Program. 1986;7(10):1–9.

75. Carr TH, Price EA. Color reactions attributed to vitamin A. *Biochem J* 1926;20:497–501.

76. Meeld JB, Pearson WN, Macro- and micromethods for the determination of serum vitamin A using trifluoroacetic acid. *J Nutr* 1963;79:454–460.

77. Bayfield RF, Cole ER. Colorimetric estimation of vitamin A with trichloroacetic acid. *Methods Enzymol* 1980;67:189–195.

78. McClaren DS, Reed WWC, Awoeh ZL, et al. Microdetermination of vitamin A and carotenoids in blood and tissues. *Methods Biochem Analy* 1967;15:1–23.

79. Henry RJ. *Vitamins: Clinical Chemistry, Principles, and Techniques.* New York: Harper & Row, 1965, p 699.

80. Hansen LG, Warwick WJ. A fluorometric micromethod for serum vitamins A and E. *Am J Clin Pathol* 1969;51:538–541.

81. Thompson JN, Erdody P, Brien R, et al. Fluorometric determination of vitamin A in human blood and liver. *Biochem Med* 1971;5:67–89.

82. Garry PJ, Pollack JD, Owen GM. Plasma vitamin A assay by fluorometry and use of a silicic acid column technique. *Clin Chem* 1970;16:766–772.

83. McClean SW, Ruddel ME, Gross EG, et al. Liquid-chromatographic assay for retinol (vitamin A) and retinol analogs in therapeutic trials. *Clin Chem* 1982;28:693–696.

84. Puglisi CV, De Silva AF. Determination of retinoic acid (13-*cis*- and all-*trans*-) and aromatic retinoic acid analogs possessing antitumour activity in biological fluids by high-performance liquid chromatography. *J Chromatogr* 1978;152:421–430.

85. Catignani GL, Bieri JG. Simultaneous determination of retinol and α-tocopherol in serum or plasma by liquid chromatography. *Clin Chem* 1983;29:708–712.

86. Driskell WJ, Neese JW, Bryant CC, Bashor MM, Measurement of vitamin A and vitamin E in human serum by high-performance liquid chromatography. *J Chromatogr* 1982;231:439–444.

87. Chow FI, Omaye ST. Use of antioxidants in the analysis of vitamins A and E in mammalian plasma by high performance liquid chromatography. *Lipids* 1983;18:837–841.

88. Frolic CA, Travela TE, Peck GL, Sporn MB. High pressure liquid chromatographic determination of 13-*cis*-retinoic acid and all-*trans*-retinoic acid in human plasma. *Anal Biochem* 1978;86:743–750.

89. Besner JG, LeClaire R, Band PR. High performance liquid chromatography of 13-*cis*-retinoic acid and of endogenous retinol in human plasma. *J Chromatogr* 1980;183:346–351.

90. DeRuyter MGM, DeLeenheer AP. Simultaneous determination of retinol and retinyl esters in serum or plasma by reversed-phase high-performance liquid chromatography. *Clin Chem* 1978;24:1920–1923.

91. Garry PJ. Vitamin A. *Clinics Lab Med* 1981;1:669–711.

92. Kaplan LA, Stein EA, Willett W, et al. Reference ranges of retinol, tocopherols, lycopene and α- and β-carotene in serum by simultaneous high performance liquid chromatographic analysis. *Clin Phys Biochem* 1987;5:297–304.

93. Smith JE, Brown ED, Smith JC. The effect of zinc deficiency on the metabolism of retinol-binding protein in the rat. *J Lab Clin Med* 1974;84:692–697.

94. McCay PB, King MM. Vitamin E: Its role as a biological free radical scavenger and its relationship to the microsomal mixed function oxidase system, in Machlin LJ (ed): *Vitamin E: A Comprehensive Treatise.* New York: Dekker, 1980, pp 289–316.

95. Catignani GL. An α-tocopherol binding protein in rat liver cytoplasm. *Biochem Biophys Res Commun* 1975;67:66–72.

96. Bieri JG, Poukka R. *In vitro* hemolysis as related to rat erythrocyte content of α-tocopherol and polyunsaturated fatty acids. *J Nutr* 1970;100:557–564.
97. Gordon HH, Nitowsky HM, Cornblath M. Studies of tocopherol deficiency in infants and children. *Am J Dis Child* 1955;90:669–681.
98. Wong SHY, Knight JA, Hopfer SM, et al. Measurement of plasma lipoperoxides by HPLC separation of malondialdehyde–thiobarbituric acid adduct. *Clin Chem* 1987;33:214–220.
99. Bieri JG, Prival EL. Serum vitamin E determined by thin layer chromatography. *Proc Soc Exp Biol Med* 1965;120:554–561.
100. Hashim SA, Schuttringer GR. Rapid determination of tocopherol in macro- and microquantities of plasma. *Am J Clin Nutr* 1966;19:137–145.
101. Hansen LG, Warwick WJ. A fluorometric micromethod for serum vitamins A and E. *Am J Clin Pathol* 1969;51:538–541.
102. Chow FI, Omaye ST. Use of antioxidants in the analysis of vitamins A and E in mammalian plasma by high performance liquid chromatography. *Lipids* 1983;18:837–841.
103. Hatam LJ, Kayden HJ, A high-performance liquid chromatographic method for the determination of tocopherol in plasma and cellular elements of blood. *J Lipid Res* 1979;20:639–645.
104. Vatassery GT, Johnson GJ, Krezowski AM. Changes in vitamin E concentration in human plasma and platelets with age. *J Am College Nutr* 1983;4:369–375.
105. Jansson L, Nilsson B, Lindgren R. Quantitation of serum tocopherols by high pressure liquid chromatography with fluorescence detection. *J Chromatogr* 1980;181:242–247.
106. Turley CP, Brewster MA, Catignani G. Administered tocopheryl acetate interferes in liquid chromatographic assay of serum tocopherol. *Clin Chem* 1985;31:1761–1762.
107. Driskell WJ, Neese JW, Bryant CC, Bashor MM. Measurement of vitamin A and vitamin E in human serum by high pressure liquid chromatography. *J. Chromatogr* 1982;231:439–444.
108. Horwitt MK, Harvey CC, Dahm CH, Searcy MT. Relationship between tocopherol and serum lipid levels for determination of nutritional adequacy. *Ann NY Acad Sci* 1972;203:223–235.
109. Farrell PM, Levine SL, Murphy MD, Adams AJ. Plasma tocopherol levels and tocopherol–lipid relationships in a normal population of children as compared to healthy adults. *Am J Clin Nutr* 1978;31:1720–1726.
110. Gutcher GR, Raynor WJ, Farrell PM. An evaluation of vitamin E status in premature infants. *Am J Clin Nutr* 1984;40:1078–1089.
111. Gutcher GR, Lax AA, Farrell PM. Tocopherol isomers in intravenous lipid emulsions and resultant plasma concentrations. *J Parent Enteral Nutr* 1984;8:269–273.
112. Herting DC, Drury EJE. Plasma tocopherol levels in man. *Am J Clin Nutr* 1965;17:351–356.

INDEX

283